Managed Mental Health Care in the Public Sector

Chronic Mental Illness

Series Editor
John A. Talbott, University of Maryland School of Medicine,
Baltimore, USA

Advisory Board
Leona Bachrach • James T. Barter • Carol Caton • David L. Cutler •
Jeffrey L. Geller • William M. Glazer • Stephen M. Goldfinger •
Howard H. Goldman • H. Richard Lamb • Harriet P. Lefley •
Anthony F. Lehman • Robert P. Lieberman • W. Walter Menninger •
Arthur T. Meyerson

Managed Mental Health Care in the Public Sector

A Survival Manual

Edited by

Kenneth Minkoff, MD

Choate Health Systems, Inc.
Woburn, Massachusetts

and

David Pollack, MD

Mental Health Services West
Portland, Oregon

harwood academic publishers

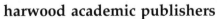

Australia Canada China France Germany India
Japan Luxembourg Malaysia The Netherlands Russia
Singapore Switzerland Thailand United Kingdom

Copyright © 1997 OPA (Overseas Publishers Association) Amsterdam B.V. Published in The Netherlands by Harwood Academic Publishers.

Amsteldijk 166
1st Floor
1079 LH Amsterdam
The Netherlands

British Library Cataloguing in Publication Data

Managed mental health care in the public sector : a
    survival manual. — (Chronic mental illness ; v. 4)
    1. Community mental health services — United States
    I. Minkoff, Kenneth   II. Pollack, David, 1942–
362.2'2'0973

ISBN 90-5702-537-X

CONTENTS

INTRODUCTION TO THE SERIES

This series on chronic mental illness is a result of both the success and failure of our efforts over the past thirty years to provide better treatment, rehabilitation and care for persons suffering from severe and persistent mental illnesses. The failure is obvious to all who walk our cities' streets, use our libraries or pass through our transportation terminals. The success is found in the enormous boost of interest in service to, research on and teaching about treatment, rehabilitation and care of those persons who, in Leona Bachrach's definition, "are, have been, or might have been, but for the deinstitutionalization movement, on the rolls of long-term mental institutions, especially state hospitals."

The first book in our modern era devoted to the subject was that by Richard Lamb in 1976, *Community Survival for Long-Term Patients*. Shortly thereafter, Leona Bachrach's unique study "Deinstitutionalization: An Analytical Review and Sociological Perspective" was published. In 1978, the American Psychiatric Association hosted a meeting on the problem that resulted in the publication *The Chronic Mental Patient*. This effort in turn spawned several texts dealing with increasingly specialized areas: *The Chronic Mentally Ill: Treatment, Programs, Systems* and *Chronic Mental Illness in Children and Adolescents*, both by John Looney; and *The Chronic Mental Patient/II* by Walter Menninger and Gerald Hannah.

Now, however, there are a host of publications devoted to various portions of the problem, e.g., the homeless mentally ill, rehabilitation of the mentally ill, families of the mentally ill, and so on. The amount of research and experience now that can be conveyed to a wide population of caregivers is exponentially greater than it was in 1955, the year that deinstitutionalization began.

This series will cover:

— types of intervention, e.g., psychopharmacology, psychotherapy, case management, social and vocational rehabilitation, and mobile and home treatment;
— settings, e.g., hospitals, ambulatory settings, nursing homes, correctional facilities and shelters;
— specific populations, e.g., alcohol and drug abusers, the homeless and those dually diagnosed;

— special issues, e.g., family intervention, psychoeducation, policy/ financing, non-compliance, forensic, cross-cultural and systems issues.

I am indebted to our hard-working editorial board as well as to our editors and authors, many of whom are involved in both activities.

This fourth volume covers a specific portion of the field, although overlapping with other books in the series; and it deals with systems-level, program management and clinical issues in managed mental health care. Its editors are both leaders in the area of community psychiatry and financing of mental health services and have the unique ability to bridge the academic and practical worlds.

Future books in this series will cover inpatient care, psychiatric rehabilitation, psychopharmacology, the homeless mentally ill, treatment compliance and the mentally ill in the correctional system. I hope you will look forward to them as eagerly as I do.

John A. Talbott, MD

PREFACE

These are difficult times in public sector mental health. Many of us, who have dedicated our careers to serving the most seriously ill and disadvantaged, are plagued by troubling questions. What is happening to our profession and the community mental health settings in which we work? Why are business managers entering the mental health system and telling us what we can and can't do with our clients? Are profit-driven mental health systems eliminating services for people with severe and persistent mental illness? Since when is community mental health care a business and when did the community mental health center (CMHC) become a "behavioral health care provider corporation"? Why can't we keep things the way they were? Can we reverse this trend? Can we hold on to community mental health as we once knew it? Can the public mental health principles that drew us into community practice survive the inclusion of managed care in the public sector? If this is what health care reform is all about, then what has been reformed and whose health is being protected?

In many public mental health settings, the sudden and dramatic changes brought about by the introduction of managed care principles and practices have caught many of us off guard. We and our colleagues may feel disoriented, frightened, insecure, angry, and discouraged. Yet, we know we can't give up. We remain committed to improving the care for the people we have traditionally served, and to continuing, as we always have (usually with inadequate resources and overburdened staff), to manage the care of the most disadvantaged clients.

In order to maintain this commitment in the face of managed care's dramatic transformation of public mental health, we must find a way to survive the onslaught. In a sense, though, mere survival is not enough. Instead, we must find a way to be successful, as clinicians and administrators, in providing quality mental health services to our communities. How do we do this? How can we be successful and feel hopeful? How do we learn the new skills that are necessary to feel competent and capable? How do we create new systems and programs that function effectively and compatibly with managed care principles?

This book is an attempt to answer these questions. It is intended to be a survival manual for mental health providers — psychiatrists, nurses, psychologists, social workers, other masters' level professionals and paraprofessionals — as well as the administrators who currently manage public mental health programs. As community psychiatrists, we approach the problem of public sector managed care (PSMC) from the perspective of clinician managers concerned about quality service delivery.

We have personally experienced this revolution in our professional roles in the past few years. Dr. Pollack has been the medical director of a large community mental health center that has been transforming its direct service and administrative approaches to adapt to increasingly risk-based payment systems and managed care contracts. He has also been involved in the development of service prioritization in the Oregon Health Plan, one of the first state efforts to shift Medicaid service delivery to managed care. Dr. Minkoff has experienced many shifts in his career, from director of a community mental health clinic to medical director of an integrated psychiatric and addiction program in a community hospital, through the hospital's bankruptcy, and into the role of medical director of a privately owned comprehensive public-private managed-care-oriented system of care. We have had to come to terms with the reality of managed care in order to succeed in our present roles. We have organized this book around the issues, ideas, and skills that we have found to be useful in our own settings.

An important basic principle of our approach is our belief that, although there is considerable controversy about the merits of managed care, success requires that we move beyond the controversy, without succumbing to the temptation to deny, ignore, or oppose the advent of managed care initiatives. For the indefinite future, managed care is with us. We feel that the best response to the managed care revolution is to involve ourselves in the planning and implementation of services so that our clients are protected and that the public mental health principles that we feel most strongly about are incorporated into the newly developing systems of care.

Our approach is to educate our colleagues about the nuts and bolts of PSMC, with specific reference to what it is and how it can be applied to the service arenas and populations with which we work. We invited experts from around the country to contribute to this book and recruited a diverse group of authors, who represent a wide range of views, areas of expertise and background experience. Some of the contributors come from the traditional public sector mental health community; some are academicians; some are former community mental health professionals who have become part of the managed behavioral health care industry; and others have come from business or private sector clinical backgrounds to their current involvement with PSMC. Many of the chapters include highlighted survival tips for clinicians and administrators.

The book begins with an overview of the history, concepts, ideology and ethics of PSMC and then proceeds in focus from system to program management to clinical program levels, with a concluding section on advocacy, evaluation, research and training issues. We feel that it is important to provide an overall view of managed care principles and how managed care is being implemented in various state systems. The systems section includes descriptions of several very different approaches to organizing care, whether through private sector managed care organizations, CMHCs, or via the development of independent provider networks, with additional attention to atypical systems such as found in the VA and rural areas.

The program management section focuses on some of the ways programs and provider agencies may need to change in order to adapt to the advent of managed care. This includes attention to managed care readiness criteria, contracting issues, networking issues, utilization management and quality monitoring.

The clinical program section identifies a number of service concepts, program innovations and skills that providers should consider developing in order to balance the need to be cost-effective with the need to meet the clinical needs of persons with severe and persistent mental illness (SPMI) and other clients. These include effective alternatives to acute hospitalization, integrated capitated case management systems for persons with SPMI, integration of primary care and mental health care, integration of addiction and psychiatric services, innovative and wrap-around services for children and effective techniques of time-sensitive psychotherapy.

The concluding section identifies key issues of advocacy, accountability and training that must be addressed. These include the need for effective and meaningful outcome evaluation, well-planned, systematic PSMC research and comprehensive professional training in PSMC skills, as well as the importance of meaningfully including family advocates and consumers in the process of planning, implementing and monitoring PSMC initiatives.

It is possible that some contributors say things that are challenging and unfamiliar to the reader. This book promotes a radical departure from the traditional perspectives of public mental health agencies; yet it retains a consistent focus on the principle of delivering high-quality, cost-effective services to the entire community. Change is bound to be stressful and threatening in some ways. Many clinicians believe that the profession should simply oppose managed care on principle. We believe, however, that we must go beyond the fear of change engendered by managed care. We must provide clinicians and administrators with the skills and preparation not just to survive, but to honor their commitment to the most disadvantaged consumers. We hope that this book will enable you to adjust to the challenges and to become effective participants and leaders in the newly emerging systems. We have tried to convey that PSMC can be approached with a positive spirit, an excitement about the potential to create dramatic and beneficial system changes, and a genuine interest in investigating the relative merits of every aspect of managed care systems.

As with any dramatic change, PSMC poses significant risks to public sector systems and clients. These include funding reductions, service dislocations, and obstacles to care imposed by financially motivated managed care organizations and politically motivated governmental entities. The more that we master the technology and skills of PSMC, the more successful we can be in preventing these risks from becoming realized and in regaining the influence required to assure that care is managed with clinical sensitivity and creativity and leads to improved outcomes.

A word about terminology. Throughout this book, the contributors describe the persons who receive mental health services variably as patients, clients, customers, consumers, survivors, persons with mental illness, or persons in recovery, sometimes using any or all of these terms in the same chapter. This practice reflects the range of terminology used throughout the public sector mental health community; in fact, many of us use these terms interchangeably, depending on the audience with whom we are dealing or the context of the discussion. As different constituents of the mental health community have different preferences, we have retained these variations to reflect this diversity, to maintain respect for the differences of opinion, and to demonstrate the identity confusion that many of us have.

We would like to acknowledge and thank the people who provided support and assistance in a variety of ways that enabled us to make this book as clear, readable, and organized as possible. Help came in the form of clerical activities, editorial advice, proofreading, indexing, support and encouragement from: Cynthia Ajilore, Jeffrey Geller, Susan Halada, Lisa Kenn, Beverly Kirkpatrick, Blanche Mulrenan, Roberta Pollack and Maureen Sullivan.

CONTRIBUTORS

Donald F. Anderson, PhD, Principal, William M. Mercer, Inc., San Francisco, California.

Jack Barbour, MD, Co-Medical Director, Barbour and Floyd Medical Associates; Co-Director, South Central Health and Rehabilitation Program, Los Angeles, California.

Allan Beigel, MD[†] Professor of Psychiatry and Psychology, Arizona Health Sciences Center, Tucson, Arizona.

Jeffrey Berlant, MD, PhD, Senior Consultant, William M. Mercer, Inc., San Francisco, California, Assistant Clinical Professor of Psychiatry, University of Washington School of Medicine.

Rod Betit, Executive Director, Utah State Departments of Health and Human Services, Salt Lake City, Utah.

James J. Callahan, Jr., PhD, Director, NIMH Training Program, Heller School, Brandeis University; Director, Policy Center on Aging, Heller School, Brandeis University, Waltham, Massachusetts.

Charles P. Carbone, BS, Senior Consultant, William M. Mercer, Inc., San Francisco, California.

Robert F. Cole, PhD, Director, National Resource Networks for Child and Family Mental Health Services, Washington Business Group on Health, Washington, DC.

Linda Connery, LCSW, MPA, Program Director, Barbour and Floyd Medical Associates, Los Angeles, California.

David Dangerfield, DSW, Executive Director, Valley Mental Health, Salt Lake City, Utah.

[†]deceased

Larry Davidson, PhD, Assistant Professor of Psychology (in Psychiatry), Yale University School of Medicine, New Haven, Connecticut.

Robert Dorwart, MD, MPH, Professor of Psychiatry, Harvard Medical School and Harvard School of Public Health; Chair, Department of Psychiatry, the Cambridge Hospital, Cambridge, Massachusetts.

Susan Essock, PhD, Director of Psychological Services, Connecticut Department of Mental Health and Addiction; Professor in Residence, A.J. Pappanikou Center, University of Connecticut, Hartford, Connecticut.

Daniel B. Fisher, MD, PhD, Director, National Empowerment Center; Medical Director, EMHS/Riverside, Wakefield, Massachusetts.

Reta Floyd, MD, Co-Medical Director, Barbour and Floyd Medical Associates; Co-Director, S. Central Health and Rehabilitation Program, Los Angeles, California.

Laurie Flynn, Executive Director, National Alliance for the Mentally Ill, Arlington, Virginia.

Rupert R. Goetz, MD, Medical Director, Mental Health and Developmental Disabilities Services Division, State of Oregon; Adjunct Assistant Professor of Psychiatry and Associate Director, Public Psychiatry Training Program, Oregon Health Sciences University, Salem and Portland, Oregon.

Howard H. Goldman, MD, PhD, Professor of Psychiatry, University of Maryland School of Medicine, Baltimore, Maryland.

Laura Lee Hall, PhD, Deputy Director of Policy and Research, National Alliance for the Mentally Ill, Arlington, Virginia.

Eunice Hartman, RN, MS, CS, Former Director of Clinical Management, MHMA/FMH; President, Hartman and Associates, Boston, Massachusetts.

William Hawthorne, PhD, Executive Director, Vista Hill Community Treatment Systems; Associate Clinical Professor, Department of Psychiatry, University of California at San Diego.

Michael A. Hoge, PhD, Associate Professor of Psychology (in Psychiatry), Yale University School of Medicine; Managing Director, Yale Behavioral Health, New Haven, Connecticut.

Richard Hough, PhD, Adjunct Professor, Department of Psychiatry, University of California at San Diego; Director of Research, Institute of Psychiatry, Children's Hospital and Health Center, San Diego, California.

Michael J. Jeffrey, MSW, Associate, William M. Mercer, Inc., San Francisco, California.

Chris Koyanagi, Director of Legislative Policy, Bazelon Center for Mental Health Law, Washington, DC.

Jeremy Lazarus, MD, Associate Clinical Professor of Psychiatry, University of Colorado Health Sciences Center, Englewood, Colorado.

Laurent Lehmann, MD, Associate Chief for Psychiatry and Coordinator for Specialized PTSD Programs, Mental Health Strategic Healthcare Group; Clinical Associate Professor of Psychiatry, Georgetown University School of Medicine, Washington, DC.

Karen Joan Ludwig, LCPC, Program Director, Child, Adult, & Family Program, Shoreline CMHS, Inc., Brunswick, Maine.

J. Jay Mackie, Open Minds, Gettysburg, Pennsylvania.

Bentson McFarland, MD, PhD, Associate Professor of Psychiatry, Oregon Health Sciences University; Adjunct Investigator, Kaiser Permanente Center for Health Research, Portland, Oregon.

Elizabeth Levy Merrick, MSW, Research Associate, Heller School, Brandeis University, Waltham, Massachusetts.

Kenneth Minkoff, MD, Medical Director, Choate Health Systems, Inc., Woburn, Massachusetts; Assistant Clinical Professor, Harvard Medical School, Boston, Massachusetts.

Dennis Mohatt, MA, Medicaid Managed Care Director, Nebraska Department of Social Services; Past President, National Association for Rural Mental Health, Lincoln, Nebraska.

David A. Moltz, MD, Medical Director, Shoreline CMHS, Inc., Brunswick, Maine.

Ann Morrison, MD, Assistant Professor of Psychiatry, Wright State University, Dayton, Ohio.

Deborah Nelson, PhD, Former Director of Quality Management, MHMA/FMH; Vice President, Beacon Health Strategies, Boston, Massachusetts.

Monica Oss, President, Open Minds, Gettysburg, Pennsylvania.

David Pollack, MD, Medical Director, Mental Health Services West; Adjunct Associate Professor of Psychiatry and Associate Director, Public Psychiatry Training Program, Oregon Health Sciences University, Portland, Oregon.

Charles Ray, MEd, Chief Executive Officer, National Community Mental Healthcare Council, Rockville, Maryland.

Brenda Roman, MD, Assistant Professor of Psychiatry, Wright State University, Dayton, Ohio.

Miles F. Shore, MD, Bullard Professor of Psychiatry, Harvard Medical School; Senior Scholar, Malcolm Weiner Center for Social Policy, Kennedy School of Government, Cambridge, Massachusetts.

Lee Ann Slayton, MS, Director of Training and Technical Assistance, National Community Mental Healthcare Council, Rockville, Maryland.

William H. Sledge, MD, Professor of Psychiatry, Yale University School of Medicine, New Haven, Connecticut.

T. Scott Stroup, MD, MPH, Assistant Professor, Department of Psychiatry, University of North Carolina at Chapel Hill; Research Fellow, Cecil G. Sheps Center for Health Services Research, Chapel Hill, North Carolina.

Allan Tasman, MD, Professor and Chairman, Department of Psychiatry and Behavioral Sciences, University of Louisville Medical School, Louisville, Kentucky.

Matthew Weinstein, BA, President, Managed Networks of America, Virginia Beach, Virginia.

Section I

Introduction and Overview

1

Overview of Public Sector Managed Mental Health Care

T. SCOTT STROUP and ROBERT A. DORWART

Cataclysmic changes taking place in the name of "managed care" threaten the foundations of public sector mental health care. Community psychiatrists worry that managed care will mean that their severely ill patients will receive inadequate treatments resulting in tragic outcomes. They fear that the arbitrary decisions of utilization managers will supersede clinical judgments. They want to know how managed care, with its emphasis on cost-containment, can be applied to the critically scarce resources of the public sector. Psychiatrists who work in public-sector settings doubt that adults with severe and persistent mental illness (SPMI), children with severe emotional disturbances (SED), and patients with disabling substance abuse disorders can be treated effectively in systems using the managed care techniques of the private sector.

Managed care is an evolving concept that refers to a variety of strategies in diverse settings. Although definitions of managed care are imprecise, the term commonly refers to techniques designed to control costs by influencing the types of care delivered and the access to these services (Well, Astrachan, Tischler, & Unutzer, 1995). Managed care should not and cannot be brought from the private to public sector without modification; it must be adapted for severely

1

mentally ill persons with a vast array of needs (Hoge, Davidson, Grimm, Sledge, & Howenstine, 1994). An ideal for public-sector managed care has been proposed that "involves the organization of an accessible and accountable service delivery system that would consolidate and flexibly deploy resources so as to provide comprehensive, continuous, cost-efficient, and effective mental health services to targeted individuals in their home communities (Hoge et al., 1994)." Although this definition may serve as a worthy model for community psychiatry, more pragmatically the term managed care, when applied to public-sector psychiatry, refers to the use of a variety of techniques to control costs and maintain adequate quality by regulating access to services, and by influencing the type, duration, and intensity of mental health and substance abuse treatments for adults with SPMI and children with SED.

The context of managed care in public-sector psychiatry is the growth of corporate medicine and privatization throughout the health care sector (Starr, 1982; Dorwart & Epstein, 1993). These trends have transformed health care into a commodity and have meant diminished professional autonomy and decreased clinical control of resources. Although familiar in the private health care sector, these impingements on professional autonomy, accompanied by diminished access to hospital beds for severely ill patients, are alarming to public-sector psychiatrists whose patients have historically been poorly served by the private sector.

This chapter willl provide an overview of managed care as it is evolving to meet the demands of public sector mental health care. First, we briefly trace the history of managed care and its involvement with public mental health services. Second, we define the terms that are commonly used to describe managed care arrangements and procedures. We conclude by briefly describing a few representative approaches to public sector managed care.

BACKGROUND OF PUBLIC SECTOR MANAGED CARE

Until the deinstitutionalization of psychiatric patients that began in the 1950s, the public mental health system was financed primarily by state and local governments. Public mental health agencies operated large psychiatric hospitals that provided treatment and housing to severely mentally ill persons with limited financial means (Hoge et al., 1994). These government agencies had little financial incentive to operate efficiently or to discharge patients in a timely fashion (Dorwart & Epstein, 1993).

Direct federal start-up funds made available through the Community Mental Health Acts of 1963 and 1965 facilitated the creation of a large number of nonprofit mental health agencies. This funding was not closely tied to the types of services offered or to the population served; the agencies had relatively low productivity demands. Since federal grants accounted for a large portion of CMHC budgets in the early years, the economic behavior of these nonprofit providers closely resembled the conduct of public providers paid by state or local governments (Clark, Dorwart, & Epstein, 1994).

The 1970s and 1980s saw political and economic pressures from a variety of sources that led to changes in financing arrangements for both nonprofit and public agencies. Efforts to reduce state and county spending that began in the late 1970s led to budget cuts that forced public agencies to improve efficiency and to seek other sources of income. Reductions in federal funding during the 1980s led to changes in the way local governments did business with the nonprofit CMHCs. Direct federal funding of CMHCs ended in 1981. Increasingly, states and counties paid for mental health care on a fee-for-service basis rather than through budgeted amounts (Clark et al., 1994). As states shifted a large portion of costs to programs such as Medicaid, where the federal government shared the expense, nonprofit and public agencies became more reliant upon payments that were based on services delivered (Hoge et al., 1994). By the end of the 1980s, nonprofit CMHCs and public agencies providing mental health services faced similar economic circumstances and incentives. Both types of agency faced pressures to increase revenues and improve efficiency while trying to provide comprehensive mental health services without regard to consumers' financial means. Both were increasingly reliant on third party payment for client services, and thus subject to conditions set by these payers (Clark et al., 1994; Dorwart & Epstein, 1993).

Meanwhile, third party payers in the private insurance market were gaining experience with utilization management, and managed care organizations (MCOs) such as health maintenance organizations (HMOs) proliferated. Multiple sources provided the impetus for managed care in the private sector. Employers who bought private insurance for their employees sought improved value, and insurers of all types sought to limit costs.

An early target of cost cutting in the private sector was mental health care. Because behavioral health costs were seen as too unpredictable and few MCOs had expertise in mental health care, mental health benefits were often "carved out" of benefit plans. They were left "unmanaged," or were managed by specialty behavioral health MCOs. By the early 1990s there were a small but growing number of these specialty behavioral health MCOs. These companies had considerable success in reducing the growth of expenditures, primarily by curtailing the expansion of inpatient treatment. However, because persons with severe mental illness often were uninsured or had exhausted their private insurance benefits, little expertise developed in managing care for these patients. Although managed care was not new to mental health care, and was not new to community psychiatrists who treated privately insured individuals, it became widespread in the public sector only in the 1990s. The advent of Medicaid managed care programs finally brought widespread capitated financing arrangements and utilization management to mental health care and substance abuse treatment for publicly funded persons.

THE METHODS OF MANAGED CARE

Strategies

By the 1990s, the public insurers Medicaid and Medicare accounted for a large portion of public mental health financing. States had taken advantage of the opportunity to shift costs to the federal government by downsizing state mental health institutions and sending patients to facilitate where their care would be paid for, in part, by federal programs. Although both payers restricted payments to psychiatric specialty hospitals (including state hospitals), Medicaid and Medicare paid for treatment in general hospitals for many with severe mental disorders.

Advocates for Medicare recipients were largely successful in their resistance to attempts to convert it to a managed care system. In 1995, Medicare remained a fee-for-service system. Its fee schedules were based on a resource-based relative value scale (RBRVS), highly controversial among physicians, that adjusted payments according to the value of labor inputs involved in providing a particular service (Dorwart, Rodriguez, Dernburg, & Braun, 1992). Implemented in 1992, the impact of RBRVS on psychiatry remained unclear in 1995. Medicare costs continued to rise, and it appeared unlikely that Medicare would remain outside the realm of managed care.

Managed care rapidly expanded for recipients of Medicaid, the joint state-federal program that financed health care for the poor. Medicaid was politically vulnerable to budget cutters on both the federal and state levels because its constituency was not politically powerful. Medicaid was the focus of numerous cost-cutting initiatives, many of which promoted managed care programs. In 1981, Congress authorized a process by which states could obtain a waiver from certain regulations of the Medicaid program. These *Medicaid waivers* required the approval of the Health Care Financing Administration (HCFA). The Clinton administration, in an effort to promote health care reform and cost-containment, acted to make the waiver process easier. By 1995, at least 40 states had received Medicaid waivers. There were two types of Medicaid waivers: 1) Section 1115 waivers were for statewide "demonstration" projects that allowed testing of innovative financing and delivery systems, and 2) Section 1915 "freedom of choice" or "program" waivers that allowed more limited changes (Intergovernmental Health Policy Project, 1994). By waiving regulations stipulating that consumers' choice of providers could not be limited, the "freedom of choice" waivers facilitated the conversion of Medicaid programs into managed systems of care. This was necessary because managed care organizations usually offer services only through a selected panel of clinicians.

Medicaid managed care programs have dealt with mental health in two ways, by mainstreaming the mentally ill or by creating carveout programs. *Mainstreaming* programs integrate mental health services with general medical care in a unified system of care. In these systems, primary care clinicians (often internists, family practitioners, or nurse practitioners) must authorize referrals to specialists and then monitor their treatments. Mainstreaming promotes improved coordination of mental health and medical services. Risks of mainstreaming include inadequate assessment and treatment of the mentally ill by primary care providers, and delayed or restricted specialty referrals. An additional risk is that funds intended for mental health services may be used for other purposes.

Carve-out programs place mental health (and often substance abuse) services in programs separate from other medical services. Advocates of carve-out systems believe that separate, dedicated mental health funding prevents money from being diverted to other services. Further, carve-out systems may allow improved access to specialty mental health treatment because referral from a primary care clinician is not always required. This improved access may, however, limit the ability of carve-out systems to control expenditures or to coordinate care with primary care clinicians.

TACTICS

Utilization management is "a set of techniques used on or behalf of purchasers of health care benefits to manage health care costs by influencing patient care decision-making through case-by-case assessments of the appropriateness of care prior to and during its provision" (Institute of Medicine, 1989). Its components include prior authorization, concurrent review, and case management. *Prior authorization* is the assessment in advance of an individual patient's need for specific treatments, as determined by a health plan's criteria for "medical necessity." Prior authorization allows a health plan to deny or restrict access to treatment, and to determine the site and intensity of the treatments it allows. *Concurrent review* assesses ongoing treatments for appropriateness and for progress toward treatment goals. Health plans use concurrent review procedures to influence treatment plans and to control the duration of treatment (Committee on Managed Care, 1992).

Case management is generally reserved for consumers who have special needs or are expected to generate large expenditures. In mental health there are two models of case management: cost containment and clinical. *Cost containment case management* is a utilization management tool that allows managed health plans to monitor and control service delivery. These case managers may be empowered to develop specialized treatment plans based on a patient's social as well as medical needs, and to authorize services beyond a health plan's coverage limits or outside its benefit design. For example, they may authorize acute residential treatment, an option that may be less costly or more appropriate than inpatient hospitalization. On the other end of the spectrum, a case manager may inflexibly enforce protocols that restrict treatment. *Clinical case managers* typically do not authorize treatments, but act as brokers who facilitate access to services. In a public mental health setting, case managers may coordinate services among housing, social service, education, criminal justice, and health care systems. They often serve as consumer advocates, seeking optimal arrays of services. Clinical case managers also work toward a goal of cost-effectiveness, by influencing the levels and types of mental health services used (Cuffel, Snowden, Masland, & Piccagli, 1994; Evashwick, 1988).

Capitation is a financing arrangement intended to provide incentives for improved efficiency. In capitated health systems, the buyers of health plans pay a predetermined, per capita fee for a defined benefit in a set period of time. The recipient of the capitated payment is at risk for the financial consequences of this arrangement. Capitated systems eliminate the incentive for overtreatment that is inherent in volume based fee-for-service plans, and minimize incentives to shift costs between service types because of the arbitrary limits specified by benefit designs (Evashwick, 1988). At best, capitated systems may promote the developmental of well-coordinated continuums of care, with improved flexibility and efficiency. At worst, capitated health plans may lead to minimal or inadequate treatments. Capitated payments and risk can be assigned to two levels: the managed care organization or the provider. If the "at-risk" entity is an MCO, the familiar elements of utilization management are employed. Clinical decisions are likely to be subject to administrative micromanagement. If providers are at risk, mental health clinicians may find themselves making unwelcome rationing decisions. On the other hand, capitated payments to providers may return to clinicians from MCOs the power to select treatments and determine their duration and intensity. *Risk adjustment* is the determination of appropriate prospective payments for the treatment of specific population groups. Risk adjustment is based on actuarial data. Arriving at accurate prospective payment levels is a significant problem in making capitated arrangements for public sector clients such as adults with SPMI, children with SED, and substance abusers. This partially accounts for the slow dissemination of managed care into the public sector.

Gatekeeping is a managed care method designed to improve service coordination and control costs. Managed health plans usually will only pay for evaluations and treatments that are authorized by gatekeepers, who control access to specialists and other expensive services. *Primary Care Case Management* (PCCM) is a gatekeeping model in which a primary care clinician (e.g. a physician or nurse practitioner) serves as a case manager, providing assessment and nonspecialty treatment in addition to authorizing specialty referrals. Although the primary clinician may be at financial risk in some capitated plans, more typically the gatekeeper is paid a fee for case management services, but has other financial incentives to keep costs low.

SETTINGS

Managed Care Organizations (MCOs) are entities that administer managed health plans; they may or may not directly provide health care services. They can adhere to any combination of numerous possible organizational structures, benefit designs, and incentive systems

(Cuffel, Snowden, Masland, & Piccagli, 1994). MCOs manage or provide a set of health services benefits to a specified population through a defined *network* of providers. Individual providers participating in these networks have usually met a set of professional qualifications. Agencies and individual providers in the networks have agreed to specific financial and operational terms for treating enrollees of the health plan. Usually the terms include acceptance of a fee schedule, utilization management procedures, and the plan's benefit design. Plan enrollees have a restricted choice of providers, although sometimes out-of-network services are authorized (Patterson, 1993).

One type of MCO, the *third party administrator*, is not a provider, but manages or administers a system for a separate panel of clinicial providers. These MCOs manage health plans, process claims, and provide utilization management (Cuffel, Snowden, Masland, & Piccagli, 1994). Their budgets may be based on fees for specific services provided, or they may have capitated contracts, with or without financial risk.

Health Maintenance Organizations (HMOs) are prototypical MCOs and have evolved into a diversity of structures. The hallmark of HMOs is that a defined benefit is provided for a prepaid, per capita fee (Broskowski & Eaddy, 1994). HMOs can be self-contained entities that employ clinicians, or can operate through contracts with an extensive network of providers. Gate keepers control referrals to specialists. Specialists may or may not have specific contractual arrangements with the HMO. Specialist providers may be paid on a capitated, per case, per episode, or discounted fee-for-service basis. Enrollees have strong financial incentives to see specialists only within the managed care network. *Point of service* (POS) plans allow enrollees to choose out of network providers at the point of service delivery, but the enrollees are liable for additional fees (Dorwart & Epstein, 1992; Patterson, 1993). Although POS plans may offer improved flexibility for enrollees in the private sector, they offer little advantage to public-sector patients without discretionary funds.

Independent Practice Associations (IPAs) are an HMO model whose clinicians practice independently and who agree to accept a prepaid rate (usually capitated) for services provided to the IPA's enrollees. IPA members have a relatively wide range of provider choice. IPA professionals usually retain other types of patients and thus maintain considerable autonomy in their practices. *Preferred Provider Organizations* (PPOs) are arrangements between payers and providers in which the payer contracts for discounted rates, sometimes in return for a guaranteed volume of referrals. Often these arrangements are administered and monitored by specialized utilization management organizations (or third party administrators) (Dorwart & Epstein, 1992).

EXAMPLES OF STATES WITH PUBLIC-SECTOR MANAGED CARE

The introduction of managed care into Medicaid programs was a primary way that states introduced managed care for public mental health services. States mixed and matched the various strategies and tactics discussed in this chapter so that each managed care Medicaid system was unique. Figure One demonstrates the diversity of a few states' approaches. The figure represents state Medicaid programs at a single point in time only, at a time when managed care systems continued to change rapidly. The following text gives a more detailed description of these representative states.

TENNESSEE

Tennessee began operating a Medicaid managed care program in 1994 after obtaining a Section 1115 demonstration waiver from HCFA. The statewide program, called TennCare, expanded health care coverage to thousands of previously uninsured people with low incomes. All of the state's Medicaid enrollees were enrolled in one of twelve MCOs that were organized as HMOs. Most users of mental health and substance abuse services were mainstreamed into a program that included inpatient and outpatient treatment limited by a specific number of treatment days. Adults with SPMI and children with SED, however, were enrolled in a carve-out system that included mandatory clinical case management. Users of the mainstream mental health system could be transferred to the case-managed system when they reached their benefit limits. The mainstream system was capitated from its beginning. The carve-out system was originally neither capitated nor run by MCOs because the MCOs objected to the proposed amount of payment (Intergovernmental, 1994). In early 1995, the MCOs agreed to accept an enhanced capitated rate for the case managed SPMI and SED populations.

TennCare was an extremely controversial program that continued to evolve well after its initiation. Initially, low fee schedules kept many physicians from signing up with the Medicaid MCOs, until they were forced to take TennCare patients in order to continue participating in the large, well funded PPO for state employees. Physician participation in TennCare increased as a result of this "cram down," but widespread dissatisfaction among providers persisted. For persons with SPMI, there were problems getting the MCOs to pay for specialized community support services (Interegovernmental, 1994). Nevertheless, consumer advocates favored the expanded coverage of TennCare, and its improved integration of mental health services with the general medical care system. By summer of 1995, however, serious problems with the allocation of mental health funds contributed to calls for major program changes. It seemed likely that program revisions would result in a completely carved-out mental health benefit.

MASSACHUSETTS

Beginning in 1992, Massachusetts operated a Medicaid system that included both a mainstreamed and a carved out mental health and

Figure 1. Selected characteristics of public-sector mental health systems in a sample of states with managed care Medicaid programs. Due to the dynamic nature of public-sector managed care, all arrangements are subject to change.

STATE	WAIVER TYPE	STATEWIDE	PRIVATE MCO	PRIVATE SPECIALTY BEHAVIORAL MCO	GATE KEEPER (Primary Care)	TARGET POPULATION	COMMENT
IOWA (Mental Health Access Plan)	1915	Yes	Yes	Yes	No	All categorically eligible	M.H. carved out into a statewide system with a single MCO.
MASSACHUSETTS (HMO option)	1915	Yes	Yes	No	Yes	All categorically eligible	M.H. mainstreamed in HMOs or carved out in a PCCM program. Higher capitated rate for disabled population.
MASSACHUSETTS (PCCM option)	1915	Yes	Yes	Yes	No	"	
N. CAROLINA (Carolina Alternatives)	1915	No	No	No	No	<= 18 y.o. only in participating areas	Area MHCs are MCOs
OREGON (Oregon Health Plan)	1115	Yes (staged)	mixed (a)	mixed (a)	mixed (a)	All in targeted areas	Regional behavioral health MCOs. Prioritized list of covered conditions.
TENNESSEE (TennCare)	1115	Yes	Yes	Yes	No	special program for SED, SPMI	Most M.H. mainstreamed; case management for SPMI, SED

(a) Contracted managed care organizations in Oregon include community mental health programs, fully capitated health plans, and two other unique nonprofit organizations ("Oregon Plan," 1995).

substance abuse program. Under the authority of a Medicaid Section 1915 freedom of choice waiver, the state compelled Medicaid recipients to enroll in one of several private HMOs, or to join the state-operated primary care case manager (PCCM) program. In the HMOs, mental health services were mainstreamed; primary care gate keepers controlled access to mental health providers. In the state's PCCM program, a private third party administrator specializing in behavioral health care managed the mental health and substance abuse benefit. The contracted MCO operated through a capitated contract that shared financial risk with the state. The PCCM program was completely separate from the mental health carve-out; the primary care provider was not a gate keeper for mental health services. Enrollees had direct access to mental health care providers that were part of the MCO's network. Benefits were subject to extensive utilization management procedures, including prior authorization for inpatient and outpatient treatment. The MCO also used concurrent review and cost containment case management. Payments to the MCO were capitated at two rates: one for disabled and another for nondisabled enrollees. Payments to providers were not capitated.

In 1995, the Massachusetts Department of Human Services revealed a plan to put all acute inpatient treatment in the public sector into a unified managed care system. Under the proposed system, Medicaid recipients as well as the uninsured, who were previously treated in state-operated facilities, would receive a benefit through a specialty MCO. If enacted, this plan would lead to a completely privatized system for acute inpatient treatment in Massachusetts, further eroding the distinction between the public and private sectors. The state DMH would continue to operate intermediate and long-stay units.

OREGON

Under the authority of a Medicaid waiver that was approved amid great controversy in 1993, Oregon began implementation of its Oregon Health Plan (OHP) (Pollack, McFarland, George, & Angell, 1994). The plan used a prioritized list of conditions to avoid expenditures for conditions without effective treatments. The state legislature was required to authorize funding for conditions above a certain rank, in effect denying treatment for conditions with low priority ratings. The prioritizing plan was criticized by some for its explicit rationing, but for persons with mental illness the plan represented a major advance toward equitable treatment. Mental illnesses were ranked on the same scale as general medical conditions, and treatments for all severe mental illnesses and most other mental conditions were expected to be funded.

The Oregon Health Plan (OHP) was designed to extend health benefits to many previously without insurance by implementing managed care techniques and using the expected savings to finance the expanded coverage. Mental health care was to be capitated in both integrated (or mainstream) and carve-out systems to be gradually phased in, initially including 25% of the Medicaid population. A variety of mental health organizations, including community mental health centers and specialty MCO, were awarded the initial contracts.

NORTH CAROLINA

In 1993 North Carolina implemented a managed care plan, called Carolina Alternatives, for Medicaid recipients under age 18. An important feature of this carve-out plan was that locally governed Area Mental Health Programs were designated to be the managed care organizations. These local agencies were responsible for the provision of all medically necessary mental health services. Carolina Alternatives initially affected about 25% of the state's Area Mental Health Programs. Expansion of the plan to services for adults and more children was planned for 1996.

IOWA

In 1995, Iowa began its Mental Health Access Plan, a behavioral health carve out for Medicaid recipients. The capitated program operated statewide through a contract with a specialty behavioral health MCO. The plan was intended for nearly all of the state's Medicaid population, with no special carve out for adults with SPMI or children with SED. The plan was similar to the carve-out component of Massachusetts' Medicaid program, but contained no option to join an HMO with a mainstreamed mental health benefit.

CONCLUSION

In the 1990s, many states converted large portions of their public mental health systems into managed systems of care. The examples discussed here illustrate that public-sector managed care is not a uniform entity, but varies widely in the specific strategies and tactics used. Other states have used other combinations of managed care approaches; each state's system is unique, based on local political and historical factors. A widespread trend is that changes associated with managed care are blurring the distinction between the private and public sectors. The impact of managed care in public sector mental health care is largely unknown and will require close monitoring to determine its various impacts. The remainder of this book addresses many critical issues raised by these monumental changes in community psychiatry.

REFERENCES

Broskowski, A., & Eaddy, M. (1994). Community mental health centers in a managed care environment. *Administration and Policy in Mental Health, 21,* 335–352.

Clark, R.E., Dorwart, R.A., & Epstein, S.S. (1994). Managing competition in public and private mental health agencies: implications for services and policy. *Milbank Quarterly, 72,* 653–678.

Committee on Managed Care of the American Psychiatric Association. (1992). *Utilization management: a handbook for clinicians.* Washington, DC: American Psychiatric Association.

Cuffel, B.J., Snowden, L., Masland, M.C., & Piccagli, G. (1994). *Managed mental health care in the public sector* (Working paper No. 6-94). Berkeley, CA: Institute for Mental Health Services Research.

Dorwart, R.A. (1990). Managed mental health care: myths and realities in the 1990s. *Hospital and Community Psychiatry, 41,* 1087–1091.

Dorwart, R.A., & Epstein, S.S. (1992). Economics and managed mental health care: the HMO as a crucible for cost-effective care. In S.L. Feldman & R.J. Fitzpatrick (Eds.), *Managed mental health care: administrative and clinical issues.* Washington, DC: American Psychiatric Press.

Dorwart, R.A., Rodriguez, E., Derburg, J., & Braun, P. (1992). Measuring the determinants of work values for psychiatrists' services in the resource-based relative value scale study. *American Journal of Psychiatry, 149,* 1654–1659.

Dorwart, R.A., & Epstein, S.S. (1993). *Privatization and mental health care: a fragile balance.* Westport, CT: Auburn House.

Evashwick, C.J. (1988). The continuum of long-term care. In S.J. Feldman & P.J. Torrens (Eds.), *Introduction to Health Services.* New York: John Wiley & Sons.

Hoge, M.A., Davidson, L., Griffith, E.E.H., Sledge, W.H., & Howenstein, R.A. (1994). Defining Managed Care in Public-Sector Psychiatry. *Hospital and Community Psychiatry, 45,* 1085–1089.

Institute of Medicine Committee on Utilization Management by Third Parties. (1989). *Controlling costs and changing patient care?: the role of utilization management.* Washington, DC: National Academy Press.

Intergovernmental Health Policy Project (1994). *Medicaid managed care and mental health: an overview of section 1115 programs.* Washington, DC: George Washington University.

Oregon Plan: Future of MH Services up in air. (1995, May 19). *Psychiatric News,* pp. 1, 30–31.

Patterson, D.Y. (1993). Twenty-first century managed mental health: point of service treatment networks. *Administration and Policy in Mental Health, 21,* 27–34.

Pollack, D.A., McFarland, B.H., George, R.A., & Angell, R.H. (1994). Prioritization of Mental Health Services in Oregon. *Milbank Quarterly, 72,* 515–550.

Starr, P. (1982). *The Social Transformation of American Medicine.* New York: Basic Books.

Wells, K.G.B., Astrachan, B.I.M., Tischler, G.L., & Unutzer, J. (1995). Issues and approaches in evaluating mental health care. *Milbank Quarterly, 73,* 57–75.

2

Public Sector Managed Care and Community Mental Health Ideology

KENNETH MINKOFF

INTRODUCTION

As public sector managed care (PSMC) spreads more widely, there is growing anxiety among public sector clinicians and managers about the perceived incompatibility of "managed care" with community mental health (CMH) ideology, and with their own deeply-held principles and ideals regarding public sector service. (See Table 1). This anxiety results, in turn, in substantial opposition to the implementation of managed-care initiatives and programs, and this may interfere significantly with the ability of their programs to respond creatively and proactively to the changes in mental health system organization and financing that managed care represents. Paradoxically, the more committed that clinicians, managers or programs become to resisting "managed care" because of the belief that it compromises their ideals of patient care in the public sector, the more likely that patient care will be adversely affected by reductions in reimbursement or loss of contracts. Successful response to managed care, therefore, requires clinicians and managers to address their ideological discomfort directly, and to explore carefully whether the *perceived* ideological incompatibility of "managed care"

13

TABLE 1: Areas of Perceived Ideological Incompatibility

1. Managed care is concerned with cost-cutting, not with quality service provision.
2. Managed care is governed by profit-oriented companies with little commitment to public sector values.
3. Managed care involves layers of intrusive control of clinical care, external to consumers, families, clinicians, and other members of the "community".
4. Managed care is insensitive to traditional community-based organization of services.
5. Managed care emphasizes short-term treatment methods which are incompatible with long-term needs of public sector clients.
6. Managed care creates disincentives to the provision of "nonreimbursable" services-such as case coordination, agency consultation, and psychosocial rehabilitation, which are so important for public-sector clients.

can be resolved. The goal of this chapter is to analyze this issue in order to determine whether PSMC can in fact be compatible with CMH ideology.

To accomplish this task, this chapter will (a) review the history, ideology, and implementation of both community mental health systems and of PSMC systems; (b) attempt to identify areas of compatibility and incompatibility in ideology and mission; and (c) discuss methods of implementation of PSMC that may enhance ideological concordance.

COMMUNITY MENTAL HEALTH IDEOLOGY REVISITED

The community mental health movement arose in response to two major problems: (a) the warehousing of large numbers of severely mentally ill individuals in remote public institutions; and (b) the lack of availability of accessible, comprehensive mental health services in most communities.

As embodied in the Community Mental Health Centers Construction Act of 1963, the goals of the movement were to develop organized systems that could address the total mental health needs of the community, and would permit services for those with psychiatric disorders to be delivered in more normative settings, closer to their natural caregivers. The movement was powerfully influenced by Gerald Caplan (1964), whose concepts of community consultation emphasized the potential for mental health professionals to serve the entire community through organizing and training community-based indigenous caregivers in crisis intervention, and in techniques of primary and secondary prevention. In the absence of widespread third-party reimbursement for health care-and especially mental health care-in the 1960's, public (federal) funding of CMHCs was conceived as seed money. These funds would stimulate the development of more permanent self-sufficiency based on multi-source funding: client fees based on ability to pay, state and local funds, and third-party insurance. (Brown & Kane, 1963).

The original ideology of the community mental health (CMH) movement, therefore, encompassed the principles outlined in Table 2:

As originally conceived, therefore, community mental health centers (CMHCs), were like capitated systems, responsible for the comprehensive mental health needs of a defined population within the constraints of a fixed budget. Over time, however, the implementation of the original community mental health vision was transformed by a number of powerful forces:

Expansion of the mental health private sector. The increase in awareness of mental health issues and in acceptability of mental health treatment spawned by the CMH movement generated a tremendous expansion of third-party reimbursement for outpatient and inpatient psychiatric services, and a corresponding expansion of private practice psychotherapists, general hospital psychiatric units, and psychiatric hospitals.

Deinstitutionalization. Simultaneous with the expansion of the mental health private sector, community-based service systems were inundated with waves of deinstitutionalized patients, whose complex needs exceeded the initial expectations of the deinstitutionalization movement (Minkoff, 1987), and whose requirement for comprehensive services became progressively more apparent (Bachrach, 1986).

TABLE 2: Original CMH Ideology

---

1. CMH should address the mental health needs of the whole community (defined by geographic "catchment area").

2. CMH services should be available to everyone, regardless of ability to pay.

3. CMH services should be provided by organized systems, responsive to the communities they serve.

4. CMH should emphasize crisis intervention and reliance on natural support systems to promote normalization and community integration.

5. CMH should emphasize the provision of community-based alternatives to institutional care.

6. CMH services are funded through provision of a fixed public budget for a defined population, and should ultimately become self-supporting, through both efficient resource utilization, and development of multiple funding sources.

Expansion of public-sector third party payment. During the 1970's and 1980's, the expansion of Medicaid and Medicare funding for community-based inpatient and outpatient services led to a major shift in the source of funding for CMH services.

These forces created a re-direction of energy within the CMH movement, characterized by the following elements:

Community mental health synonymous with public sector mental health. From the perspective of assessing the needs of the population, CMH programs became focused on identifying underserved populations-usually those without private resources-and diverting private-paying patients elsewhere. Continuation of funding for CMHCs largely came from state departments of mental health, whose major priority was deinstitutionalization. The focus of CMHC services thus became (slowly, and often with great resistance from CMHCs themselves), the chronically mentally ill.

Community mental health services no longer delivered primarily by CMHCs. Deinstitutionalization resulted in an expansion of need for CMH services in every catchment area, as well as an expansion of the range of services required (e.g., housing, vocational rehabilitation, socialization support). This expansion, plus the resistance of many CMHCs to prioritize services for the chronically mentally ill, led to a proliferation of vendors, with multiple public funding streams, providing CMH services. The expansion of services was consequently accompanied by a reduction of coordination of care, including "lack of coordination among multiple providers, lack of continuity in treatment planning over time, reimbursement systems that contain disincentives for community-based and rehabilitative treatments, minimal incentives for efficiency or cost-saving, and poorly developed systems for monitoring the necessity, appropriateness, and effectiveness of care." (Hoge, Davidson, Griffith, Sledge, & Howenstine, 1994, p. 1086).

Community mental health services increasingly dependent upon third-party fee-for-service reimbursement. The expansion of availability of Medicaid payments for community-based inpatient and outpatient services enabled CMH service expansion and state hospital diversion to private inpatient units with less direct reliance of state and local funding. However, as noted above, the idiosyncrasies of Medicaid and Medicare reimbursement have often included disincentives for development of hospital diversion programs and for utilization of "non-medical" services like psychosocial rehabilitation and case management.

The ideology of community mental health service delivery has been somewhat realigned by these changes, as described in Table 3.

This revised ideology has largely governed the operation of "unmanaged" public sector community mental health systems, and has resulted, nationwide, in a broad expansion of community-based inpatient and outpatient services for the seriously mentally ill which may represent the demonstrable success of the CMH movement (Ozarin, 1995). Nonetheless, within this ideology are the roots of three major problems that have led to the emergence of "managed care".

TABLE 3: Public Sector Community Mental Health Ideology

1. Within the two-tiered system of care, CMH should focus primarily on public-sector supported patients.

2. CMH is not "all things to all people", but focuses limited resources on those most in need and least able to pay (Stern & Minkoff, 1979).

3. CMH emphasizes the provision of community-based services to *seriously mentally ill* individuals (as opposed to substance abusers, for example), as alternatives to *public-sector* institutional care (i.e. utilizing private community hospitals is an acceptable alternative).

4. CMH services to seriously mentally ill clients should be provided by organized community support systems, encompassing multiple public and private providers.

5. CMH should emphasize crisis intervention primarily as a form of *triage and pre-screening* to reduce inappropriate access to institutional care, and enhance development of *professionalized* service systems as institutional alternatives, rather than rely on indigenous caregivers.

6. CMH programs should advocate for expanded public resources to fund needed programs, both through legislative advocacy and through expansion of third-party revenue.

Lack of incentives for cost control. Unmanaged Medicaid benefits have been associated with an explosion of utilization, justified by the unarguable needs of the clients served. Yet, there has been no mechanism to ensure that Medicaid expenditures are being utilized cost-effectively. The needs have justified the means, as it were, but cost-based and outcome-based accountability have been lacking.

Lack of systems coordination. As noted in the comments by Hoge et al. (1994), cited earlier, the ideal coordination of community support systems has rarely been achieved, resulting in observable service fragmentation. Awareness of service gaps has become particularly acute in recent years with the expanded visibility of the homeless mentally ill.

Lack of service integration. Focus on services in the public-sector to persons with SPMI has resulted in unanticipated barriers to service to other populations: substance-disordered patients (especially those with dual diagnosis); children and families; geriatric patients; uninsured patients without serious mental illness; and even patients with SPMI with private insurance (who may be unable to access publicly funded community support services). The CMH system has evolved in such a way that the ability to *plan* resource allocation for the *total* community has been lost.

THE IDEOLOGY OF PUBLIC SECTOR MANAGED CARE

PSMC has emerged as a mechanism to address these problems. But, what is PSMC? Although a clear consensus definition has not yet been established, existing definitions in the literature reflect two major themes, which derive directly from the problems listed above.

Systems coordination and service integration. Hoge et al.'s (1994) excellent analysis of PSMC as a solution to poor integration and coordination attendant to "unmanaged public mental health systems" led to the following definition:

> Public sector managed care involves the organization of an *accessible* and *accountable* service delivery system that is designed to *consolidate* and *flexibly deploy* resources so as to provide *comprehensive, continuous, cost-efficient* and *effective* mental health services to *targeted* individuals in their home communities" (Hoge et al., 1994, p. 1087).

Cost containment. Charles Ray, Executive Director of the National Council of Community Mental Health Centers, has described managed care as much more payer-driven or cost-focused:

> "Managed care is the action by any payer, public or private, to contain costs while maintaining an established or negotiated standard for care." (National Council of Community Mental Health Centers [NCCMHC], 1992).

In reality, PSMC represents an attempt to fuse these two elements. Hoge et al.'s (1994) definition implies that managed care primarily involves *service reorganization* to improve cost-effectiveness, citing the Robert Wood Johnson Foundation project on chronic mental illness (Shore & Cohen, 1990; Goldman, Morrissey, & Ridgely, 1990) as an example:

> "By combining administrative, fiscal, and clinical responsibility in one local [mental health authority] ... this strategy functions to consolidate ... funding so that scarce resources can be efficiently and flexibly deployed...." (Hoge et al., 1994, p. 1086).

Yet, true managed care is inevitably payer-driven and requires *payment reorganization*: the creation of a payment *mechanism* to *incentivize* the careful clinical and financial management of the cost and outcome of each episode of care, which in turn drives the service reorganization described above.

Understanding the purpose of managed care leads to the following major point: *Managed Care ≠ Managed Care Companies*. Managed care is a *function* that can be performed by many different types of agencies, in many different ways.

Thus, the cost/care management described above can be performed by an *external* managed care company incentivized (by capitation or other means) to conserve costs while adhering to negotiated outcome measures required by the public sector payer (e.g.,

Medicaid) with which the Managed Care Organization is contracted. Alternatively, however, the same care management can be performed by public sector *providers* or by public agencies, which can be *directly* incentivized to manage their own care and outcome by capitation or other risk-based contracting directly with the payer, without a "managed care company" as intermediary. (See chapter by Dangerfield and Betit).

The ideology of PSMC, therefore, emphasizes the *function* of managed care, not who performs the function, and embodies *both* the fiscal value of cost containment and enhanced efficiency of resource utilization *and* the clinical value of enhanced service coordination and clinical outcome. The principles of this PSMC ideology are outlined in Table 4.

TABLE 4: Principles of PSMC Ideology

1. PSMC should address the mental health needs of the whole community. *The "community" is defined by the public-sector payer, not by geography.*

2. PSMC must make services potentially accessible to the population as a whole, not just to the seriously mentally ill.

3. PSMC requires the creation of organized systems of care management, responsible for providing comprehensive, continuous, efficient, and cost-effective services, that are responsible to the customers' needs: payers, consumers, and families.

4. PSMC emphasizes the development of targeted interventions that enhance reliance on consumer empowerment, client strengths, and the development of more normative support systems (like clubhouses) rather than foster overdependence on professional care.

5. PSMC emphasizes the development of triage systems that offer a comprehensive spectrum of community-based alternatives to *any* hospitalization (public or private) for patients with *any* diagnosis (mental health, substance abuse, etc.).

6. PSMC, through provision of fixed dollars for a defined population (per capita), encourages providers to manage those dollars through efficient resource utilization and to evaluate resource needs through outcome evaluation.

7. PSMC supports the elimination of the two-tiered system of care. By funding private providers to provide services to public-funded clients, and by encouraging public providers to develop services that can compete for private dollars, PSMC promotes the belief that *all* programs should provide services to targeted clients regardless of payer source.

COMPARATIVE IDEOLOGY

The ideology of PSMC, therefore, even though it may be inconsistently implemented, is strikingly similar to the original ideology of the community mental health movement. Community mental health centers were the original capitated providers, and community mental health professionals have always believed in providing *equal* services regardless of ability to pay, even though we have participated in a two-tiered system in which private and public services differ markedly (Minkoff, 1994). Yet the breakdown of our traditional boundaries and concepts is enormously stressful, and leaves us without many familiar guideposts for evaluating the value of services and service systems. Bachrach (1981) has noted the tendency of community mental health professionals to become hypnotized by certain affect-laden concepts. According to Hoge et al. (1994, p. 1088), "we then judge systems and initiatives in the context of those value-laden terms. Thus, systems with 'case management' and 'assertive community treatment' are judged favorably, without reference to the actual implementation of these concepts, and 'privatized' systems are summarily dismissed because they evoke the notion of profit, which many consider anathema to the public-sector environment."

We must be prepared, therefore, to move beyond simple judgments of "good" vs. "evil" to develop a practical understanding of how to implement PSMC in a way that is truly consistent with our shared ideology. Charles Ray wrote that as managed care evolves, it will not matter whether or not providers believe they are primarily public or private. (NCCMHC, 1992). This prediction is definitely coming true. Managed care is not equivalent to private for-profit managed care companies; PSMC represents a larger systems change in which managed care companies may play a role. This will only happen if we, the public purchasers of their services, believe that they deliver what we want-or what we are unable-as providers- to deliver ourselves. Clearly public-sector agencies that wish to see the implementation of PSMC conform to CMH ideology would be well advised to develop the capacity to truly "manage" care and cost in a responsible manner.

Further, in evaluating the implementation of the CMH/PSMC ideology, we need to evaluate performance in relationship to principles, as follows:

Cost-cutting vs. quality improvement. PSMC encompasses values of enhanced service coordination at reduced cost. The key question in implementation is, how are the cost/quality trade-offs made, and who monitors them? If cost savings can occur without reduction in quality, as in Massachusetts (Callahan, Shepard, Beinecke, Larson, & Cavanaugh, 1994), should the money saved be retained in the general fund or be utilized to expand services? Massachusetts chose the former course; New York, on the other hand, has made an effort to demand community reinvestment (Swidler & Tauriello, 1995).

Incentivization vs. quality monitoring. Regardless of whether PSMC is in the hands of the public or private sector, incentives for cost containment must be balanced by external quality monitoring. Capitation arrangements where the managed care provider keeps all the savings may adversely affect access to services, compared to an arrangement where there is a narrow shared-risk corridor with quality based incentives. That is, the managed care company is not at full risk; it may get paid a flat (e.g., 5%) management fee plus a small percentage of savings, and be at risk for only a small percentage of losses. There may also be incentive payments based on quality and outcome measures like consumer satisfaction, or rate of readmission.

Community Involvement and Oversight. One major change that has occurred between traditional CMH ideology and PSMC is the change in our definition of community. Communities, in general, are less local and more "global" than they were thirty years ago. Community membership is now defined by payer rather than geography, and local responsiveness is less of a concern as we move to larger regional and statewide systems of care organization.

Nevertheless, mechanisms for "community control" of PSMC arrangements are vitally important; oversight should not be the sole province of public bureaucracies. Thus, in locally organized managed care programs, such as the county-based models described elsewhere in this volume, community oversight can be accomplished by the empowerment of community advisory boards, incorporating representation from local consumers, families, mental health advocates, and providers. Similar advisory boards (e.g., state psychiatric society, statewide provider organizations, state Alliances for the Mentally Ill, and consumer coalitions) with representation from larger and more powerful constituencies, should be constructed to monitor the performance of regional or statewide managed care programs.

Focused Treatment vs. Long-Term Care. Appropriate PSMC creates both financial and quality incentives to continue to provide ongoing care management to the long-term mentally ill. As the results of the Monroe-Livingston capitation study indicate (Reed, Hennessy, Mitchell, & Babigian, 1994), quality of service for the most serious mentally ill was maintained, at reduction of cost, through enhanced case management and psychosocial rehabilitation resulting in reduction of inpatient utilization. Managed care may result in more clearly focused use of psychotherapy, for patients at every level of severity (See chapter by Ludwig and Moltz), but can retain the capacity to develop individualized care management to offer *enhanced* psychotherapy to the small number of patients who require that level of intervention to maintain stability and to make progress.

CONCLUSION

In conclusion, the ideological incompatibility between community mental health and PSMC is more apparent than real; substantial ideological concordance *in principle* is present. The challenge for us, as providers and advocates, is to develop our skills and our energy to insure that the implementation of managed care conforms to those principles in a way that truly enhances service delivery. We, in community mental health, are involved in "a radical transformation" of the public mental health system; but we must act quickly to make these changes occur in the way we want (Minkoff, 1994). We need to be prepared to learn new concepts, new skills, and new program models. More importantly, we need to advocate for quality and standards, incorporating principles of accessibility, continuity, comprehensiveness, adequacy of funding, outreach, incentivization of quality, maximization of choice, and community/consumer accountability (Minkoff, 1994).

At its best, PSMC has the potential to help us attain a more equitable, integrated, and efficient service system. Let us all work together to make that vision more of a reality.

REFERENCES

Bachrach, L.L. (1981). Continuity of care for chronic mental patients: A conceptual analysis. *American Journal Of Psychiatry, 138,* 1449–1456.

Bachrach, L.L. (1986). The challenge of service planning for chronic mental patients. *Community Mental Health Journal, 22,* 170–174.

Brown, B., & Kane, H.P. (1963). The many meanings of comprehensive: underlying issues in implementing the community mental health program. *American Journal Of Orthopsychiatry, 34,* 834–839.

Callahan Jr., J.J., Shepard, D.S., Beinecke, R.H., Larson, M.J., & Cavanaugh, D. (1994). *Evaluation Of The Massachusetts Medicaid Mental Health/ Substance Abuse Program.* Unpublished manuscript. Brandeis University, Heller School for Advanced Studies in Social Welfare, Waltham, MA.

Caplan, G. (1964). *Principles Of Preventive Psychiatry.* New York: Basic Books.

Goldman, H.H., Morrissey, J.P., & Ridgely, M.S. (1990). Form and function of mental health authorities at RWJ Foundation program sites: preliminary observations. *Hospital & Community Psychiatry, 41,* 1222–1230.

Hoge, M.A., Davidson, L., Griffith, E.E.H., Sledge, W.H., & Howenstine, R.A. (1994). Defining managed care in public-sector psychiatry. *Hospital & Community Psychiatry, 45,* 1085–1089.

Minkoff, K. (1987). Beyond deinstitutionalization: a new ideology for the post-institutional era. *Hospital & Community Psychiatry, 38,* 945–950.

Minkoff, K. (1994). Community mental health in the nineties: PSMC. *Community Mental Health Journal, 30,* 317–321.

National Council of Community Mental Health Centers (1992). *Managed Mental Health Care – The Manual.* Rockville, MD.

Ozarin, L.D. (1995). Community mental health centers: success or failure? (taking issue). *Psychiatric Services, 431.*

Reed, S.K., Hennessey, K.D., Mitchell, O.S., & Babigian, H.M. A mental-health capitation program: II. Cost-benefit analysis. *Hospital & Community Psychiatry, 45,* 1097–1103.

Shore, M.F., & Cohen, M.D. (1990). The Robert Wood Johnson Foundation program on chronic mental illness: an overview. *Hospital & Community Psychiatry, 41,* 1212–1216.

Stern, R., & Minkoff, K. (1979). Paradoxes in programming for chronic patients in a community clinic. *Hospital & Community Psychiatry, 30,* 613–617.

Swidler, R.N., & Tauriello, J.V. (1995). New York's State Community Mental Health Reinvestment Act. *Psychiatric Services, May,* 496–500.

3

Ethical Aspects of Public Sector Managed Care

JEREMY LAZARUS and DAVID POLLACK

INTRODUCTION

In many respects the public sector has always "managed" populations of patients under fixed budgets. The vagaries of state and/or
federal funding have traditionally influenced the extent to which public systems could meet mental health needs. Ethical dilemmas about
financing and allocation of resources under public sector managed
care (PSMC) have been experienced for decades. Nevertheless, the
broad range and diversity of PSMC initiatives with varying models
of delivery, cost consciousness, and profit motives have created new
sets of ethical dilemmas and intensified others. This chapter will focus on how the current ethical dilemmas may manifest themselves
and how we might deal effectively with them.

ETHICAL THEORY

Modern medical ethics essentially began with Hippocrates, then
moved to Percival's code in the late nineteenth century, and finally
was codified by the AMA in the twentieth century. The American
Psychiatric Association (APA) and other mental health professional
associations' codes are in large part derived from these ethical principles (AMA, 1994). The APA, while following the seven AMA ethical

25

principles, added its own annotated code to add specificity to unique problems encountered in psychiatry (APA, 1993). Specific ethical issues in managed care have been addressed in additional AMA publications and by others (AMA, 1993, 1995; Lazarus & Sharfstein, 1994). Because the health and mental health care landscape is changing so dramatically, there are questions about whether medical ethics will survive (Pellegrino, 1993). The bioethical principles of autonomy, beneficence, nonmaleficence and justice are being strongly pressured by the current forces of the market.

Medical ethics define responsibilities to patient, society and self. The responsibility towards individual patient advocacy has always taken priority and has been reaffirmed by the AMA. In the public sector, however, the responsibility to society or community has always played an important role in that the need to allocate resources across a population and to rely on principles of social or distributive justice are essential and beneficial to effective public health care. Innovative application of justice principles (Daniels, 1985) have also been applied in the private sector (e.g., Harvard Community Health Plan and Group Health of Puget Sound). It is ethically sound in this type of system with a limited budget to balance cost and outcome by providing effective and beneficial services and by limiting or excluding services which are only marginally beneficial. The articulation of this type of social contract needs to be made explicit to the public system. Unfortunately the definitions of marginally beneficial care are not clear. A fair review of these definitions may only be possible with scientifically validated outcome studies.

The influence of managed care on ethics has been most apparent in the private sector. However, the latest trend toward public/private partnerships, bidding for public mental health services, and increased numbers of Medicaid waiver demonstration projects puts many public systems into a turmoil of potential change. Some have questioned whether state mental health agencies will survive health care reform (Glover & Petrila, 1994). The ethical obligation to individual patient advocacy is being challenged by a population or social justice based model of patient advocacy (Sabin & Daniels, 1994) and the pressures of economic constraints and demands for outcome accountability. While some of these forces may have a salutary effect on patient treatment, many in the health care community are doubtful that cost savings or improved health care will be obtained. This is a crucial time to carefully examine and deal with these changing and troubling ethical scenarios.

ETHICAL ISSUES

The ethical issues facing PSMC include dilemmas regarding confidentiality, informed consent, full disclosure, conflicts of interest, double agentry, honesty, financial incentives, interference with the clinical relationship, and altered relationships with other mental health clinicians. We will focus on how these dilemmas impact the ethical delivery of services under PSMC.

Survival Tips

Ethical Issues in PSMC
    Confidentiality
    Informed consent
    Full disclosure
    Double-agentry and conflicts of interest
    Honesty
    Financial incentives and disincentives
    Outcomes
    Interference in the clinical relationship
    Relationships among mental health professionals
    Consumers as providers
    Telemedicine
    Formulary restrictions
    Leverage
    Inadequate experience of PSMC systems
    Organizational issues

Confidentiality. If a public system is managed by an external entity, there may be additional exposure of client information to EAPs, employers, public regulators, and large data banks. Employers may be interested in the health care status of current or future employees or whether employees are utilizing benefits from the employer (Wise, 1995). Insurance companies and health plans might be concerned about adverse selection risks posed by those with serious psychiatric illness. Certain business entities might utilize confidential information for marketing purposes. The extent to which there will be inappropriate disclosure of information will depend on the confidentiality protocols built into an internal or external managed care system. Human error and limitations on the amount and nature of information that is released out of the consulting room will also play a role. Health plans or their agents, such as primary care gatekeepers, may insist on certain information about clients in order to authorize payment for services rendered by the mental health provider (See chapter by Pollack and Goetz). Clear guidelines defining what needs to be released and for what purpose need to be developed. While there have been unintended leaks of confidential information in managed care systems, there does not appear to be any wholesale or epidemic disregard of most client confidentiality restrictions.

Public systems need to create additional safeguards, training programs, and quality monitors to assure effective confidentiality in managed care systems. If these are not in place and respected, the potential for distrust of the public system and resistance to seek needed services will increase. This would lead to undertreatment of persons with SPMI with significant negative social and health consequences.

Informed consent. Clients have a right to know the types of treatment available to them and the factors which may influence their treatment. To the extent that PSMC affects any of those factors, clients should be adequately informed. There are already significant constraints on informed consent in public systems because of time constraints, language barriers and acuity of illness. In addition, cost factors may exclude some services which may be beneficial to clients. If this is the case, the system or mental health clinician is obliged to inform the client.

If managed care systems involve priority setting, there should be public disclosure of the service priorities. In the Oregon Health Plan, for example, the prioritized benefit package is explicit about which health care services are covered (Pollack, McFarland, George, & Angell, 1994). For the sake of fairness, PSMC programs and plans without such a legislated informed consent should develop informed consent provisions for their clients.

Full disclosure. A similar ethical dilemma relates to the obligation of a mental health clinician to fully disclose any factors which might interfere with client treatment. This includes budgetary limits and the availability of clinicians within the system able to treat specific problems. The special areas of concern related to managed care include allocating resources towards profit and administrative costs. If the individual clinician is part of a team providing care or has no financial conflict of interest, it should be the obligation of the public agency itself or the clinician with team leadership to make such disclosure. This principle also holds true for informed consent. In private managed care, funds provided for client care are called "medical loss" and it is a goal of the business to minimize that "loss" and to produce increased profit. Administrative expenses and profits may reach forty percent. In some states (e.g. Knox-Keene Act provisions in California), public disclosure of these amounts is required. PSMC disclosure obligations could most easily be met by the public agency in a standard format. However, mental health providers should make such disclosures if the agency itself does not. The competitive nature of managed care markets may lead to troubling "proprietary" restrictions of the disclosure of such information in public systems. Providers should remain alert to and resist such restrictions, if at all possible.

Double-agentry and conflicts of interest. The population based nature of public sector mental health systems divides clinician loyalties between their clients and the community. This potential for conflict of interest between advocacy for the individual client and for the system can be termed double-agentry. By adding managed care into this equation there may be additional layers of double-agentry or conflicts of interest. For example, under managed care there may be financial incentives or disincentives which affect decisions regarding treatment. Insofar as these treatment decisions do not limit access to care or detract from needed treatment there is no ethical problem. If, on the other hand, incentives or disincentives provide some direct benefit for the clinician, system, or managed care entity, there is a substantial double-agent or conflict of interest problem.

While public systems have traditionally returned budget savings from efficient care to clients in the form of improved or expanded programming, managed care systems may return these savings to clinicians, administrators, or the managed care organization (MCO). Depending on the incentives and methods of distribution of these budget savings there may be multiple conflicts of interest which may have effects on client care. In keeping with the principle of full disclosure, any such conflicts of interest or double agent situations created by managed care should be disclosed to the client and the public which funds the system. Depending on the circumstances, the client should have the freedom to participate knowing of these conflicts. The choices of clients seeking care in the public system are usually very limited. Nevertheless, the client should be given the opportunity to be informed and to choose.

The potential diversion of revenues or budgeted funds away from needed client services and into MCO profits is a serious concern. However, there have already been several reports about successful Medicaid managed care programs which have not resulted in increased client morbidity or mortality. The published reports so far indicate substantial cost savings (Cole et al., 1994; McFarland, 1994; Reed, Hennessy, Mitchell, & Babigian, 1994). Unfortunately, these reports do not show much improvement in clinical outcome. The cost savings have come primarily from decreased hospital utilization.

Whether managed care will support social and rehabilitative programs for persons with SPMI remains to be seen. These programs, which have become integrated in public systems for decades, have not been a part of managed care in the past. Whether for-profit managed care will support such programs is unknown. Perhaps the demonstration of outcome enhancement and cost savings for such programs will lead to increased support. The public sector is a major new opportunity for growth of the larger for-profit managed behavioral healthcare companies. It will be in their best interest to recognize these issues and have highly qualified experts to assist them. The possibility of continued stigma against the mentally ill, engendered by managed care benefit limitations is a significant concern. Active client advocacy supported by professional groups will hopefully address those concerns.

Honesty. "Gaming" the system to obtain service payments is a troubling aspect of both fee-for-service and managed care systems. Clinicians often feel caught between the need to provide necessary services and an external system which is insensitive or cost driven. If these conflicts invade PSMC systems, clinicians will need to advocate for beneficial care for clients in an honest and direct manner. If the same forces which produce conflicts in private managed care systems lead to dilemmas about honesty, a vicious cycle of dishonest beneficence followed by intrusive micromanagement could occur. These conflicts can be minimized if the medical necessity or level of care criteria and professional guidelines for treatment are explicit, clinically based, and clear to all parties involved, especially the provider, the utilization manager (whether internal or external), and to the client (See chapter by McFarland, Minkoff, Morrison, and

Roman). Clinical decisions must be made in a fair and scientific manner and not solely for cost containment reasons.

Financial incentives and disincentives. Since managed care uses numerous methods to control costs, financial incentives applied to programs or individual clinicians are sometimes used to achieve that goal. For example, clinicians may be paid a bonus for providing less care; administrators may derive increased income by achieving more revenues; capitated systems may derive increased income by providing fewer services; and cost savings may be taken out of the client care system. From a business perspective these financial motivaters can be quite powerful. In private managed care, incentives have contributed to dramatic changes in the way mental health services are delivered. Egregious utilization review practices in which reviewers were paid bonuses for denying or limiting service authorization are fortunately becoming less frequent. More common are arrangements which either place financial risk on the provider group or incentivize clinicians to give only "necessary" care e.g. case rates, retainers for fixed numbers of clients, and progressively decreasing reimbursement to the clinician for longer courses of treatment. These financial incentives, especially those linked to individual client decisions, place the clinician or system in a significant conflict of interest situation.

These dilemmas may be less common in public systems, if the clinicians are salaried employees and thus less subject to incentives. For-profit or non-profit managed care companies that compete for large public contracts may obtain financial benefits by excessively limiting services. However, if hospital services are diminished, with no adverse effect on clients, there is less of a problem. If savings are returned to the public system in a fair manner, instead of being converted to company profits, there is even less of a problem. If the PSMC program uses internal utilization management and savings are funneled back to client care, there is less ethical concern. Some have proposed caps or limits on profit and/or administrative costs in PSMC systems, establishing a reasonable rate of return, similar to a public utility model. Such a model would limit any potential conflicts of interest related to financial incentives.

Outcomes. There are concerns that the primary purpose of managed care is cost containment over improved quality or access. When improved quality or access, as defined by scientifically valid measures, results in cost containment, a PSMC system will be on solid ethical ground. The question of funding services which produce only marginal versus material improvement is a societal issue related to the whole issue of universal access and health care reform. Unfortunately, scientifically valid outcome studies are limited (Wells, 1992). Many managed care systems rely on client satisfaction surveys, anecdotal reports, and a few validated but limited functional outcome measures.

Fortunately, there have been no published outcome studies indicating poor outcomes in PSMC. We are in a market driven period without the benefit of carefully monitored and controlled scientific studies utilizing valid measures to compare clinical outcomes over time. PSMC systems should pool their efforts towards adequate outcome measures specific to the most vulnerable populations. It is especially important that outcome measures go beyond the short term and recognize the chronicity and relapse potential in many psychiatric disorders. While it is difficult to prove that financial incentives will actually improve care, effective and strategic administrative management can lead to cost savings, some of which should be reinvested in client care or other system improvements, such as MIS upgrades, quality improvement efforts, or training.

Interference in the clinical relationship. PSMC brings increased reporting and accountability requirements, including outcome or client satisfaction measures. Each time an external third party gathers information from the client and the clinician, there is the possibility of intrusion and interference in the therapeutic relationship. The extent to which cost containment factors influence care decisions may determine the extent of this problem. When the form and methods of these requirements are primarily for client benefit and scientifically justified, they are ethically and clinically appropriate. Clinicians have an ethical obligation to participate in peer review. The extent of these "valid" peer review mechanisms should be done in a manner that minimizes interference in the therapeutic relationship. Intrusive and repetitive micromanagement of clinical decisions for cost containment has little justification. In fact, more advanced MCOs are dropping intensive inspection models and promoting effective process development.

Too often external utilization reviewers have less experience or training than the care provider. When services are denied or limited, the denial should come from a mental health clinician with credentials comparable to the provider's. Capitation offers some solutions to this external review problem, since clinical decision making is an internal process of the provider organization, which has a vested interest in managing the care.

One justifiable addition to the clinical relationship is in the area of case management of high utilizing clients. This provides not only improved quality of treatment in the least restrictive setting but will also tend to decrease cost of treatment. This type of case management is most effective with unstable and seriously ill clients, who need the coordination of treating clinicians, social service and family support systems. Clinicians treating such clients should welcome the additional help of a good case manager. Such case managers are already an integral part of many community mental health systems and external case management would, therefore, be superfluous.

Relationships among mental health professionals. There is considerable debate about the benefits and risks of dividing treatment between a psychiatrist providing medications and another clinician providing psychotherapy or other supportive services (Woodward, 1993). This is less controversial in public systems where collaborative treatment is the norm and where there is regular and ongoing supervision. The extent to which PSMC would increase or decrease such collaborative treatment needs attention. Clinicians should endeavor to provide the most competent treatment which can be rendered with existing resources. The critical factor in public systems is the adequacy of the operating budget. Inadequate funding, compounded by potential profit motives, could create systems with less well trained clinicians treating the sickest clients, and the marginalization of psychiatrists into more isolated roles, limited to writing prescriptions and signing treatment documents. Adequate staffing patterns in PSMC systems should allow for sufficient staff interface, in particular for psychiatrists to fulfill teaching, supervision, and consultation roles, when appropriate.

OTHER ETHICAL PROBLEMS UNIQUE TO PSMC

Consumers as providers. Public systems have developed innovative systems using clients as providers. The primary rehabilitation goal of such programs is augmented by additional benefits for other clients who benefit from the consumer-provided services and the identification and shared experiences with their peers. The potential for PSMC systems to expand these programs primarily for cost considerations needs cautious review. PSMC systems have tended to refer to groups of providers who agree to lower reimbursement rates. Using clients as providers (or as employees) has many inherent ethical problems including; (1) concerns about boundary problems, especially if the client is being treated in the same program in which he or she is working, (2) concerns about who is benefiting most from the consumer's work, i.e., does the work fit with the rehabilitation goals for the consumer-employee or is the consumer being exploited as cheaper labor, and (3) concerns about fair and reasonable compensation for the consumer-employee. Introducing potential cost savings by using lower cost consumer-employees, raises the specter of exploitation of such clients for profit.

In general, MCOs follow strict credentialling protocols for their clinicians in order to provide competent services and to avoid legal risks. Adequate ethical safeguards and consultation should be considered prior to developing or expanding internal consumer employment programs under managed care. These safeguards should be contained in personnel policies establishing the parameters of both the employment and client role and with full informed consent for potential consumer/employees.

Telemedicine. The use of telemedicine services offers a unique opportunity to expand public services in underserved rural areas. Ethical concerns associated with telemedicine should be addressed. These concerns relate to cost factors which may create disincentives to provide telemedicine services. If priority setting for public systems utilizing managed care includes access to rural areas through telemedicine there may be improved service to these populations. Whether MCOs would be willing to invest in a potentially revenue negative activity remains to be seen. If telemedicine services were included in contract requirements, there would be less concern. The ethical issue is whether innovative public system development can be improved or stifled by cost centered motives. Savings derived from effective managed care practices in rural systems should be funneled into innovative programs, such as telemedicine (See chapter by Mohatt).

Formulary restrictions. Psychiatrists in managed care systems are concerned about prescribing restrictions for expensive medications. This is especially true for the newer antidepressant and antipsychotic medications. Budgetary constraints are already affecting state hospital systems (APA, 1995). The rationale is that the newer medications are not more efficacious than older, less expensive ones. On the other hand, clinicians recognize that some of the newer medications may benefit clients by reducing side effects and promoting better compliance. Because antidepressants and antipsychotics are so widely used in public systems, their use should be driven by good clinical practice and not solely by cost factors. The authorization of newer medications should not require absolute evidence of improved efficacy, but should be made by clinical or peer review entities.

Leverage. In the private sector some clients who are either noncompliant with treatment or "chronic" do not fall within the contracted benefit plan and are either dropped from the plan for contractual reasons or are denied services. This contributes to what is called patient "skimming" or attempts to limit "adverse selection" for purposes of cost containment. The public sector serves many of these difficult clients. It is ethically essential for PSMC programs to continue to treat clients who, because of their psychiatric illness, are ambivalent, resistant and noncompliant, and who may require lifelong treatment. The appropriate and clinically justified use of coercion or leverage (e.g., access to housing or financial resources) with some clients may result in improved client compliance. This requires appropriate budgeting and advocacy by administrators and clinicians to prevent profit motives from subverting medically necessary treatment decisions. Expedience is not sufficient justification for using leverage.

Inadequate experience of PSMC systems. With the increase in competition for PSMC programs, there are concerns that the market will attract HMOs or other private sector managed care entities, which may be ill prepared to deal with a public system population. If there are not adequately trained clinical staff, case managers familiar with public system clients, well developed continuum of care programs, outreach and rehabilitation programs, and adequate funding, there may be a significant decrease in the long term quality of care for these clients.

As some private MCOs become better prepared and willing to handle persons with SPMI, there will be less concern about the delivery of competent and compassionate care. The risk that for-profit MCOs might abandon these public contracts if profits decrease needs to be addressed. Safeguards such as length of contract, service regulation, and caps on profits and administrative costs would help to avoid major treatment disruptions in the lives of the most vulnerable client populations.

Organizational Issues. Because there is no clearly articulated managed care ethic, such systems and clients need to rely on the ethics of the clinicians within them. Managed care systems may, because of the competitive nature of the business, become embroiled in fierce legal battles (including litigation over contract disputes). Such an atmosphere does not lend itself to an organizational ethic which will adequately support professional ethics. For example, if one company sues another or the state over alleged unfair advantages in the procurement process, there may be delays in the availability of treatment to the population covered. Because MCOs may not follow a professional ethic (i.e., they may have the legal right to sue, but is it right to do so, if access to care is affected?), the only redress at the state or national policy level is through legislation prohibiting the abandonment or delay in program start-up by procurement litigation. This may also be averted by prohibiting such litigation in the process of competition for contracts.

The entry of non-profit providers into for-profit managed care subsidiaries has raised ethical issues. Making a profit is not by itself unethical. The underlying ethical problems of conflicts of interest and full disclosure place a high burden on MCOs to protect public systems from losing needed resources to profit and administrative expenses. Because there is no legislation or regulation that provides protection, public systems are subject to the same market forces which have caused deep concerns in the private sector. Until there is appropriate regulation, safeguards need to be implemented to protect the integrity of the delivery system from unethical financial practices. Capping profits or administrative costs from the onset would be one solution to this dilemma.

The competitive environment has increased the "brain drain" phenomenon, siphoning off public sector experts into private MCOS, creating a vacuum in some systems and concern in others. Potential conflicts of interest, especially when the former public official brings "inside" knowledge to the MCO, possibly giving the MCO unfair advantage over its competitors, must be addressed.

CONCLUSION

Ethical issues which have caused significant difficulty in the private sector are being replicated in PSMC programs. Concerns about reductions in historically insufficient funding, and staffing uncertainties add to the ethical conflicts experienced in the private sector. Benefits derived from managed care programs such as decreased reliance on inpatient hospital treatment, increased availability of a continuum of care, better information and tracking systems, and high utilizer case management will benefit public systems even as managed care may evolve into other forms. Since cost factors have driven much of the current managed care movement, it is unclear whether cost or quality of treatment will be the main force affecting system changes into the next century. Whether the new trend to privatize Medicaid markets will result in stability in the service systems for the mentally ill remains an open and vexing question. Because the driving force in managed care has been cost containment more than altruistic commitment to treatment of persons with SPMI, the stability and dependability of privatized systems, especially if profits decrease, remains uncertain.

With 41 million uninsured in the U.S. in 1996, the need for universal access remains an ethical priority. The need to provide universal access may lead to renewed public discussions about comprehensive health care reform, especially if PSMC systems fail to adequately serve their mandated populations. Since there is no evidence that managed care or incremental insurance reform will decrease administrative costs (Office of Technology Assessment, 1994), there continues to be support for a single payer system. Whatever happens on the larger stage of health and economics policy debates, the public must be assured that the most vulnerable psychiatric patients, who are largely treated in the public sector, will continue to receive compassionate, competent, and ethical treatment driven by professional ethics to do what is best for patients and not primarily for cost containment or profit. Clinicians and client advocacy groups will need a strong and unified voice to continue to push for parity for the mentally ill under any health reform scenario. This will provide more choices for clients and clinicians to develop systems of care, whether public or private, that can adequately serve our patients in a fair and ethical manner.

REFERENCES

American Medical Association (1994). *Code of medical ethics*. Chicago IL, American Medical Association.

American Medical Association (1993). *Guidelines for the conduct of managed care*. Chicago, IL, American Medical Association.

American Medical Association (1995). Ethical issues in managed care. *Journal of the American Medical Association, 273*, 330–335.

American Psychiatric Association (1993). The principles of medical ethics with annotations especially applicable to psychiatry. Washington, D.C., American Psychiatric Association.

Glover, R., & Petrila J. (1994). Can state mental health agencies survive health care reform. *Hospital and Community Psychiatry, 45*(9), 911–913.

Cole, R. et al. (1994). A mental health capitation program: patient outcomes. *Hospital and Community Psychiatry, 45*(11), 1090–1096.

Daniels, N. (1985). *Just Health Care*. Cambridge, MA, Cambridge University Press.

Lazarus, J., & Sharfstein, S. (1994). Changes in the economics and ethics of health and mental health care. In J. Oldham & Riba M. (Eds.) *Review of Psychiatry, 13*, 389–411.

McFarland, B. (1994). Health maintenance organizations and persons with severe mental illness. *Community Mental Health Journal, 30*(3), 221–242.

Office of Technology Assessment, Congressional Budget Office (1994). Understanding estimates of national health expenditures under health reform. Washington DC. Publication OTA-H-594, GPO stock 052-003-01374-6.

Pellegrino, E.D. (1993). The metamorphosis of medical ethics: a 30-year retrospective. *JAMA, 269*, 1158–1162.

Pollack, D.A., McFarland, B.H., George, R.A., & Angell, R.H. (1994). Prioritization of mental health services in Oregon. *Milbank Quarterly, 72*, 515–550.

Reed, S.K., Hennessy, K.D., Mitchell, O.S., & Babigian, H.M. (1994). A mental health capitation program: II. Cost-benefit analysis. *Hospital and Community Psychiatry, 45*(11), 1097–1103.

Sabin, J., Daniels, N. (1994). Determining "medical necessity" in mental health practice. *Hastings Center Report, 24*(6), 5–14.

Staff. (1995). Budget deficit leads New York to restrict Clozapine use. *Psychiatric News.*

Wells, K.B., Burnam, M.A., Rogers, W.H., Camp, P. (1992). The course of depression in adult outpatients: Results from the medical outcomes study. *Archives of General Psychiatry, 49*, 788–794.

Wise, D. (1995). Private matters. *Business & Health, February*, 22–28.

Woodward, B., Duckworth, K., Gutheil, T.G. (1993). The pharmacotherapist/ psychotherapist collaboration. In Oldham, J., Riba, M., & Tasman, A., (Eds.) *Review of Psychiatry, 12*, 631–650.

4

Principles and Values for Advocates and Policymakers*

CHRIS KOYANAGI

Is "managed care" of publicly funded mental health services only an attempt to rationalize major cuts? Or could it enable the public mental health system to develop successful, widespread organized systems of care? Should mental health policymakers and advocates eschew managed care or embrace it?

Managed care systems that agree to provide all necessary care for a fixed payment have an incentive to deny services or to coerce people into accepting services they may not want. This creates the potential for great harm to individuals with high-cost needs. On the other hand, some aspects of managed care arrangements have the potential to improve the public mental health system significantly. These include controlling the use of inpatient and residential services, increasing the emphasis on care in the least restrictive setting of the consumer's choice, substituting support services for

---

*Editors' Note: This chapter is a slightly modified version of the Executive Summary of "Managing Managed Care", a report published by the Bazelon Center for Mental Health Law. The full report can be obtained from the center at: 1101 Fifteenth St NW, #1212, Washington, D.C. 20005-5002.

expensive clinical care, fostering greater efficiency among provider agencies, and improving service quality and outcomes.

Serving people in the public mental health system is different in many ways than providing care through employer-based health insurance. In general, the population in the public system has more serious disability and mental health needs, often compounded by extreme poverty, than the privately insured population. Furthermore, there is a public responsibility; states are and must remain the agents of last resort for people with no other means of accessing services. When states contract for managed care, that responsibility must be built into the contract.

LESSONS FROM THE PUBLIC MENTAL HEALTH SYSTEM

Although there are important issues concerning mental health services for people with less severe disorders, the real challenge is to ensure that managed care approaches do not result in inappropriate or insufficient services for adults with serious mental illness and children with serious emotional disturbance who rely for their care on the public sector.

It is crucial, therefore, for managed care arrangements to adopt the basic values of a good public mental health system. Merging the advantages of managed care with the strengths of good public systems can enable policymakers to:

- create a flexible system that provides funds for meeting the needs of an identified population, in place of a rigid funding system directed to providers;

- move from a provider-driven system that tends not to individualize services to one that creates the opportunity to consider the consumer a customer;

- shift resources from politically popular line items, such as state hospitals, to programmatically valuable services, such as psychiatric rehabilitation; shift from a system relying on volatile fee-for-service and underfunded grants to one providing relatively stable and predictable levels of funding more closely allied to real costs; and

- overcome the pervasive problems in public mental health systems, such as difficulty in finding and accessing services, lack of coordination and accountability, disincentives for community-based and rehabilitative treatments, and poor monitoring.

There is evidence that, with careful planning, diligent oversight and the active involvement of consumers, families and mental health advocates, these goals could be achieved. Evaluations of small-scale managed care and capitated programs in the mental health system have generally found encouraging results, and most of the consumers and families enrolled in these programs have been satisfied with their care.

PRINCIPLES AND VALUES

The public mental health system has developed a set of values and approaches to care that have proven effective for adults with serious mental illness and children with serious emotional disturbance. Good public mental health systems focus on the individual's recovery and consider consumers to be partners in treatment and rehabilitation. Service plans are driven by consumers' goals and build on their strengths. These values and approaches should be incorporated in managed care.

For adults, this philosophy and approach is articulated in the principles of the federal Community Support Program and, for children, through the Child and Adolescent Service System Program's system of care.

This book assumes that a decision has already been made to move to managed care. In this case, specifications (in law, regulations or contracts) are needed to guard against limitations on access, to maintain the quality of care and to establish and protect consumers' rights and ensure that the system respects their wishes. "Managing" managed care in this manner increases the likelihood that states can obtain the cost-efficiency they want while ensuring appropriate access and quality of care and giving consumers real choices.

Any managed care arrangement must include the following elements:

Consumer and family involvement in design, implementation and evaluation of the managed care plan

- Include consumers, families and advocates in the planning group (commission, task force, workgroup, etc.) that will write the draft plan.

- Set up a state-level consumer-oversight board to review implementation of managed care.

- Require the managed care entity to conduct regularly scheduled consumer-satisfaction surveys and to use the results to improve its services.

Protection of consumer rights

- Assure consumers of the right to be fully involved in all treatment decisions, to participate in the development of their service plan and to refuse any treatment they do not feel is appropriate.

- Guarantee consumers' right to file a grievance at any time and to receive a response within a reasonable time, with the goal of resolving the grievance (if it can be resolved to the consumer's satisfaction) within 15 business days.

- Prohibit disenrollment because an individual refuses treatment, misses appointments or presents other challenges to implementing the service plan.

Provision of a full array of services that are truly accessible

- Make available psychiatric rehabilitation, case management, assertive community treatment, intensive in-home services for children, school-based day treatment, consumer-run self-help and other services necessary to achieve positive outcomes.

- Allow flexibility to use funds for alternatives to inpatient care and ensure that any "savings" generated remain in the managed care system to be reinvested in community alternatives or to expand eligibility to an uninsured population.

Access to and effective use of community services

- Include, for a transition period (five years, for example), community public-sector agencies that are identified by the state mental health authority as essential providers and are willing to work to meet the same standards as other providers in the network. At the end of the transition period, these agencies should be expected to compete on the same terms as others.

- In addition to providing geographically and culturally accessible services, conduct targeted outreach to potential and current enrollees, particularly to individuals who are homeless, who live in isolated areas or who face other barriers to enrollment or the provision of services. Such outreach is most effective when done regularly by consumers or family members and can be conducted under the auspices of the managed care entity, the state agency or both.

Implementation of strategies to limit involuntary treatment

- Focus on providing a full array of acceptable treatment alternatives in order to reduce involuntary commitment.

- Work with police on appropriate diversionary procedures to ensure that people are given access to alternative services.

- Hold the managed care entity financially responsible for mental health care for any consumer committed to an inpatient facility, eliminating any incentive to shift costs to the state by seeking commitment.

Appropriate structuring of the managed care system

- Consider the advantages and disadvantages of a full or partial carve-out of mental health services, particularly for adults with serious mental illness and children with serious emotional disturbance.

- Consider an integrated benefit for those whose mental health needs are not as extensive. Since there is less need for concern about undertreatment for those with less severe disorders, such an option allows integration of basic mental health services for the general Medicaid population with the basic physical health care benefit.

Measures to ensure that financial issues do not undermine the system

- In states without the resources to finance the system adequately, consider leaving the public-sector mental health services out of any capitated managed Medicaid plan for the time being.

- Develop blended-funding arrangements whereby all child-serving agencies that now fund mental health services pool resources to develop a single coordinated system. These state agencies typically include child welfare, education/special education, juvenile justice, substance abuse, health and mental health.

- Consider a "soft capitation" rate, which allows some risk-sharing between the managed care entity and the state to cover expected additional costs. Soft capitation pays the company more if needed services exceed a specified level. This helps to remove incentives to dump consumers with more costly care needs into the public system, but it also attenuates cost-containment.

- Do not cut too deeply. Medicaid agencies may hope to reduce current expenditures by moving to managed care, but generally capitation rates for a given population should be at least 90–95% of cost history.

Quality assurance and inclusion of outcome measures

- Establish as a goal for any managed care plan that it improve consumers' outcomes and set specific requirements for outcome measures to evaluate access to services, utilization, consumer satisfaction and potential problems (such as incarceration rates).

- Make assessments and monitoring information available to the public.

The imposition of standards for managed care organizations

- Select issues and items in the managed care contract to serve as triggers for sanctions, making it clear what constitutes a violation leading to sanction. It is particularly important that sanctions be imposed quickly on plans that violate individual rights or have excess utilization of their grievance and appeals systems.

- Establish well-defined review criteria that are clearly understood by all providers and made available to the public.

- Routinely distribute educational materials about the managed care plan, including details of how to access services.

Advocates and policymakers should be assertive. Corporations purchasing managed behavioral health care make clear exactly what they want; those who purchase on behalf of the public should be expected to do the same.

————— **Section II** —————

Systems Level Issues: Introduction

KENNETH MINKOFF

This section begins with an analysis of the various factors which contribute to the design of a PSMC program for any particular state or region. It then continues with a series of examples of different types of managed care arrangements, as described by the managed care authority in each case. These include:

1. Statewide capitated Medicaid managed care by a private MCO: Massachusetts

2. Regional capitated PSMC by a CMHC: Utah

3. Local capitated PSMC by community psychiatrists: South Central Los Angeles County

4. Managed care by the public agency itself: The Veterans Administration

5. Rural PSMC systems

5

Designing Public Sector Managed Care Systems

JAMES J. CALLAHAN, JR. and
ELIZABETH LEVY MERRICK

This chapter addresses systems level issues that community mental health professionals need to understand in order to evaluate the pros and cons of various managed care models and to develop effective strategies for designing optimal PSMC systems. While there is probably no "best" system in the real world, different models have different consequences for patients/consumers, mental health professionals, third-party payers such as Medicaid, and managed care companies. Trade-offs are involved in selecting any particular approach.

The Chapter by Stroup and Dorwart provided an outline of the strategies, tactics, and settings for PSMC. This chapter discusses these issues in greater depth, with emphasis on how to select a specific managed care program structure in relation to the goals and objectives of key stakeholders.

Implementing and evaluating PSMC in any particular state or region involves making decisions along each of the following dimensions:

1. The "make versus buy" decision

2. For-profit MCOs versus non-profit agencies

3. Total population versus subpopulation coverage

4. Statewide versus sub-state coverage

5. Carve-out versus integration with general health care services

6. Selection of strategies for limiting utilization: demand versus supply side controls

7. Capitation versus non-capitated payment

8. Managed care networks versus HMOs

9. Selection of methodologies for accountability and quality control

These dimensions can be combined in a variety of ways to create a specific mental health managed care program. Each of the design features has consequences for the various players in managed care: clients, providers, payers, and managed care organizations.

THE "MAKE VERSUS BUY" DECISION

The make or buy decision is the choice of providing managed care through public employees or contracting with an outside party. There is no reason theoretically why a public agency could not hire appropriate staff and conduct managed care activities; practically, however, there are serious problems. Public personnel hiring requirements make it difficult to hire the most qualified persons quickly. Salary amounts may be behind the market. Funds cannot be shifted from one purpose to another without a trail of approvals. Finally, political intervention may make it impossible to select some providers for a network while not selecting some that are politically connected. As a result, Medicaid agencies usually "buy" managed care services.

For consumers, "buying" services rather than "making" them does not necessarily imply a difference in access to or quality of services. The nature of coverage and service delivery depends in large part on the terms of the contract developed between the public agency and the MCO. Range of services to be offered, size of network in relation to enrolled population, gatekeeping mechanisms, type of financial incentives built in, and customer service operations are among the many important contract terms. Operational management of services is delegated to the managed care company or other provider organization, thus creating increased distance between government agency payers and actual service delivery oversight. In terms of accountability, the managed care organization is an additional layer between the consumer and government. For providers, in some instances, the managed care company may appear to drive a harder bargain since, as noted, the company may operate under somewhat fewer constraints than the government agency itself. Both consumers and providers may find private managed care companies or other vendors more impervious to political pressure, complaints, and other input; on the other hand, they may also be more flexible and customer-focused than entrenched public bureaucracies (See chapter by Lehmann for further discussion of the difficulties of implementing managed care flexibility within a public bureaucracy).

FOR-PROFIT MCOs VERSUS NON-PROFIT AGENCIES

The expanding role of profit-oriented managed care companies doing business in the public sector is a controversial aspect of PSMC and challenges an ideology that promotes non-profit or public auspices exclusively. There are, however, sound reasons for considering profit-oriented MCOs. The first is that these organizations have the capacity to provide managed care because they are currently doing so for about 103 million people in both risk based and non-risk based programs, employee assistance programs, utilization review programs, and various network arrangements (Open Minds, 1994). The management, data processing and clinical infrastructure is there to be applied to public enrollees. They also have access to capital and retained earnings, two attributes not available to non-profit or public agencies (Brown, 1986). Revenue for behavioral MCOs was about $2 billion in 1993 (Open Minds, 1994). Finally, profit-oriented MCOs do not face the legal and bureaucratic constraints faced by public agencies in purchasing and hiring, thus allowing more flexibility and immediate action. On the other hand, while the profit motive may drive creativity and efficiency, it may result in mindless cost cutting and denial of access to achieve its profit targets. PSMC planners must be alert to insure that this does not happen. Other potential disadvantages of profit-oriented MCOs are: public mistrust of the profit motive, lack of experience with and sensitivity to public sector client needs and to consumer and family advocacy groups, and lack of awareness of unique local community needs.

Non-profit agencies, by contrast, may be better equipped to manage more local and regional projects with greater understanding of both clinical and community need, but possibly with less effective cost reduction or containment (See chapter by Dangerfield and Betit). Non-profits are likely to be more familiar with the long term needs of consumers and to have had experience in involving consumer and family groups in planning and program development (See chapter by Fisher). Non-profits also have the advantage that they are owned by their "members", usually local people, presumably with a commitment to the community, rather than to remote stockholders. If a non-profit dissolves, its resources go to another non-profit (Brown, 1986), thus staying in the community. In some states, non-profit agencies are forming into large regional or statewide behavioral health networks to compete or collaborate with private MCOs to obtain large managed care contracts (See chapter by Weinstein).

Many of the concerns raised about for-profit MCOs can be addressed by using public payers or networks of non-profit agencies to manage care (Elias, Leadholm, Kerzner, & Kravitz, 1993). However, as PSMC has evolved, the search for the best possible approaches has led to the development of managed care models which attempt to integrate the advantages of both sectors.

There are several ways to attempt to capture the benefits of both types of organizations while minimizing their drawbacks. The most common model is the public/private partnership capitation model, in which a state or county pays a private MCO a fixed amount for each person covered and the firm is at full or partial (shared) risk for the cost of services and administration of the program. The MCO is responsible for development and oversight of the provider network, utilization management, claims payment, case coordination, quality assurance, and provision of data for program evaluation. The state or county is responsible for monitoring the program, ensuring quality and access for public clients, and monitoring adherence to public sector values and appropriate involvement of advocacy groups, using standards developed with the MCO. Although there are not yet sufficient findings, at least the early results in Massachusetts, one of the first states to use this model, appear to be encouraging (Callahan, Shepard, Beinecke, Larson, & Cavanaugh, 1994; Beinecke, Goodman, & Rivera, 1995). The Massachusetts program is discussed in depth in the next chapter.

The extent to which the potential negative consequences of such a capitation arrangement are avoided depends on the contract design and monitoring. The degree of risk sharing is one crucial component. In addition, performance standards which specify levels of access, quality, and other measurable parameters, tied to financial rewards or penalties, must be crafted carefully to encourage the right balance of cost reduction and adequate service provision. Contract compliance must be monitored effectively.

There are other models which utilize the strengths of private MCOs while limiting their disadvantages, most notably the diversion of funds to profits. Two such models are the flat management fee model, in which the MCO is paid a management fee to manage care, and the enabling model, in which the MCO is a consultant to the public organization, enabling the public entity to manage the care itself. These are alternatives to private/public partnership models, in which the MCO is at risk through capitation. U.S. Behavioral Health has been a leader in the development of these alternative approaches. The flat management fee model has been used in Solano County, California, and the enabling model in King County (Seattle), Washington (Feldman, Baler, & Penner, 1995).

TOTAL POPULATION VERSUS SUBPOPULATION COVERAGE

In any state system, there are a number of categories of public beneficiaries that could be included or excluded in a PSMC program: AFDC parents and children, children with severe emotional disturbances (SED), SSI disabled persons, state mental health authority clients. The needs, and hence services, vary among these groups and pose particular challenges to a managed care company. Covering the entire population can result in a greater degree of risk spreading, since there will be a wider spectrum of low- to high-cost enrollees. Broader program coverage may also result in broader support (politically and among the public) as well as reduced stigma for some groups, although not necessarily. On the other hand, separate coverage for subpopulations can facilitate better matching of expertise and services for distinct groups of enrollees. For instance, services to children involve engaging parents in the care plan, the recruitment of scarce specialists, significant coordination with schools and social service agencies, and perhaps the creation of new residential options. For services to seriously mentally ill disabled persons, new outreach and tracking systems may be required as well as coordination with a range of social services. For poorer populations location of services and transportation costs become significant issues.

STATEWIDE VERSUS SUB-STATE COVERAGE

A PSMC plan can be implemented on a statewide basis or, with the appropriate federal Health Care Financing Administration (HCFA) waiver, at a sub-state level, such as a county or catchment area. The values of a statewide program are equity for the citizens of the state, elimination of the possibility of cost shifting among catchment areas, the potential to capture large amounts of savings and gaining actual experience of implementing a statewide program. Conversely, a catchment area approach will reduce exposure to big mistakes in quality, access and costs and provide the opportunity to conduct well designed research before expanding an untested program statewide. A catchment area approach also offers the opportunity to tightly organize the providers in a smaller area to manage care to enrollees on a risk sharing basis. The value of one approach may be the downside of the other.

From the consumer standpoint, statewide coverage offers a guarantee of similar benefits regardless of where one resides, but quality may be easier to monitor in a smaller geographic area. For providers, a catchment area approach offers more control over the design of the local system and reduces competition from outside vendors. Payer oversight may be facilitated by the smaller scale of a sub-state program. The catchment area approach also facilitates involvement of smaller public sector agencies in "care management"; statewide coverage is more likely to require the resources of a large private MCO (See chapter by Dangerfield and Betit).

CARVE-OUT VERSUS INTEGRATION WITH GENERAL HEALTH CARE SERVICES

Public agencies such as Medicaid may choose a managed care plan design that integrates mental health benefits with other medical benefits, or may set up mental health services as a separate system. It can be argued that comorbidity of health and mental health problems, the "offset" effect of mental health services on general health care utilization, and the need for coordination of care suggest the need for a mainstreamed approach. Supporters of a carve-out, however, believe that the need for specialized knowledge and unique programs (e.g., residential treatment, emergency service, involuntary commitment, etc.) require a group of providers who are specialists in mental health. There is little research to settle which approach is the best.

For consumers, it is important to recognize that whether mental health coverage is carved out or left in a comprehensive benefit package, there is the question of how well mental health and other health care services will be coordinated. Carving out mental health does not necessarily mean a lower level of coordination and consultation with medical care. Conversely, in many plans that include both mental health and health benefits, there is nonetheless very little integration at the service level. Furthermore, there are concerns about which professionals are best able to identify mental health needs. Research has shown, for instance, that primary care physicians frequently fail to diagnose and/or properly treat common mental health problems such as depression and anxiety (Eisenberg, 1992). Thus, the potential benefit of using specialized personnel as gatekeepers and of utilizing a company that specializes in delivery of mental health services (as in a carve-out) must be balanced against the possible facilitation of integration with general health care that might occur in an inclusive plan.

Of importance to both consumers and payers is the fact that the carve-out approach lends itself to enabling the payer to specify the level of expenditures and type of incentives for mental health service provision (Frank, McGuire, & Newhouse, 1995). This is particularly important considering that in mainstreamed plans such as general HMOs, there may be disincentives to providing high-quality mental health services for the severely ill due to fear of attracting high-cost consumers (Mechanic, 1994). The choice of a carve-out versus mainstreamed approach does not predictably determine the clinical sensitivity or adequacy of reimbursement provided by mental health care managers, but some specialized behavioral health care companies that manage carve-outs may better understand the interests and concerns of mental health providers.

SELECTION OF STRATEGIES FOR LIMITING UTILIZATION: DEMAND VERSUS SUPPLY SIDE CONTROLS

Demand side controls attempt to influence the consumer's behavior, while supply side controls aim at influencing the provider.

A. Demand side controls

1. *Eligibility restriction.* The basic control of client demand used by payers is to establish eligibility for a particular set of individuals. For Medicaid, an individual must both belong to a covered category (e.g., disabled, parent with dependent child, elderly) and meet defined low income requirements. To be eligible for specific services (e.g., hospital care), additional criteria such as severity and acuity of illness may be imposed.

2. *Benefit restriction.* Payers also define the *type* of benefit (e.g., inpatient, outpatient, day treatment) and its *duration*. Duration of treatment may be defined as limits on the number of visits, days of hospitalization, lifetime maximum benefits, and so on.

3. *Cost-sharing.* Additional demand side controls include requirements that an individual share in the cost of care by paying a flat amount or percentage of the cost of their visits, procedures, days of care, or hospital admission (co-insurance) and/or expend a certain amount out of pocket before the payer makes any payments (deductible).

4. *Gatekeeping.* Finally, administrative controls featuring gatekeeping may be imposed. Gatekeeping refers to the need for special authorization by an agent for the payer for certain services. Gatekeeping functions may be performed by primary care physicians, payers' case management program personnel, or utilization review staff. Examples of gatekeeping include requiring primary care physician referral in order to be covered for specialist care, prior approval before initiating particular procedures or continuation of treatment, or participation in the payers' case management program for high-risk/high-cost patients. Each version of gatekeeping places a potential barrier between the patient and sought-after care, while attempting to eliminate inappropriate or unnecessary care.

B. Supply side controls

1. *Limitations on size of network.* Payers limit in various ways the supply of providers with whom they do business. The basic control is determining which providers will be eligible to provide the covered benefits. Provider eligibility requirements range from minimally restrictive to highly specific. The least restrictive is that a provider must be licensed. A second step might require additional certification by relevant professional organizations (e.g., board certification, Joint Commission). Additionally, provider contracts may be contingent on meeting certain practice pattern requirements. Finally, payers may limit the absolute number of providers of various types (e.g., hospital beds, outpatient clinics, psychiatrists, psychologists, social workers), based on predetermined need formulas, to reduce the perceived pressure to overutilize services due to oversupply.

2. *Payment controls.* Payers also attempt to influence provider behavior and supply of services through methods of payment — paying usual and customary fees, paying discounted fees as part of a referral agreement, or paying on the basis of prospective payment or risk sharing.

3. *Utilization management.* Payers may enhance cost containment without reducing service quality by reducing the availability of high cost services (e.g., hospitalization) and employing aggressive utilization management protocols to encourage the development and utilization of less expensive and possibly more effective alternatives, such as intensive outpatient crisis intervention, day hospitalization, crisis residential services, and outpatient detoxification. Reduction

in expensive hospital utilization and expansion of community treatment alternatives can be one of the most positive supply-side effects of public sector managed care.

4. *Administrative controls.* Finally, payers may restrict supply of services by imposing administrative controls on providers, including: prior approval of service, retrospective and/or concurrent review of claims, treatment protocols, and care planning. These techniques involve monitoring and determining care to be received on a case-by-case basis. This category encompasses: 1) gatekeeping measures, since these affect providers as well as consumers, 2) retrospective review, in which payment for services judged to be inappropriate or unnecessary may be refused, and 3) treatment protocols which determine standard procedures or treatments for specific clinical scenarios and which require special authorization for services that exceed the service limits in the protocols.

Although the MCO generally has wide latitude in determining the types of demand or supply side controls to utilize (usually, emphasis is placed on limiting the provider network, obtaining rate discounts, and reducing inpatient utilization), the public payer has wide latitude in designing the managed care program itself and in determining which controls should be especially emphasized and which ones should be avoided. For example, demand side controls, such as benefit restriction and cost sharing, may be easy to administer, but may be politically or clinically untenable for impoverished person with SPMI. Limitations on network size or bed capacity may be politically influenced by professional societies or hospital associations, which can be important stakeholders in determining the success of managed care efforts. Administrative controls run the risk of leading to payment delays, which can also be a devastating blow to the perceived success of the PSMC initiative. As a consequence, gatekeeping, utilization management, and payment discounts are often the more preferred methods for controlling supply or demand.

CAPITATION VERSUS NON-CAPITATED PAYMENT MECHANISMS

Prospective payment can be used broadly to refer to financing systems in which a pre-set fee is paid for some bundle of services. Unlike fee-for-service payment, additional services or costs do not result in additional reimbursement. Thus, financial risk is placed on the provider rather than the payer.

There are two main types of prospective payment. In the first, payment is made on a per-case or per-episode basis. For example, hospital stays may be paid at a flat rate regardless of actual costs, services delivered, or length of stay for a particular individual. The second type is capitation, in which a set fee is pre-paid for each individual, to a provider who agrees to provide any care needed within the defined scope of services over a fixed duration (typically one year). With pure capitation, the provider assumes full financial risk;

the provider is liable for expenses if care provided exceeds the capitation payment (and stands to profit if costs are below the capitation payment). In addition to the capitation payment, which is generally based on past utilization and is designed to cover patient service costs, an administrative fee may also be paid if not otherwise included. Both types of prospective payment are viewed generally as offering incentives to the provider to increase efficiency, but also risking potential under-provision of services and/or avoidance of high-cost patients due to the pressure to cut costs.

Risk-sharing payment mechanisms involve the sharing of financial risk between payer and provider. This is accomplished through payment that is only partially independent of the actual costs of current treatment for a given individual. For example, both per-case prospective payment and capitation can be modified to allow for only partial risk. For example, "soft" capitation limits the degree to which actual costs result in losses or profits. Soft capitation contracts feature a target or base capitation payment, but unlike pure capitation costs are shared according to a chosen formula. Such contracts often set a risk corridor in which costs within a chosen percentage above and/or below the target are borne by the provider. Outside of this zone the payer may assume all or part of the risk. It could, for instance, be specified that if costs fall within 10% above or below the target, these profits or losses will be assumed by the provider. Profit or loss outside the 10% corridor could either accrue to the payer or could be shared by payer and provider in the proportion specified in the contract.

The purpose of such risk-sharing clauses would be to moderate the incentives to under-provide services, avoid costly patients, or other problematic aspects of pure capitation incentives. Incentives to keep costs in an appropriate range could further be bolstered by measures such as designing a cost-based system up to a determined cost level, thus discouraging excessive cost-cutting. Protection for the managed care company or other provider could be built in by guaranteeing some level of payment at the highest-cost levels to serve as a stop-loss of disastrously high expenses.

Capitation frequently involves HMOs, but capitation payments can also be made to other providers such as mental health clinics, group practices, and primary care physicians. Capitation can cover health and mental health together, or mental health services can be carved out. Individual providers within a capitated plan may be paid in various ways, from salary to discounted fee-for-service to sub-contracted capitation. With fee-for-service financing, the incentives to the provider are to do more, not less, thus avoiding the incentive to provide insufficient services, but potentially driving up costs and allowing unnecessary or inappropriate service delivery. Conversely, capitation, as noted earlier, may create an incentive to undertreat, but may also increase clinical discretion and flexibility.

Flat management fee with fee-for-service payment to providers. Continuation of fee-for-service payment means that enrollees are not exposed to a system in which the incentive is to undertreat. Although a flat management fee does not provide the MCO with a strong financial incentive to be as efficient as possible, the MCO will presumably be motivated to keep costs down given that its performance will certainly be evaluated in large part by how well it constrains costs, which, in turn, will strongly influence contract renewal.

MANAGED CARE NETWORKS VERSUS HMOs

The financing and organization of health services is changing so rapidly and in so many ways that it is difficult to establish mutually exclusive categories to fit their reality. Despite this difficulty, public agencies may choose to contract with different entities which will have varying consequences for clients.

In Massachusetts, for example, Medicaid recipients were given the option of joining a full practice HMO where they would receive all their health care including mental health services, or enrolling in the primary care case management system (PCCM). Individuals enrolled in PCCM must use the primary care physician to access medical services. For mental health and substance abuse services, however, there is a carve-out and they are the responsibility of a private managed care company, Mental Health Management of America (See chapter by Hartman and Nelson). In a carve-out, the public agency may limit its financial risk totally by payment of a capitated amount per enrollee with a ceiling or limit its risk partially by establishing risk corridors outside of which it would be responsible for expenditures.

The implications for consumers of a choice between HMO or MCN revolve around integration with general health care, expertise in mental health service organization and delivery, and ensuring an adequate level of quality, volume, and comprehensiveness in mental health services.

HMO models range from a closed staff model with salaried physicians exclusively seeing HMO members in HMO offices to an independent practice association (IPA) model with individual physicians seeing both member and non-member patients under a variety of payment arrangements. For this discussion, an HMO will be the staff model type.

There are several potential advantages of using full-practice HMOs for persons with mental disorders (either staff-model or IPA). Integration of mental health and other health care services may be facilitated, provider incentives are present to maximize the offset effect (reduction in medical services due to use of mental health services), and the stigma of using mental health services may be reduced (Lehman, 1987).

There are, however, reasons why an HMO may not be the best choice for servicing public clients. Both Lehman (1987) and Mechanic (1994) note significant obstacles to successful application of this model to persons with chronic, disabling conditions. To avoid adverse selection of the more seriously disabled an HMO may give short shrift to mental health services. In addition, HMOs may not have the exper-

tise to provide the needed services to public patients. It is likely that
an HMO would use its existing mental health resources, designed for
private patients, and not have available some of the specialized and
long term services (e.g., day treatment) a public patient requires. Finally, most HMOs have geographic limitations (although they are beginning to cover larger areas) which can result in parts of the state
being uncovered.

A managed care network has the advantage of being able to
create and apply specialized knowledge and services. It can attract
highly qualified professionals who will be recognized in mental
health care and not have to compete with medical specialists. It will
be able to implement appropriate client tracking and management
information systems.

The most obvious disadvantage of the MCN is the delinking of
general health care from mental health services, with the potential
of a perverse incentive to define some mental health problems as
physical in order to cost shift to the PCP or general health plan.

A public payer has to make a prudent judgment as to which
course to take: HMO, MCN, or a combination of the two. In doing
so, it will have to weigh client needs and convenience, range and
quality of services available, costs, geographic factors, and political
considerations.

SELECTION OF METHODOLOGIES FOR ACCOUNTABILITY
AND QUALITY CONTROL

Accountability and quality control are difficult to achieve in either a
fee-for-service or managed care environment. Under public law it is
clear that the accountable entity for Medicaid is the single state
agency designated in the state plan approved by the Federal government. The accountable agency for mental health services is that
named in state statutes — usually the Department of Mental or
Behavioral Health. As the accountable entities they have the responsibility of supervising and monitoring the managed care contract.
While establishing lines of accountability may be easy, assuring
good performance of the accountable entity requires vigilance. The
Federal government will be monitoring Medicaid. State legislative
committees will monitor state agencies. Providers, consumers, and
advocates must also be closely involved in the monitoring process
(See chapters by Flynn & Hall, and Fisher).

Methods of quality control and systems level performance indicators need to be established by Medicaid and DMH working in
conjunction with consumer groups, provider organizations, other
state agencies, and the managed care entity. Methods of quality control include claims review, record review, on site observation, and
client/family/provider interviews and surveys. These should be
carried out by the managed care contractor with verification surveys conducted by state Medicaid and mental health authorities
(See chapters by Berlant et al., and Essock and Goldman). There can

be a range of indicators at different levels of organization. Below are examples of some major areas with some specific questions:

Access to services: Has overall access expanded or declined? Has access shifted by type of service? Are services located to facilitate access? Are sufficient minority providers enrolled in the network? Is there a formalized outreach program? Is enrollment information available, understandable, and available in different languages?

Adequacy of providers: Are there enough providers for the enrolled populations, is the array of specialties appropriate, is there certification of their professional training, do providers have input into system design?

Efficient administration: Are requests for prior approval handled quickly and appropriately, are service authorizations honored, are payments to providers made on a timely basis, are complaints resolved expeditiously?

Program creativity: Are new services created if needed, is outreach imaginative, are funds used for services not usually covered by Medicaid, are new ways sought to involve and empower clients, are in-home services offered, are families involved?

Clinical care: Are clinical care protocols in effect and followed, do services match patient need, is medication appropriate and monitored, are consumers fully informed?

Costs: Are providers being overpaid or underpaid by the capitation formula, are payments adequate for services expected, are lower cost services being appropriately substituted for higher cost services?

CONCLUSIONS

The increasing prevalence of managed care in the public mental health sector presents both challenges and opportunities. Clinicians must be informed and vigilant in order to advance the well-being of their clients and their own professional standards. At the same time, it is important to recognize the potential benefits and weaknesses of various managed care arrangements in order to advocate most effectively for optimal PSMC system design.

There are numerous ways to influence public sector managed care system design. First, involvement by professional organizations can have some influence on the development of managed care plans. Initial involvement as well as organized feedback once a system is in place are important. Second, if problems arise with individual cases it is important to take the time and trouble to pursue any complaint or appeals process available; documenting these incidents may provide valuable information that can be used to push for changes. Finally, it would be desirable for provider groups within any state to join forces with consumer and family organizations to advocate jointly for mutually acceptable PSMC models, ones which would appear to lead to the best outcomes with regard to access, quality, and cost.

Survival Tips

Designing Public Sector Managed Care Systems

There is no one superior type of PSMC system or program. Each PSMC program is a unique combination of various settings, strategies, and tactics.

Effective advocacy for optimal systems design involves making decisions along eight dimensions:

1. The "make versus buy" decision

2. For-profit MCOs versus non-profit agencies

3. Total population versus subpopulation coverage

4. Statewide versus sub-state coverage

5. Carve-out versus integration with general health care services

6. Selection of strategies for limiting utilization: demand versus supply side controls

7. Capitation versus non-capitated payment

8. Managed care networks versus HMOs

9. Selection of methodologies for accountability and quality control

Models which utilize the strengths of private MCOs, while limiting their disadvantages, include the flat management fee model, in which the MCO is paid a management fee to manage care, and the enabling model, in which the MCO is a consultant to the public organization, enabling the public entity to manage the care itself. These are alternatives to private/public partnership models, in which the MCO is at risk through capitation.

Choice of the "best" system for a particular state or region depends on the characteristics of the existing service system and the needs, goals, and political influence of the various stakeholders.

REFERENCES

Beinecke, R.H., Goodman, M., & Rivera, M. (1995). *An assessment of the Massachusetts managed mental health/substance abuse program: year three.* Unpublished manuscript. Suffolk University, Department of Public Management.

Brown, P.C. (1986). The complete guide to money making ventures for nonprofit organizations. Washington, D.C. The Taft Group.

Callahan Jr., J.J., Shepard, D.S., Beinecke, R.H., Larson, M.J., & Cavanaugh, D. (1994). *Evaluation of the Massachusetts Medicaid Mental Health/ Substance Abuse Program.* Unpublished Manuscript. Brandeis University, Heller School for Advanced Studies in Social Welfare.

Eisenberg, L. (1992). Treating depression and anxiety in the primary care setting, *Health Affairs, 11*:3:149–156.

Elias, E., Leadholm, B.A., Kerzner, J.P., & Kravitz, M.D. (1993). Paving the road to recovery in mental illness: beyond good intentions to a comprehensive system design. Unpublished manuscript.

Feldman, S., Baler, S., & Penner, S. (1995). *Roles for private managed care companies in the public sector.* Unpublished manuscript.

Frank, R.G., McGuire, T.G., & Newhouse, J.P. (1995). Risk contracts in managed mental health care, *Health Affairs, 14*(3), 50–64.

Lehman, A.F. (1987). Capitation payment and mental health care: a review of the opportunities and risks. *Hospital and Community Psychiatry, 38*(1), 31–38.

Mechanic, D. (1994). Integrating mental health into a general health care system. *Hospital and Community Psychiatry, 45*(9), 893–897.

Open Minds (1994). Vol. 8, Issue 3, p. 10.

6

A Case Study of
Statewide Capitation:
The Massachusetts
Experience

EUNICE HARTMAN and DEBORAH NELSON

BRIEF HISTORY OF THE MENTAL HEALTH/SUBSTANCE ABUSE PROGRAM

In this chapter we describe the experience to date of the Massachusetts Mental Health/Substance Abuse (MH/SA) Program. Since it was the first statewide managed care carve out, there are now over three years of experience, with positive and negative examples from which we think others can benefit. We summarize throughout the chapter the evaluative voices of various stakeholders.

The Massachusetts Medicaid Program, since its inception in 1967, has been one of the most extensive in the U.S. with respect to both eligibility and services provided. The cost of providing this program grew from $1.5 billion in FY 1988 to $2.7 billion in FY 1990. Massachusetts faced the dilemma that the expansion of the cost of providing the Medicaid Program was creating a fiscal crisis which threatened the provision of social welfare programs, and other needed services.

Options under consideration by Massachusetts to "tame the cost beast" included restricting the Medicaid benefit (perhaps eliminating outpatient benefits), restricting eligibility and income guidelines, or managing the care.

The Division of Medical Assistance (DMA) opted for managing the care and applied for and obtained a Health Care Finance Administration (HCFA) waiver to enroll Medicaid recipients in a Managed Care Program. One component of the Managed Care initiative was to "carve out" and contract with a private company for the management of the mental health and substance abuse services provided to recipients enrolled in the Primary Care Clinician Program. In this model, the managed care organization (MCO) became the capitated entity, while providers continued to be reimbursed on a fee-for-service basis.

In January of 1992, DMA entered into a contract with Mental Health Management of America Health (MHMA) to manage the MH/SA Program for about 380,000 Medicaid recipients, including the aid categories of SSI/Disabled, AFDC, Refugee, and Psych under 21 Programs. The MCO became responsible for the provision of acute services, while DMH and other state agencies retained responsibility for the provision of long-term and intermediate care. The objective of DMA's contract with MHMA was to contain the increasing costs and to measure and improve access and quality, while retaining consumer freedom of choice. The DMA/MHMA contract specified that the contractor would demonstrate ability to establish baseline measures of quality for the population and demonstrate improvements in access and quality. The state also required the contractor to develop a management information system which would integrate clinical case management functions with claims payment functions. In order to meet the systems development and claims payment requirements of the RFP, MHMA partnered with one of the largest Medicaid claims payers, First Health Systems. As this was the nation's first "shared risk" public sector capitated contract, the contractor had to demonstrate fiscal stability.

An independent evaluation of the program was included as a condition of the HCFA waiver. "The Federal government granted the waiver for a two year period. At the end of this period a two year extension could be sought if the program had reduced costs without significantly reducing enrollee access to services and quality" (Callahan, Shepard, Beinecke, Larson, & Cavanaugh, 1994). MHMA obtained the two year extension, and a new Request For Proposals (RFP) was issued in September, 1995. A second independent evaluation was released in April, 1995. Excerpts from both evaluations will be cited throughout this chapter regarding the impact and results of the first three years of this ambitious endeavor.

"Managed care companies bring strong expertise in how to manage care efficiently, but CMHC and other public treatment facilities have the experience working with the needs of the seriously mentally ill and lower income populations. Together they have the potential for synergistic public-private collaboration.... It is not surprising that many leaders of the CMHC "movement" went on to become executives of the private sector managed behavioral healthcare companies ... the parallels between community mental health and managed behavioral healthcare are striking." (Freeman & Trabin, 1994). MHMA is an early example of this phenomenon: the company was founded by persons with many years of experience in the public sector, and who felt that the integration of managed care methods and public sector treatment would result in improved treatment while generating cost savings.

Before the RFP, MHMA staff spent months in Massachusetts to obtain provider opinion about what would work for this population: identifying what services were in place, what services were needed, and seeking provider recommendations about how to implement managed care in Massachusetts. MHMA was confident of three things: 1) Treatment was being delivered in inpatient settings that could more efficiently and effectively be delivered in community based settings if the services were available. 2) The provider community would work collaboratively with MHMA to develop needed services if funding was made available. 3) The state's capitation rate, which reflected a 20% savings over unmanaged projected costs, was feasible.

Once the contract was awarded, the MHMA team moved quickly to hire "locals" to implement and manage the MH/SA Program. The Executive team is comprised of professionals with strong public sector service experience. Regional Managers hired to manage the network in the six regions of the state brought a wealth of state and local experience, as did the clinicians and physicians. "Many informants reported that having locally recruited professionals managing the MHMA program was a positive element. Knowledge of the local human service system, pre-existing relationships with others in the mental health/substance abuse system and personal incentives to maintain a good reputation can be important elements in making a program work well." (Callahan et al., 1994). The management team held the belief that managing care within a full continuum of services, and "doing the right thing for each recipient" would result in improved treatment and outcomes, while creating a fiscally sound program.

KEY PROGRAM ELEMENTS

The MHMA approach to managing care was to develop a comprehensive continuum of care which links the client with the level of care that is consistent with level of functioning. The aim was to maintain community mental health principles and to develop standards of care and quality measures to evaluate the effectiveness of treatment delivered. The five crucial program elements include: Network Development and Management, Clinical Management, Information Management, Functional Partnerships (including collaborative agreements), and Quality Management which drives the integration of continuous quality improvement throughout the organization and the network.

PROVIDER NETWORK DEVELOPMENT AND MANAGEMENT

Prior to managed care, patients had freedom of choice of providers but choice was among very limited treatment modalities. There were few integrated or comprehensive systems of care to address the complex needs of the recipients in this fee-for-service system. Network development was implemented on a regional basis, and was headed by Regional Managers who were not only familiar with provider services, but also with the regional management and services provided by state agencies.

The HCFA waiver allowed for expansion of care by the purchase of alternative or diversionary services, which were previously not Medicaid reimbursable, as long as the MCO could demonstrate that these services would enhance care at no increase in cost and would decrease hospitalization costs. After a needs analysis, a plan for the procurement of alternative services was presented to DMA. An ambitious process for the procurement of alternative services required written applications, site visits, record reviews and collateral contacts with entities such as consumer advocacy groups, state agencies, and crisis teams. Approximately 300 providers of alternative services were credentialed and added to the continuum of care. (See Table 1).

While the procurement of alternative services focused on the expansion of available community based treatment options, the inpatient procurement process was designed to decrease overall inpatient bed capacity in the system, through the development of a selected network. "Under DMA supervision, written criteria were developed.... The five general criteria were 1) accessibility, 2) managed care experience, 3) clinical quality, 4) quality improvement programs, and 5) competitive pricing.... Important additional criteria included an analysis of capacity, experience with Medicaid (consumers), cultural competency and geographic distribution...." (Callahan et al., 1994). The procurement process was similar to that described for alternative services. "As a result of this process ... MHMA had established a statewide network of hospitals,"

TABLE 1: MHMA Provider Network

Continuum of Care for Medicaid Recipients	
Acute Inpatient Hospital	Methadone Maintenance
Observation Beds	School Based Services
Crisis Stabilization Beds	Outpatient Services (Multiple
Acute Residential Treatment	Modalities)
Level III (Medically Monitored)	Cultural and Linguistic
Detox	Consultation
Partial and Day Programs	Enhanced Substance Abuse
Structured Outpatient	Services for Women
Addictions Programs	Intensive Clinical
Family Stabilization Teams	Management
Intensive Outpatient Treatment	Community Support Services

(Callahan et al., 1994) with the final selection including 46 facilities (55 Units), a reduction from the previous 96 facilities who were Medicaid reimbursable. As a provision of the waiver, MHMA included private psychiatric hospitals in the network, making this a new option for adult Medicaid patients.

Medicaid providers had previously been reimbursed on a per discharge rate. Hospitals which had been reimbursed on this basis "would often transfer the patient ... to another hospital, where the patient would appear as a new admission" thus obscuring total length of stay for the complete illness episode (Callahan et al., 1994). Not only was it difficult to obtain utilization data, but comprehensiveness, continuity and overall quality of care suffered. To address this problem, the procurement process established an all inclusive per-diem rate payment methodology.

The procurement of outpatient services was an inclusive process, with a few providers being excluded based on quality of care concerns. MHMA wanted to maintain convenient access to outpatient services, without disrupting existing provider/client relationships.

In procuring this contracted network, MHMA established provider performance specifications for the delivery of services. Initial network management efforts focused on compliance with performance specifications. Network profiling and additional quality measures were identified for each provider type. Based upon profiling results, quality improvement plans were implemented. All provider types are now on a semi-annual profiling and quality improvement schedule for network management.

CLINICAL MANAGEMENT

In developing the Clinical Management Program, MHMA recruited local experienced professionals. Eight years of clinical experience, a masters degree (or equivalent) and licensure were minimum requirements for MHMA clinicians (12–14 years of experience per clinician was the norm). Multi-disciplinary teams of clinicians with experience and with demonstrated empathy and understanding of the complex and multifaceted needs of this population in a variety of settings, were selected. A physician advisory team was selected through a process of provider recommendations, including board certified adult, child and adolescent, addictions, forensics, consultation-liaison, and geropsychiatry psychiatrists. To have credibility with the provider community, the clinicians and physician advisors need to be experienced and respected professionals.

The purpose of clinical management is to monitor the process of care. The clinical management function facilitates access to care, treatment in the most effective level of care, timely and comprehensive treatment, aftercare planning, service linkage and continuity of care, provider compliance with standards of care, and timely payment for care through service authorization.

Clinical criteria, along with clearly defined policies and procedures, are the guidelines by which clinical management is effective. Criteria drive the system toward a more standardized approach to assessment and treatment. A Provider Manual was published which defines level of care and medical necessity criteria for the expanded continuum of care. American Society of Addictions Medicine (ASAM) criteria were adapted to define levels of care for substance abuse services. As new services were procured, MHMA clinicians and physicians assisted in teaching and guiding providers in the criteria and utilization of the expanded services.

The MHMA clinical teams work from a data rich on-line case management system that integrates clinical, authorization and claims data. The recipient file identifies Medicaid eligibility, MHMA enrollment, third party payers, demographic information, as well as the recipient's primary provider(s), and clinical "Alerts". The previous clinical reviews (from all levels of care) are easily accessed, as are the aftercare plans and claims history. The availability of this data enables any MHMA clinician to assist the provider in formulating informed treatment decisions.

To promote collaborative working relationships with providers, a model was implemented in which the MHMA clinicians work consistently as care managers with assigned providers, matching area of clinical expertise to program and service type. Care managers develop provider specific plans to address improvement goals. The intent is to work with each provider in such a manner that a trusting relationship is developed. As the relationship develops, the care manager becomes utilized as a consultant and client advocate for difficult cases, and the need for individual case review can be minimized. Providers who demonstrated delivery of high quality care were advanced to a retrospective "clinical indicator" review model, which increased the responsibility of the providers while maintaining MHMA's quality management function.

In 1994, an Intensive Clinical Management (ICM) Program was implemented to better assess and meet the needs of the highest risk recipients. The ICM program incorporated concepts of case management from both the private managed care field and CMHC models. Clinical and claims data were analyzed to identify ICM patients. The ICM clinicians work collaboratively with the consumer, the consumer's family, providers, and other agencies to develop an integrated, comprehensive treatment plan. The ICM program developed provider delivered Community Support Services which could be purchased for consumers who need "hands-on" community-based support. The ICM program has quality measures in place which are evaluated quarterly. These include: 1) days spent in the community, 2) number and length of acute admissions, 3) utilization of community based services, 4) medical cost offset and primary care physician visits, 5) cost of treatment, 6) level of functioning, and 7) consumer satisfaction.

To manage outpatient services, MHMA began with a program of open access to outpatient treatment with eight "initial encounter" sessions. After eight sessions, providers submitted a written treatment plan requesting authorization for additional sessions. In 1993, MHMA developed and published Outpatient Treatment Guidelines based on age, diagnoses, severity of illness, and phase of treatment. In 1994, these guidelines were reviewed and revised through feedback from stakeholders. This prior review and authorization process, although relatively easy and generous, was difficult to administer and created delays in timely payment to providers. Therefore, in 1995 MHMA began a privileging process to "exempt" providers who practiced within the guidelines from the prior authorization process. Approximately one half of all outpatient treatment is now provided without prior approval. MHMA is assisting providers to establish internal systems of utilization and quality management, and plans to eliminate the prior authorization process completely, as providers demonstrate internal management capabilities.

In addition, the Clinical Department established a retrospective Quality Review Program for all levels of care. The retrospective review of medical records is utilized to measure the quality of care being provided in the network, and is combined with claims profiling data for incorporation into Provider Improvement Plans.

INFORMATION MANAGEMENT: INTEGRATION OF DATA

The MHMA information system is composed of health data analysis, claims payment, and client management subsystems. The central transactions/claims database and client management system integrates on-line utilization management with real time linkage to Medicaid eligibility files, transmits authorization data to the claims processing system, and generates custom designed reports.

A variety of information is shared with the state and other agencies. The current technology allows for partial integration, but there is not yet a shared data base. However, there is on-line eligibility data, service authorization, claims payment, case management, provider profiling, utilization and financial reporting, and the analysis of outcomes data.

PUBLIC AGENCY COOPERATIVE AGREEMENTS AND PARTNERSHIPS

As stated earlier, the MH/SA program was responsible for the provision of acute services, while long-term residential and intermediate care remained the responsibility of state agencies. "MHMA supported by Medicaid ... worked cooperatively with state agencies to develop relations which facilitate client care.... Interagency Agreements have been signed with the Departments of Mental Health, Social Service, Public Health, Youth Services and Mental Retardation.... A clinical task force has done extensive work on operationalizing the agreements with the Department of Mental Health. Major emphasis has been placed on differentiating responsibility for shared DMH/MHMA clients and developing clinical criteria and protocols for decision making and transfers ... the objective is to promote seamless access to quality and efficient mental health services." (Callahan et al., 1994).

To succeed in a public/private environment, a managed care company must work collaboratively with others invested in the delivery of services. These include consumers and families, providers, trade and professional organization representatives, legal advocates, and the state agencies which are frequently involved in the provision of other services to this population. An Advisory Council consisting of about 25 stakeholders was established at the inception of the program. This Advisory Council meets every six weeks and advises on policy, reviews new services before they are implemented, and reviews quality and access.

In order to improve consumer input, a separate Consumer Advisory Council was developed to keep MHMA and DMA advised of recommendations, concerns and issues identified by the consumer network. Of equal importance have been the recommendations and feedback from the provider community. Attention to these partnerships, although challenging by increasing the number of "cooks" wanting to stir the "broth", unequivocally results in better service for consumers.

MANAGING FOR QUALITY WITH CQI PRINCIPLES

In 1994, MHMA went forward with adopting tenets of continuous quality improvement (CQI) in the running of its business. A director level quality position was added to the management team, while the services of an experienced CQI consultant provided guidance in the implementation. The emphasis throughout the CQI initiative and Quality Management program is on pragmatism. These initiatives are fully integrated into the business plan, and are critical to the measurement of the organization's success.

Initially, some 60 topic areas were identified as well suited for measurement and improvement. Eight key Quality Measurement activities were ultimately selected: 1) reducing unplanned readmissions responsibly; 2) improving the processes of acute care for children; 3) improving access to services for non-English speaking patients, 4) profiling and improving service delivery to substance affected individuals; 5) measuring and improving access to outpatient services; 6) measuring variation in the top five diagnoses in outpatient services; 7) measuring and improving continuity of care and variation in service linkage from detoxification facilities; and 8) measuring and improving telephone access to MHMA clinicians. The Quality Management Council arranged for CQI training for staff, and then chartered eight problem solving (CQI) teams to work on these key concerns.

THE IMPACT OF RAPID IMPLEMENTATION

The implementation of the managed care program was ambitious. Although much time was spent laying the groundwork, once the contract was awarded, DMA defined an aggressive timeline. DMA and MHMA have been criticized for the speed with which the changes were made. However, DMA took great care to announce the plans, contractual obligations and program goals prior to the start of the program, so that there were few surprises.

The contract was awarded in January, 1992, the HCFA waiver granted in February, the start of clinical management for inpatient services was in April, and procurement of the network began in June. Clinical management and claims payment for all services with the on-line integrated case-management and claims payment system, and the capitated shared-risk contract began in July. The inpatient network was selected by October. An expanded network of services was procured in approximately one year.

The rapid implementation of this program made it difficult to meet the requirements of the contract in the allotted time, and represented a large amount of change for consumers. Staff had to be hired and trained quickly and internal processes developed by both MHMA and providers. Providers had to allocate resources to respond to the Application for Affiliation proposals and the clinical review process. Although provider organizations approved the procurement process, this resulted in a decrease in revenue for the hospitals not selected. In some cases, this contributed to the closure of some acute inpatient units.

Managed care causes change in providers, provider types, services, and payment methodologies, which results in MIS changes and requirements which are difficult to accommodate. MHMA added approximately 300 new alternative service programs, but many of these providers did not have the infrastructure to support authorization and claims submission processes. As a result, while patients began to receive new and creative treatment alternatives, MHMA and providers struggled to keep up with the changes, and timely payment for services frequently suffered. The later corrections of the internal processes and the introduction of CQI management principles refined and improved the systems created in the first two years. "Nearly all providers reported that much more time was being spent administratively managing the MHMA clients than before ... the primary criticisms of MHMA were its bureaucratic administrative procedures and the difficulties reaching staff by phone." (Callahan et al., 1994).

A longer time line would have allowed for increased stakeholder involvement in the implementation phase. However, the state's fiscal crisis threatened its economy and the rapid implementation allowed the state to begin generating cost savings in the first year. Adherence to the timelines may have prevented "special interest" groups from organizing lawsuits and other delays in the implementation of the program. Some difficult questions remain unanswered: Would it have been better to have a more moderately paced implementation? Was there a better way to address the fiscal crisis?

SPECIAL CHALLENGES

As a pioneer in PSMC, MHMA faced challenges unique to managing the care for the Medicaid population. The following are some of MHMA's responses to these problems.

INFORMATION SYSTEMS

To comprehensively manage public sector care, more system integration is required than for the private sector. An internal MIS is needed which integrates claims, clinical management, and quality management (e.g., outcomes, satisfaction) information. The ability to integrate these data with the Medicaid data base and other state agencies data bases is also essential.

Different agencies collect information in different ways and often define or code it differently. Standard data definitions, such as level of functioning or treatment encounter or episode of treatment, need to be developed. Even when such definitions are developed, many provider information systems do not easily allow for such changes. "Documenting the care provided the most seriously mentally ill is difficult because that care is funded by two different state agencies with different, but overlapping responsibilities. Merging large data bases from different state agencies is difficult technically and politically." (Eisen & Dickey, 1994). MHMA currently shares data with other state agencies. Because recipient involvement with other state agencies is indicated in the MHMA case management system, clinicians are alerted to coordinate care with other involved agencies. However, much more work needs to be done to improve data sharing for this vulnerable population while remaining alert to the need to respect confidentiality issues.

The whole area of medical cost offset is controversial and difficult to measure. MHMA shares information on paid claims for Medical services via tapes with DMA. Medical cost offset studies are being developed.

Merging family unit data for behavioral health and medical information is also an enormous problem. Family members may have become eligible for Medicaid and enrolled through different agencies, with no link to other family members (i.e., a mother may be eligible for AFDC while her child may have been enrolled in Medicaid by DSS). Having a medically ill family member is associated with more behavioral health care utilization in other family members, and vice versa. The need to merge family unit data is great, requiring MCOs to design better integrated systems. However as systems become integrated, the challenges of confidentiality and how to create system security arise.

Behavioral healthcare systems need better and more fluid systems to capture multiple domains of information for purposes of measuring value and quality. The key to improving processes of care is to first measure and understand them. More integrated systems will help us better understand patients and their needs, the practice patterns of providers, and treatment outcomes.

MEASURING OUTCOMES

"Recipients, consumer advocates, and purchasers expect managed care companies, in partnership with their providers, to measure and continuously improve quality of care. This task can prove especially challenging when the beneficiaries of that care are covered by a publicly funded program." (Nelson, Hartman, Ojemann, & Wilcox, 1995). Medicaid patients are poorer, often do not speak English well, and encounter more life stressors than the private sector population. As more states contract with MCOs for the care for their Medicaid populations, the need to measure the quality of services will be inevitable. MHMA's outcomes measurement and management efforts have been created through collaboration with DMA, patients, providers, and other stakeholders. The outcomes program's principles may be helpful to others considering similar public/private partnerships.

The Quality Management program provides a coordinated, comprehensive and systematic framework for the measurement of processes and outcomes. A key aspect is measurement of outcomes and tying those outcomes back to processes of care. Much work has been done on measuring functional status and satisfaction.

Level of functioning. MHMA has investigated and tested a number of level of functioning tools with the Medicaid population. The aim has been to find tools that: 1) are feasible to administer to various populations (e.g., inpatient, outpatient, adult, children); 2) provide clinically useful information; 3) are sensitive to change; 4) are available in and relevant to different languages and cultures, and 5) use consumer self report.

MHMA has developed a modular outcomes measurement system for adults, comprised of the SF-12 (Ware & Sherbourne, 1992), and the BASIS-32 (Eisen & Dickey, 1994), which should be useful for ongoing, routinized use across populations and treatment modalities, and the Child Health Questionnaire (CHQ) for children.

Satisfaction. Patient satisfaction is a critically important outcome, one which is associated with better functional outcomes. As with functional status tools, existing customer satisfaction tools designed for other populations do not often reflect the unique needs of the Medicaid population. Consequently, MHMA adapted items from some existing surveys (Eisen & Dickey, 1994; Cleary et al., 1991), and created some new ones. The survey was developed with input from consumers, advocacy groups, state agencies, and subject matter experts, and was focus group tested.

The outpatient satisfaction survey yielded a response rate of approximately 38%, which is relatively high for a vulnerable and transient population. Respondents report being generally satisfied with their treatment (86%); better able to handle their day to day responsibilities (functioning) (72%); and satisfied with access to outpatient services. The survey has been adapted and administered in outpatient mental health and substance abuse settings.

The most important predictors of overall satisfaction appear to be respect from staff, good treatment outcomes, confidence in staff and one's own abilities, and the quality of staff communication. Predictors of dissatisfaction are staff not being friendly/courteous, staff and recipient not working together on goals, and the clinic not being clean.

The results also showed much variation among the clinics. Interestingly, the clinic with the best satisfaction and good access is also a clinic which provides treatment within utilization parameters. This suggests that it is possible to deliver satisfactory and accessible care which is also efficient and effective. The variation among clinics has led to the development of quality improvement plans among those with lower performance, and an analysis of "best practices" of the clinics which consistently outperformed others. Continuous measurement leads to continuous improvement efforts, and provides us an early warning, should satisfaction with services decline.

CULTURAL/LINGUISTIC ISSUES IN TREATMENT

The Medicaid population differs from a private sector population, in that many recipients do not speak English as a first language. More than 40 languages are represented in the MH/SA programs. Communicating with these consumers and measuring how they are doing poses unique challenges.

Our Quality Management Council initiated a CQI team to improve access to linguistic and culturally competent services. The team has determined and verified root causes to problematic access to services, and implemented corrective actions, which will be periodically reassessed. MHMA has also developed a Cultural Linguistic Enhancement program of outpatient clinicians who are culturally and linguistically competent available to acute treatment settings.

SUBSTANCE ABUSE COMORBIDITY

The preponderance of substance abuse comorbidity has been recognized as a significant problem, costly in terms of human lives, suffering, and dollars. The Quality Management Council created a CQI team to address this issue. The team has profiled the extent of the problem: approximately 70% of recipients who receive inpatient MH services have coexisting mental health and substance use problems. The team has focused on the under-diagnosis, minimal outpatient treatment, and the overuse of inpatient stays with these individuals, who may be better served in community based settings. A valid and reliable screening tool has been implemented, and clinical pathways for referral and treatment are in operation.

COORDINATION WITH PRIMARY CARE CLINICIANS

It is incumbent upon care providers in the behavioral health field to actively promote linkage between MH/SA clinicians and primary care providers (PCP). Whether a patient is in a carve out or an integrated (carve-in) system, PCPs seldom make referrals to MH/SA providers. Coordination between the MH/SA providers and the

PCP is a primary thrust of the ICM program, with PCPs frequently attending treatment planning meetings. ICM clinicians encourage and assist patients to keep primary care appointments. MHMA is in the process of developing a program to enhance communication and coordination between primary and behavioral health care for all recipients. Electronic linkage may improve communications and provide a better sense about the treatment each may be providing.

COORDINATION OF CARE WITH MULTIPLE AGENCIES

Although the goal of managed care is to have "seamless" systems for service delivery across agencies, it takes an incredible amount of time and energy to coordinate care for Medicaid patients. Many have multi-agency involvement. As many of the other agencies have their own budgetary cutbacks, resources are frequently limited. MHMA has often continued to provide services in the acute system while patients are awaiting other agency residential placements. Although this has improved, the state has not yet achieved a "seamless" system.

RESULTS TO DATE: ACCESS, QUALITY AND COST

The relative value and success of any managed care initiative needs to be based of the impact of the program on *access, quality, and cost.* "We finally have proof that a carefully implemented program of managed care can improve the service delivery system while simultaneously saving money. We still have work to do, but we are pleased with the evolution of the program thus far." (Medicaid Commissioner Bruce Bullen, 1994).

A second independent evaluation states that "Overall, providers and stakeholders consider access and quality of care to have remained the same or improved each year under the managed care program," and that providers report that "integration of care between state agencies and coordination of care and planning among providers to be improved." (Beinecke, Goodman, & Rivera, 1995).

Access. The percentage of "unduplicated" recipients who receive MH/SA services has increased from 21.3 to 23.5% under managed care. Also, recipients now have access to greater range of services. "The changes keep people out of hospitals and give clients faster access to the specific care they need at any time in appropriate facilities" (Beinecke et al., 1995).

Quality. Prior to managed care, quality measurement received little attention. "While it is desirable to know whether quality has changed, this cannot be determined directly because there are no studies of the quality of the (unmanaged) fee for service system" (Callahan et al., 1994). Therefore the independent evaluation relied heavily on provider interviews to evaluate the quality of the MH/SA Program. By provider report, quality of care has improved under the managed care program (Callahan et al.; Beinecke et al., 1995).

MH/SA Program is increasingly driven by data, which is used to manage for quality. MHMA has surveyed patient, provider and employee satisfaction and developed management action plans to improve key indicators. CQI teams are working to implement improvement measures for our key quality indicators. Provider profiling through claims analysis and clinical indicator record review are assisting providers in targeting areas for improvement. Functional assessment tools have been incorporated in measuring outcomes for this population. MHMA has been able to identify and target "high risk" recipients for intensive clinical management, and measures functional outcomes and satisfaction on an ongoing basis for these most vulnerable consumers. Four quarterly administrations of the SF-36 provide preliminary evidence that consumers are reporting better functioning. They report that community support services are helping them to function better. Finally, MHMA's pilot program to reduce readmissions has done so in 4 out 6 hospitals, and halted an increasing readmission rate in one hospital. Predictors of readmission are being used to manage our system to promote more time in the community.

Cost. In the first year, MHMA met and slightly exceeded the state's targeted goal of 20% savings over projected unmanaged costs. This represented a $46 million savings. In year two, the goal was to allow for 4% growth over the savings generated in 1993. For the following two years, modest growth in cost are projected.

To date, the program has resulted in preserving an unlimited benefit for behavioral health services. MHMA's purchasing power has increased attention paid this disenfranchised population. "A number of organizations ... found that the new system forced clinicians to think more sharply about treatment. MHMA's requirements had triggered discussions about what was going on and what needed to be done, and had made diagnosis and treatment planning linked to it more critical, and was leading to a more rational approach to treatment. It was the view of most, although not all ... that the potential for improvement over the largely unlimited system of the past was great." (Callahan et al., 1994).

FUTURE DIRECTIONS

In the fall of 1995, DMA issued an RFP for the next three years of the MH/SA program. DMA decided to contract with a different MCO, a partnership created between Value Behavioral Health and FHC Options, Inc. MHMA apparently lost the contract because the Value-Options partnership submitted a "more competitive bid." It was reported that quality of care was not at issue in the decision to change vendors. The transition was scheduled for July, 1996.

MHMA will work collaboratively with the new vendor to facilitate a smooth transition. It is expected that many of the initiatives created by MHMA will be continued and that many of the MHMA staff will be retained.

MHMA will recommend the continuation of collaboration between the MCO and providers to integrate utilization data into a continuous quality improvement model. Provider profiling based on the integration of claims and medical record review data, along with consumer satisfaction and outcomes data, is the means by which a comprehensive quality picture is obtained. Such integrated data can be used to define improvement goals for the structure and processess of care.

The managed care vendor must ensure that access and quality of services can be measured prior to subcapitating payment to providers. MHMA worked to encourage and assist providers to develop internal quality and utilization management processess and management information systems. This effort should be continued under the new contract.

Survival Tips

Statewide Capitation

- Do your homework prior to contract award and implementation.
- A longer timeline for implementation is desirable.
- Hire local, well-respected professionals.
- Listen to stakeholders.
- Interagency agreements are crucial.
- Develop internal expertise on managing by CQI principles.
- Maximize integration between primary care and mental health, substance abuse and mental health, and acute care and long-term care.
- Develop functional provider partnerships.
- Use existing level of functioning and satisfaction tools as a starting point, but refine them.
- Obtain flexible relational data base technology.
- It is not necessary to implement programs with first generation managed care techniques.
- Be flexible and learn from mistakes.
- Be aware of the risks of competitive and proprietary behavior.

SURVIVAL TIPS

As other MCOs and traditional provider systems consider initiatives in managing Medicaid funded care, we offer the following survival tips from the leassons we've learned:

- Do your homework prior to contract award and implementation. Define goals and implementation plans, and develop grassroots support.

- A longer timeline for implementation is desirable, if that is at all possible.

- Hire local, well-respected professionals with representation from providers and state agencies. Do careful and thorough interviewing to ascertain their empathy and respect for the patient population.

- Listen to stakeholders and keep them informed, but stay true to the goal of implementing meaningful system changes.

- Interagency agreements are a crucial part of ensuring that care is coordinated for this population. Make this a contractual responsibility and include merging or sharing data as part of the agreement.

- Develop internal expertise on managing by CQI principles and make this a central part of the organization.

- Develop policies and strategies to maximize integration between primary care and mental health, substance abuse and mental health, and acute care and long-term care.

- Develop functional provider partnerships. A MCO is only as good as the providers in its panel.

- Use existing level of functioning and satisfaction tools as a starting point, but refine them to meet the needs of the specific population.

- Obtain flexible relational data base technology. Ensure that the MIS allows an open format that can merge data from medical claims and other agencies. Invest in continued improvement and advancement of MIS technology.

- It is not necessary to implement programs with first generation managed care techniques as was done in Massachusetts. Many states already have better defined systems of care in place that will allow management through provider networks and subcapitation contracts.

- Be flexible and learn from mistakes. When changing paradigms of services delivery, it is not always possible to be right on the first try.

- Be aware of the risks of competitive and proprietary behavior. The current trend of procurement litigation is troublesome. Competition must not prevent providers and MCOs from working together to improve the technologies which will enhance our profession and improve care. "It is critical that in this emerging field decision makers learn to support one another and understand that successful programs built city by city, state by state, are the elements that will allow this industry to grow. As movement into public markets increases, there is less and less room for a proprietary approach to protocols, strategies or measurement tools. Let our profession celebrate that, and take advantage of the opportunity to build on the experience that has gone before, taking giant steps into the future" (Pattullo, 1995).

REFERENCES

Beinecke, R.H., Goodman, M., & Rivera, M. (1995). *An assessment of the Massachusetts managed mental health/substance abuse program: year three.* Unpublished manuscript. Boston: Suffolk University, Department of Public Management.

Callahan Jr., J.J., Shepard, D.S., Beinecke, R.H., Larson, M.J., & Cavanaugh, D. (1994). *Evaluation of the Massachusetts Medicaid Mental Health/ Substance Abuse Program.* Unpublished Manuscript. Waltham, Massachusetts: Brandeis University, Heller School for Advanced Studies in Social Welfare.

Cleary, P., Edgmen-Levitan, S., Roberts, M., Moloney, T.W., McMullen, W., Walker, J.D., & Delbanco, T.L. (1991). Patients evaluate their hospital care: A national survey: *Health Affairs.*

Eisen, S., & Dickey, B. (1994). *Perceptions of care.* Unpublished manuscript. Belmont, Massachusetts: McLean Hospital.

Eisen, S.V., Dill, D.L., & Grob, M.C. (1994). Reliability and validity of a brief patient-report instrument for outcome evaluation. *Hospital and Community Psychiatry, 45*(3), 242–247.

Freeman, M.A., & Trabin, T. (1994). *Managed behavioral healthcare: History, models, key issues, and future course.* Unpublished Manuscript.

Massachusetts nixes Medicaid contract. (March 1, 1996). *Managed Medicare and Medicaid.* p. 8.

Nelson, D.C., Hartman, E.M., Ojemann, P.G., & Wilcox, M. (1995). Outcomes measurement and management with a large Medicaid population: A public/private collaboration. *Behavioral Healthcare Tomorrow, 4,* 31–37.

Pattullo, E.A. (1995). Is believing you have a case a good enough reason to sue? *Behavioral Healthcare Tomorrow, 4,* 40–41.

Ware, J., & Sherbourne, C. (1992). The MOS 36-item short-form health survey (SF-36). *Medical Care, 30*(6).

7

Care Management by Public Sector Provider Organizations: Salt Lake City

DAVID DANGERFIELD and ROD BETIT

INTRODUCTION

The emergence of public sector managed care has usually been associated with private proprietary managed care firms which develop contracts to manage services in what has traditionally been the public domain. This trend toward privatized managed care and services in the public sector has created intense feelings for many public mental health providers, recipients, and advocates. Public sector managed care is not, however, the exclusive province of private MCOs.

This chapter describes a risk based capitated model for managing mental health services to the Medicaid population of much of the state of Utah. The model is financially and clinically operated by a public sector community mental health center (CMHC) that has had a long-term commitment to the Medicaid population, as well as to other public mental health recipients.

The elements of this model will be analyzed from four perspectives. First is the history and basis of the decision to capitate all the Medicaid mental health services to a public CMHC, in lieu of contracting with a private managed care firm or a larger inclusive health care system. Second, we describe the necessary skills, both clinically and administratively, for a CMHC to successfully operate a risk-based capitated system. Third, we address the challenges faced in the operation of this model and how they were dealt with and overcome will be detailed. And finally, we provide a description of specific lessons learned and recommendations for CMHCS, and others interested in serving public recipients of mental health services in a managed care environment.

HISTORY AND ELEMENTS OF THE MODEL

Testing an Experimental Model: On July 1, 1991, the State of Utah Medicaid Agency began partial risk capitated contracts with three separate CMHCs. Each was to be the sole mental health provider for the Medicaid population within geographical areas they traditionally serve. This project was designed as an experimental model to compare differences in mental health services for the Medicaid population. This comparison was between a managed care approach with the provider being at-risk and the traditional fee-for-service models. The experimental and control groups were established by the geographical location of the Medicaid recipient. The three centers in the capitated managed care experimental side would have approximately one-half of the Medicaid population enrolled in their capitated payment. The control group would be the other half of the Medicaid population, who would remain in the traditional fee-for-service system. One of the test CMHCs is in the most populous area of the state, while the other two test sites serve rural Utah.

The experience of Valley Mental Health, the urban test site, will be the basis from which material for this chapter is drawn. Valley Mental Health (VMH) is a nonprofit corporation contracting with Salt Lake and Summit counties as the sole provider and administrator of public mental health services. The operating budget is $45 million with 700 staff serving 20,000 people per year. Over one-third of these 20,000 people are Medicaid recipients. The total Medicaid population in the two counties is just over 50,000 people. VMH primarily operates a staff model out of 37 locations. Service sites include traditional outpatient, partial hospitalization, and residential programs. In addition, programs are in schools, correctional facilities, and in the homeless community. Case managers help clients at multiple-supported housing complexes owned and operated by Valley Mental Health. The center also contracts with 50 therapeutic foster homes. In-house employment screening, employment placement, and job-coaching are part of the service system. VMH operates a separate company hiring the mentally ill in supported employment positions and employment contracts with private businesses for temporary work placements of clients are available.

Since the experimental program was established, over four years ago, the State of Utah has determined that there were positive results from the project and have decided to institute managed care capitated contracts in the rest of the state. The Medicaid agency has now contracted throughout the state with each of the CMHCs through local county mental health authorities.

Why a CMHC? There are a number of reasons that the CMHCs were selected as the provider and manager for a risk based capitated program. First and foremost, the centers were already firmly established in the communities and had developed a continuum of services with emphasis upon least restrictive treatment interventions. The centers had a long tradition of working with the Medicaid population and had established priority services for seriously mentally ill children, adolescents, and adults. Many of these clients are enrolled in the Medicaid program.

In Utah, the county commissioners are, by statute, the local mental health authorities. As such, they have the obligation to set the size and scope of the public mental health program in their local communities. State general fund mental health dollars are allocated and then distributed to the counties on a formula basis. Each county is obligated to match at least 20 percent of the state dollars. By tradition, most counties in Utah have exceeded the match requirements to further public mental health services. The local mental health authorities were involved in the early discussions about the capitation experiment and were part of the decision making process.

The local mental health authorities (county commissioners) had to be part of the discussions. Not only are they the local authorities, but a large part of the Medicaid outpatient services were partially funded with local dollars allocated to mental health. The reason for this is that the federal requirement for local matching dollars on Medicaid was met by the contribution from the county's mental health allocation. Thus, there was an already established pattern that Medicaid dollars were heavily used in the county mental health programs. The CMHCs were established by the counties to operate their public mental health programs. There was strong interest in not disrupting this established funding pattern.

A third reason for the model selected by the State Medicaid agency was the concern, which was shared by the State Mental Health Department, as well as the county mental health authorities, that the infrastructure for the seriously mentally ill needed to be enhanced. Through their local county mental health authorities, the CMHCs had responsibility for the county and state general mental health dollars. Therefore, this was an opportunity to pool capitated Medicaid, state and county dollars to continue to enhance the infrastructure and services for the seriously mentally ill.

Model Selected: In addition to the CMHC being the sole responsible provider of Medicaid mental health services for its geographical region, there are three additional key structural elements in the contracts between the Utah State Medicaid agency and the CMHCs:

(1) *Mental Health Carve-out*: The Medicaid population obtains its general health care from fee-for-service physicians, or are enrolled in HMOs. Medicaid enrollees in the capitated system obtain their mental health services, both inpatient or outpatient, from the CMHC. The

center, as the managed care provider, either arranges for or directly provides the services.

(2) *Phase-in of Risk*: During the first two years, the three centers were at-risk for inpatient care, including physician visits and all ancillary charges. Although the centers were prepaid a per-member per-month capitated amount for inpatient and outpatient services, the centers were initially not at-risk for outpatient care. There was a settlement at the end of each of the two years for the outpatient portion. This settlement was for actual services provided, at the standard rate of reimbursement for fee-for-service, compared to the gross amount prepaid in the outpatient capitated rate. During the third year of the demonstration project, the three community mental health providers were to be at-risk for both inpatient and outpatient benefits.

This phase-in of risk provided an incentive for the contractors to build their service system capacity. Major concerns regarding managed care for the public sector recipient are unmet need and inadequate service capacity. This plan provided an avenue under which the contractors could: (1) build traditional outpatient services with no financial liability, and (2) build non-traditional services from the inpatient savings.

(3) *Inclusion of Entire Medicaid Population*: The Utah project, unlike other Medicaid managed behavioral health care programs, included the high risk disabled population. The only exceptions were patients in the Utah State Hospital and children in state custody. Children in state custody who needed inpatient services were, however, a part of the capitation agreement. Two per-member per-month rates were established for each Medicaid eligibility category, one for inpatient and one for outpatient. Each rate was set to accommodate the unique risk projected for the different subgroups of the Medicaid population.

REQUIRED SKILLS

Our experience as a CMHC responsible for a capitated system suggests that certain skills are necessary to manage the risk and provide quality services. First and foremost is the development of a consistent clinical model. The model must be easy to articulate to the staff responsible for implementing it and congruent with the overall philosophy of community mental health. The basic philosophy of providing "least restrictive treatment in natural environments" has been the strength of community mental health programs for years. This philosophy is the one most necessary for managing a capitated system. Once the clinical model is established, the model must be communicated to the staff, recipients, advocacy groups, and payers. The second needed skill is the development of a training curriculum for the staff and community. The third skill is the development of the administrative capacity to monitor the outcome of services provided and the financial goals within which the program is to operate. A fourth needed skill is the development and maintenance of collaborative relationships with the payer and regulators.

CLINICAL PRACTICE MODEL

To assume the clinical, administrative, and fiscal responsibility, it was important to clearly define the Clinical Practice Model. Although there are similarities between managed mental health services in the private sector and the public sector, there are clear and significant differences to address in developing a Clinical Practice Model for the public sector recipient. One of these differences is the level of expected demand. For some Medicaid recipients their use is not episodic, but continuous. In addition, the Medicaid population is involved in a variety of other related social, health, and legal service agencies. To accommodate for heavy demand and the need to closely connect with multiple social service agencies, there are certain basic principles and methods of managed care required to be successful. The most critical ones are as follows:

(1) *Inclusive System of Integrated Services*: If the delivery system is to be cost-effective, of sound quality, and clinically efficient, there are a whole host of important wrap-around services that the recipient of public mental health services requires. They are diagrammed in Figure 1.

To treat a recipient of mental health services in the public sector effectively, attention must be paid to the full range of social service system supports. For example, supported housing is a critical component in the array of available services. Not only is housing critical

An Integrated Mental Health Service System

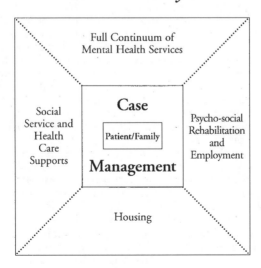

Figure 1

clinically, but also financially. All too often hospitals and residential treatment stays are prolonged for public patients simply because they do not have an acceptable place to reside. Since the beginning of the managed care program in Utah, the supported housing arrangements have been significantly expanded.

Housing needs are not unique to the adult population. Many children in the Medicaid program are in need of substitute family care. The mental health provider operating a public managed care system must plan for and have a network of therapeutic foster care or other residential options available. As VMH took on the clinical and financial risk of the public child and adolescent patient, it became clear that crisis foster home and long-term out-of-natural home placement options were critical.

Employment is also necessary for the public mental health recipient. The public managed care provider must ensure that there are opportunities for pre-job skill training, temporary employment placements for confidence-building, opportunities for job coaching, and supported employment placement options. It is not sufficient to refer clients to the Department of Vocational Rehabilitation or other employment programs. The mentally ill are often overlooked in these programs. Valley Mental Health's experience is that capacity for employment training and placement must be a part of the managed integrated system. Developing the employment training and placement capacity can be accomplished by reallocating dollars from the capitation rate.

The provider of managed care in the public system must ensure that services are integrated both horizontally across the traditional treatment continuum and vertically across the community support systems. Important connections must be maintained with primary health care and educational systems catering to the public recipient of services. Merely having referral procedures in place to social service, health, and vocational agencies is not enough. In a public managed care system, it is not a matter of creating a network of providers authorized to provide care but in creating a broad-based delivery system, that is coordinated and easily accessible. All elements of the service plan must be responsive to each other. Therefore, it is imperative that there is rapid and accurate communication across the service system. It is VMH's experience that to truly establish coordination and integration, many of these supportive non-traditional services must be directly managed and operated by the mental health provider.

(2) *Understand and Collaborate with Community Support Systems*: The Medicaid population has a significantly different social environment and level of disability than most other populations enrolled in managed care programs. They are frequently involved with a wide range of community services and social service agencies. It is imperative, therefore, that the managed care provider takes the time and allocates funds to coordinate liaison meetings to establish and maintain positive working relationships with these agencies. Treatment plan development must not occur in a vacuum, but result through collaboration with other important partners. Respectful collaboration is

the rule; these agencies must be seen as "sister" agencies to the mental health provider, not as subordinates, competitors, or opponents.

It is also imperative that efforts be made to enlist the support and involvement of the client's natural support systems. In contrast to traditional funding arrangements, in which the involvement of natural support systems tends to be more of an afterthought or is even discouraged, active development of strategies to strengthen the natural support systems, and thereby to reduce excessive reliance on professional supports, is a central component of risk-based PSMC.

(3) *Mobile Outreach*: To be effective, the public sector provider must provide mobile outreach for case finding and to engage clients when access to services would ordinarily not occur until a severe crisis has developed. Deployment of staff from the managed care provider to work in organizations and institutions with a high prevalence of Medicaid recipients can help to reduce more expensive service utilization through earlier intervention and enhanced service coordination.

As VMH attempted to provide services in these settings, other ways to provide services were discovered. For example, we increased staff time available in schools, correctional agencies, and welfare departments. We also reallocated dollars from the capitation payment to subcontract with the child welfare system to provide intensive in-home family preservation services for mental health clients. This subcontracted service is closely coordinated with our own in-home services: intensive case management, medication monitoring, and crisis outreach.

A number of positive things have been accomplished through this sub-contracting. It has significantly enhanced the relationship between mental health and child welfare, decreased the number of emergency referrals from the child welfare system for psychiatric hospitalization, and shortened the average length of stay for children in hospitals and acute residential services.

(4) *Up-Front Utilization Management*: One of the most important managed care principles is to meet the client's needs quickly. Therefore, mechanisms need to be available to ensure active and aggressive outreach to potential mental health users. The more pro-active the treatment, the less likely costly intensive services will be required. Public mental health recipients, particularly those with SPMI disorders, tend to be resistant to treatment interventions and non-compliant with medications. We found it essential, both from a clinical and a financial perspective, to have mobile intensive case management teams empowered to provide immediate and flexible interventions for these difficult-to-manage individuals.

(5) *Pre-Certification and Utilization Review*: In this model, pre-certification is required for care in intensive 24-hour programs. A separate and distinct unit of the provider organization has the responsibility to authorize these services. The pre-certification team is comprised of some of the most experienced nurses and physicians on the VMH staff. In order to make the level of care decisions, the team uses adult and child clinical practice guidelines, developed at Valley Mental Health.

When a request is received to place an adult in intensive services, the pre-certification team can give approval by telephone. If there is a request for a youth to go into an intensive placement, approval cannot be made until a face-to-face assessment is completed by a member of a specialized mobile children's team. For both adults and children, approval is for initial admission only because immediately upon admission, the reviewer begins to make community placement plans. Reviewers are in the treating facility within 24-hours after admission to meet with the client and staff to begin a 72-hour onsite review process.

Reviewers are more than brokers or approvers of service. Their mission is to be seen by the client and the client's family as advocates for proper care. Reviewers have the clinical authority to move clients from one level of care to another or to assign acute care case managers if needed to serve the client. Although reviewers have this authority, it is critical that they consult with the primary therapist in the decision making. If there is a clinical dispute between the reviewer and the primary therapist, that dispute is resolved by the VMH Medical Director.

At VMH it is not necessary to receive prior approval for entry into outpatient programs and other less intensive levels of care. This facilitates ease of access into less intensive services, which is critical for program success. If access is made too difficult, clients are more likely to decompensate, requiring more costly treatment or long-term hospitalizations.

(6) *Differential Levels of Care Management*: In traditional definitions of case management, the acronym C.A.L.M. (Coordinating, Advocating, Linking, and Monitoring) is often used. In a public sector managed care environment, much more is required. VMH's managed care model is a three-tier case management system. The first tier is provided for all clients by a primary service coordinator assigned at the time of enrollment. On this tier the C.A.L.M. functions are provided.

If the client requires more case management activities than the primary service coordinator can provide, a second tier of case management is available. This tier is called "acute care case management" (maximum 60 to 90 days) and can be requested by the primary service coordinator, intensive service staff, or the pre-certification team. The most highly trained case managers, housed in our outpatient units or with the pre-certification team, are assigned as service providers on this tier.

A third tier of case management is reserved for a clients who are more chronic and require continuous services, not merely episodic care. In this tier, case managers are more than brokers of service and provide more than the C.A.L.M. functions. The case managers are, in fact, in-home psycho-social rehabilitation practitioners. This role includes the direct provision of daily skill development services, including cognitive and behavioral-oriented interventions. The success of our PSMC program is in large part predicated on the third tier of case management being included in the service component.

(7) *Single Clinical Authority*: In a PSMC environment, there is a critical need to coordinate care across a vertically and horizontally

integrated service delivery system. Because of this, there must be a mechanism for resolving legitimate clinical differences. In a managed care environment, clinical disagreements are more likely to occur than in the traditional fee-for-service mode. This is because of the emphasis on nontraditional services, short-term and goal-oriented treatment, and increased demands for coordination with many social service, educational, vocational and health care agencies.

VMH places the responsibility for dispute resolution on our Medical Director, who is assisted by three senior management clinical staff, one for adult mental health services, one for children's mental health services, and one for the client support and wraparound services. These individuals have ultimate clinical authority and their decisions are binding on all treating parties.

(8) *Accessible Grievance System*: One of the primary impacts of managed care is that the recipient has a limited choice of providers. In a staff model of service delivery the degree of freedom of choice is even more restricted, therefore, it is important that clients feel they have legitimate avenues to express their concerns regarding the services they are receiving. At VMH there is a readily available grievance system where second opinions are encouraged and arranged at the expense of the managed care system.

ELEMENTS OF STAFF TRAINING

The mental health organization that is both a provider and manager must be efficient. Any duplication of effort or inconsistency of purpose is costly and can add to the financial strain in a capitated environment. Our experience suggests that the best way to guarantee efficiency is to allocate time and money for staff training. VMH spent considerable time repeatedly presenting the clinical practice model selected by the organization, the underlying philosophy supporting the model and specific examples of its implementation. VMH included its "sister" agencies in this training as well, in order to promote good will and to facilitate their efforts to provide a total treatment environment.

VMH believes the most important message to give to staff in the course of the training is the following: "Provide what the client needs, when the client needs it, and the finances will take care of themselves." This must not only be said but believed and acted upon by the administration. The goal is to create a flexible system of care that provides a full range of cost-effective service options so that clinicians can make utilization decisions based on clinical need without exceeding the financial limits of the capitation.

ADMINISTRATIVE AND DATA MANAGEMENT

In the past, attention to administrative controls, data collection and information management have too often been overlooked by public sector providers. However, in a risk-based capitated system, these functions are critical to success. One of the keys to a successful system is to use data to self-correct. At the beginning of the capitation experiment, VMH engaged staff, clients, advocates and Medicaid in a process to identify three critical areas for data collection: access, quality, and cost. This group of stakeholders determined key indicators for each area that would be consensually validated outcome measures for the project. These would be monitored and regularly reported to managers and staff.

PARTNERSHIPS WITH PAYER

If a provider assumes increased financial risk through managed care, it is necessary to work in partnership with the payer. The more the financial risk is shifted from payer to provider, the greater the need for agreement on objectives and outcomes. If the payer is only interested in cost containment, and not in quality service, there is not a basis for a true partnership. In the Utah model, VMH and the Medicaid agency formulated specific objectives that were to be accomplished by moving from fee-for-service to managed care. Those objectives included cost containment, flexibility in resource management, focused accountability, innovation and quality improvement in community-based care.

CHALLENGES

In any new venture, there are potential gains and losses. The experience at VMH in the managed care environment suggests an overall improved quality of care and increased efficiency. The penetration rate of services to the Medicaid enrollees has increased from below 10 percent to 18 percent. A system of care has been developed and client satisfaction has been maintained at high levels. All of this did not come without some very big challenges.

CLINICAL BARRIERS EXPERIENCED BY THE CMHC

At the beginning of the capitation experiment it was important for VMH to quickly identify what the potential clinical barriers to success would be in this new managed care environment. The following barriers were considered to be the most significant:

(1) *Passive System of Care*: As a traditional CMHC in a fee-for-service environment there was little effort at outreach to clients. If clients failed to keep their appointments, it was the client's problem, not ours. Waiting lists were common and lengths of stay in the more intensive services like residential treatment and day treatment were long. Many long-term clients were clearly dependent on the intensive treatment units for ongoing support.

(2) *Fragmentation and Duplication of Effort*: Prior to the capitation, each program element was a unit unto itself with little need to coordinate efforts on behalf of a client. In the fee-for-service system, pro-

grams tend to use increased services as a method to generate more dollars for the agency, sometimes in order to subsidize less revenue generating services, but also without the awareness of the need to maximize efficiency of resource utilization for the system as a whole.

(3) *Lack of a Systems Approach*: Prior to capitation, VMH had relationships with a number of other social and health care institutions in the community. However, these relationships, although cordial, could best be described as promoting coordination and sharing of general information on community health and social welfare issues, rather than facilitating collaboration regarding specific clients or programs. VMH needed to develop partnerships with multiple agencies as specific client treatment plans were formulated and implemented. Changing the nature of past interagency relationships took a great deal of effort and special attention.

(4) *Lack of Flexible Treatment Options*: VMH had developed a set of standard treatment interventions for its clients. Flexibility was not encouraged under a traditional fee-for-service system.

The process of dealing with the clinical barriers began months prior to the implementation of the capitation contract and remains an ongoing challenge. VMH had a number of staff retreats and planning meetings to identify what were considered our strengths and weaknesses if we were to survive in a managed care environment. Out of that process the basic clinical practice model and managed care principles identified in earlier sections of this chapter were developed. There followed an extensive process to analyze what the barriers were in our system that would prevent these principles from being implemented. Out of these discussions of barriers came the identification of needed changes. The entire process was summarized in writing and kept in front of staff and administration as decisions were made.

The clinical practice model and managed care principles were reinforced in every large gathering of the staff. The overriding belief was that consistency of approach was the most critical element in moving our system into a successfully managed care arena. A staff taskforce, through a quality improvement process, changed the medical record format used for assessments and initial treatment planning. The assessment was changed to become a managed care plan, which contained a number of very specific and time-limited goals that clients could achieve. At intake, the client and the primary service coordinator (therapist) rank the client on a five point scale, indicating the client's current status and anticipated outcome with regard to each of the goal statements. The document is then signed by the client and therapist and becomes the working treatment plan for the mental health intervention. At each scheduled review, goals are evaluated and rated as to any progress made. The advantage of these changes for VMH is that the assessment process itself began to reinforce very important managed care principles of time, specificity, practicality, and monitoring the impact on changed behavior.

If staff are to be empowered to provide more flexible treatment options, then those treatment options need to be available. With the support of funding agencies and the governing board, specific steps were taken up front to allocate dollars, energy, and staff resources to increase the number of flexible treatment options and supportive services within the agency.

ADMINISTRATIVE BARRIERS FACED BY THE CMHC

In the administrative and financial arena, there were four major challenges to face in converting from fee-for-service system to a managed care system.

(1) The negotiation and final determination of the capitated rate is crucial. Understanding how the state or county developed actuarial projections in setting rates is important, but more important is being able to correlate these projections with the perceived need in the community.

(2) Once the rate is determined, the mental health center as manager has to determine how much of the capitation payment will be allocated to inpatient services, outpatient services, treatment collaboration, other needed wrap-around services, and training.

(3) In a managed care system, the data monitored is characteristically different from what is monitored under fee-for-service. The quantity of direct service hours in outpatient services is important in a fee-for-service organization. However, in a capitated system, this data may be less important than data reflecting penetration rates, recidivism, lengths of stay, and actual services by Medicaid eligibility category. In addition, more emphasis must be placed on client and family satisfaction, as well as data that measures clinical outcome.

Another important challenge is to accurately predict Medicaid population growth and fluctuation by category and the likely utilization by service type for each category. Budgets are set based on these projections. Capacity must be developed to verify enrollments, and monitor actual revenues by eligibility category against expenditures.

A provider who intends to participate in the managed care environment not just as a provider, but also as a manager and financial risk-taker, must be willing to develop new data systems, budgeting methods, and actuarial expertise. This is an area that cannot be overlooked, because the financial risk is far too great. Fortunately, VMH had the governing board's commitment, and the financial ability, to make the long-term commitment to develop this capacity.

PUBLIC RELATIONS BARRIERS FACED BY THE CMHC

There were two significant issues that VMH faced from a public relations standpoint. The first was the broad expectation that since VMH was now capitated, we had to provide mental health services to everyone, regardless of need. Several social service agencies looked to us for assistance with any of their clients. It took a great deal of time and energy on the part of administrators and program managers in continuing discussions with these agencies to help clarify and define a more realistic expectation that we could provide agency consultation, but would limit services to specific clients, based on assessment results and prioritization of need.

A second problem was the concern expressed by VMH's staff, Board, and clients, that if savings were generated by our successful managing of the capitated Medicaid contract, the state and county payer might reduce their contribution of general fund mental health money. Although, this has not occurred, nevertheless, it is a worry that persists. Our success in not losing dollars is a result of our established partnerships with funding organizations and "sister" agencies. VMH staff have made conscientious efforts to keep these partners informed about the success of the capitated managed care system, the advantages of pooled funding, and the need to have collaborative treatment planning. The concept that managed care in the public sector benefits many, including: the client receiving services, the multiple public funding agents, other providers and the community as a whole, must be believed and communicated. In addition, savings have been put into building the support services infrastructure and in providing increased services to unfunded public clients.

For example, there were significant reductions in inpatient care for children and adolescents. As this occurred, savings were diverted to provide more residential treatment beds for seriously ill youth who had no health insurance. With these savings, more treatment staff were placed on site at high-risk schools.

Survival Tips

Care Management by Public Sector Provider Organizations

The basic philosophy of community-based treatment in the least restrictive settings is critical in managed care environments. CMHCs can effectively satisfy this philosophical mandate and provide quality PSMC services. To do so, they must attend to the following issues:

- **Keep up with private and public sector managed behavioral health care initiatives.**

- **Monitoring client outcomes is necessary.**

- **Public sector clinicians must become proficient in continuous case monitoring and utilization management.**

- **Attention must be paid to the financial strength of the manager/provider.**

- **Track utilization of all services for each subcategory of the enrolled population.**

- **The provider must have well-developed clinical utilization review criteria.**

- **The provider must have clearly stated and easily accessible processes for resolving clinical controversies.**

SURVIVAL TIPS AND RECOMMENDATIONS

Due to strong market forces and payer concerns in the private sector
and the governmental arena, a shakedown in the mental health industry is taking place. There will be a change in the landscape of providers of mental health services. The survivors and leaders in this
mental health revolution need to be innovators and risk-takers. In this
evolving environment, there is opportunity to provide improved
mental health care, and CMHCs can bring experience to this new
landscape. The basic philosophy of community-based treatment in
the least restrictive settings is critical in managed care environments.
Who better than CMHCs can demonstrate this philosophy through
the work they have been doing for years?

The most important lesson is that it is possible and profitable
for a CMHC to independently administer and clinically operate a
capitated risk-based PSMC system. If the principles detailed in this
chapter are implemented, the potential for success increases. To survive and thrive under managed care systems, CMHCs and other
public mental health providers need to adhere to the following
"readiness criteria":

1. Keep up with private and public sector managed behavioral health
   care initiatives. The traditional CMHC needs to adopt an aggressive "market-oriented" approach, but one that is geared to the entire community. The provider must consistently assess the needs
   of clients, families, payers, and referral sources and address those
   needs with flexible and innovative treatment programs and with
   creative interagency collaborations.

2. Monitoring client outcomes is necessary. Key indicators of
   performance must be measurable and meaningful to the four
   stakeholders (client, family, payer, and referral source). It is not
   enough to track inputs, outputs or encounters, but to measure the
   actual impact of service. In a continuous quality improvement
   model, data from key indicators are fed back into the provider's
   integrated service delivery system so that the system becomes
   continuously self-correcting.

3. Public sector clinicians must become proficient in continuous case
   monitoring and utilization management. This monitoring function helps to ensure that the assessment of client needs is accurate, that services are provided when they are needed, and that
   the desired impact is achieved.

4. In risk-based managed care programs, attention must be paid
   to the financial strength of the manager/provider. If financial
   strength is lacking, staff and management may become overly
   concerned with financial risk in such a way as to negatively affect
   treatment decisions. To engage in PSMC without financial
   strength is a disservice to clients and increases the likelihood of
   failure. A financially strong organization can sustain a risk and
   be more willing to allow innovative program development. The
   message presented to the clinicians is: "If you give clients what

they need, when they need it, you do not have to worry about the organization being financially stable. If you begin to worry or make your decisions solely because of finances, then clients will not receive appropriate care." Inappropriate care results in the poor clinical outcomes which, in turn, lowers quality and increases long-term costs.

5. Under PSMC, it is important to track utilization of all services for each subcategory of the enrolled population. The data system must have the capacity to track actual use against standards that were previously set for each client subgroup.

6. The provider must have well-developed clinical utilization review criteria, that are understood and accepted throughout the system, and must assure that initial assessments and ongoing care management are based on these clearly established criteria.

7. The provider must have clearly stated and easily accessible processes for resolving clinical controversies. Clinicians must be aware of the standards used to judge their performance and the process to resolve clinical disagreements.

CONCLUSION

Capitated PSMC programs are developing in various forms across the country. Mental health providers need to be aware of these developments. They must recognize that these programs provide hope for public sector providers. Public dollars need to be used efficiently and managed care has potential for increased cost-efficiency. If done correctly, a Medicaid mental health program managed by a public sector provider will not only be cost-effective, but can provide an opportunity for financial stability for CMHCs and other public sector providers. The more important outcome will be the improved quality of care for public sector recipients brought about by the creation of integrated mental health service delivery systems.

8

Capitated Care Management by Community Psychiatrists: LA County

JACK BARBOUR, RETA FLOYD, and LINDA CONNERY

BACKGROUND

Several states and other governmental entities have decided that capitation may be the most desirable method of providing managed mental health care for persons with SPMI. Capitation has been described as the best payment mechanism since it includes "an increase in service flexibility, particularly in outpatient services; new configurations of services that are broader, better coordinated and less redundant and reduced financial barriers that make earlier intervention possible. A system that integrates services under a single agency and provides patients with a case manager to guide them through the system could ensure more appropriate and cost-effective care. Capitation funding is believed to produce incentives to intervene early in acute episodes of chronic illness to alleviate more serious consequences" (Rothbard, Hadley, Schinnar, Morton, & Whitehill, 1989).

In the past five years, Los Angeles (LA) County has begun to experiment with capitated payment approaches to fund services for selected individuals with SPMI. For a variety of political, economic, and social policy reasons, historically LA County has had no coherent system of treating the mentally ill, especially the adult population with SPMI. Instead, a fragmented system has evolved, which has inadvertently encouraged discontinuity in care and expensive over-utilization of emergency and in-patient services. This configuration has been described as a "system in shambles" (Weisburd, 1988). The president of the local Alliance for the Mentally Ill (AMI) referred to the system as being "crazier" than the individuals it purports to serve. In response to pressure from AMI and other advocacy groups, legislation was passed (Wright, Bronzan, & McCorquodale, 1988) which enabled the state Department of Mental Health to fund two pilot capitated Integrated Services Agencies (ISAs). The goal was to demonstrate that one agency having financial and clinical responsibility for coordinating integrated services for persons with SPMI could be cost effective and could improve quality.

As a result of the success of the two pilot ISAs, the Director of the LA County Department of Mental Health (DMH) issued a Request for Proposals (RFP) in early 1991, with the goal of funding four to six additional ISAs to serve specific geographic areas of this large, diverse county. DMH preferred to develop these new capitation programs rather than to develop clubhouses and case management programs utilizing existing payment mechanisms (i.e., cost reimbursement, fee-for-service), because of the success of earlier state-funded ISAs and capitation experiences in other parts of the country. Los Angeles offered the opportunity to test capitation in a major urban center. These capitated ISAs were to be based on the following principles: integrated and coordinated services, client-driven services, client empowerment, continuity of care in and out of the hospital, and cultural relevancy. Barbour and Floyd Medical Associates, a partnership formed by two African American community psychiatrists, who had long been working in the community with long-term state hospital patients, came into being in response to the RFP.

COMMUNITY PSYCHIATRISTS AS CARE MANAGERS

As two community psychiatrists who had worked in a CMHC in South Central LA, we had become acutely aware of the need for an improved method of delivering services to patients with SPMI. Our in-patient experience made us familiar with the revolving door phenomenon: clients who regularly cycled through the hospital as a result of not using the out-patient services offered to them at the point of discharge. We had also had experience providing services and consultation to community-based agencies that had a rehabilitation focus, that provided case management, and that were involved in all aspects of their clients' lives. We were impressed with the reduced need for hospitalization that resulted from the use of these services.

As a result of this experience, we had met with the DMH Medical Director in 1991 with our own proposal (independent from the RFP) to develop a program that would move patients from the state hospital to the community, where they would be provided with intensive services. Our intent was that these services would be comprehensive, addressing all of the client's needs and providing a seamless system of care. While DMH expressed some interest in this proposal they were not willing to commit to such a project at that time. However, this set the stage for us to develop the concept that we, ourselves, could provide a single point of responsibility and a community model of treatment, utilizing a flat fee payment schedule. It was obvious to us that a single agency with central responsibility for a finite number of high service utilizers could "manage" care more effectively and efficiently than the existing agencies.

By the time the RFP was released, we had resigned as Medical Directors of the CMHC in-patient service and were working in community-based clubhouse and case management programs, one of which was located in South Central LA. South Central LA is an area historically lacking in mental health and social service resources. The clients of this ISA have suffered not only from the devastating impact of mental illness on them and their families, but also from poverty, substandard housing, uncaring educational institutions, crime, drugs, police harassment and brutality, and all the other corollaries of racism and minority status. We found ourselves in an excellent position to submit a competitive proposal to develop the South Central ISA.

There were two major reasons for this. First, the limited services already in South Central (a comprehensive CMHC and two out-patient clinics) were traditional county-operated facilities and were excluded from competing for the RFP.

Second, our experiences in community settings and our lack of bureaucratic baggage positioned us to better respond to the RFP than many of the large independent CMHCs and other mental health agencies. We didn't have to contend with the problem of incorporating a managed care model within the structure of other payment approaches.

Thus, although we were competing against the large CMHCs and other mental health entities in the county, we (Barbour & Floyd) were awarded a capitated contract to serve 50 high utilizers of mental health services in South Central LA. Once funded, we immediately became immersed in the business of starting an agency. We decided to incorporate as a for-profit partnership (to take on a non-profit contract) for the sake of expediency and to keep our future options open. We later established a non-profit entity which would provide us with more opportunities for growth.

Due to our previous management roles, as inpatient Medical Directors, which required autonomy and accountability, we moved naturally into our roles as Co-Directors of the new ISA. We came with awareness of the need for policies and procedures, accounting practices, personnel management, program development, quality improvement, a team approach, and the need to provide leadership.

Starting a new agency entailed locating and leasing a site, obtaining all the necessary equipment and supplies, and hiring and training staff. We developed a line item budget to cover these expenses. One necessary decision was how we would pay ourselves. We decided to view ourselves as salaried employees of this newly formed entity; therefore, we determined our salaries based on the resources available to us. Since we had worked within the local mental health community, we were able to hire most of our clinical staff based on our prior relationships with them. We hired staff who, first, had expertise in areas such as case management and psychosocial rehabilitation and, second, had enthusiasm for the project, since they had to "hit the ground running" in order to enroll the 50 clients assigned to this ISA.

CLIENT REIMBURSEMENT

Our new agency requested, and was awarded, 50 clients, also referred to as "slots," at a capitation rate of approximately $16,000. We received a quarterly "slot dollar" advance for program start-up, which has continued to be the major payment mechanism. The other source of revenue is through billing for services, especially Medi-Cal reimbursable services, wherein the county slot dollar money is used as the required county match in the Medi-Cal formula.

Medi-Cal is the California version of Medicaid. Private Medi-Cal (or fee-for-service) is utilized by private and general hospitals, physicians, psychologists, and clinics, billing the Medicaid program directly. Public Medi-Cal is administered through the County and State Departments of Mental Health and requires a county match of 50%. For the ISAs, county general fund slot dollars are utilized for the match. If the client does not have Medi-Cal, the full cost of services provided by the ISA is billed against the county dollars. This provides an incentive for ensuring that all clients who are eligible get enrolled in Medi-Cal, since the Medi-Cal billing saves county (and ISA) funds.

Medicare and other insurance carriers can also be billed for the services they cover, but, in most cases, they have limited mental health benefits and don't cover the services which these high utilizers require. Most of the clients do not have other coverage, so these are very minor revenue sources. Therefore, there is an incentive to provide as many services as possible and to provide them directly rather than to pay for clients to receive services from another source. When services are purchased from outside sources, the ISA is obligated to pay the rates established by DMH or a rate negotiated with the provider.

There are two payment mechanisms for purchased services. All county-operated or DMH contract agencies bill for the services that have been approved by the ISA through the DMH Management Information System (MIS) as is done with any other client. DMH pays the agencies directly and the ISA then reimburses DMH. When services are purchased from a vendor who does not receive funding from the DMH for services rendered, the ISA makes direct payment to that facility.

It therefore made sense for our new ISA to become Medi-Cal certified to provide a range of services (e.g., crisis intervention, case management, outpatient treatment, medication management, alcohol and drug rehabilitation, and psychosocial rehabilitation day services). The agency therefore rapidly developed its infrastructure of programmatic and administrative policies and procedures, job descriptions, personnel policies, and all other requirements for Medi-Cal certification. Once this certification was obtained, the agency was positioned to maximize its contract through the combination of county general funds and Medi-Cal reimbursements.

Services are purchased from the outside only under specific circumstances, such as when a client has been seeing a psychiatrist in another facility for an extended period of time or if the client has a positive transference and insists on continuing with the psychiatrist. In regard to the purchase of outside services, an individualized services planning process comes into play. Both the ISA staff and the client must agree, as partners, on which ISA services will be utilized and what services need to be obtained from another provider. These critical issues relate directly to clinical care, encompassing such concerns as quality of care and ethical treatment, and are not made lightly. The ISA team members must agree, and then must hold clinical meetings with the prospective provider to clarify the ISA's authorization and contract for specific expectations of services purchased. This calls for creativity on the part of the ISA staff to utilize the latitude of the capitation to develop quality service plans that are also cost-effective. Thus, in the example of a client wishing to continue with the current psychiatrist, a contract would be established which covers the frequency and duration of visits and the duration of the reimbursement agreement. Such services are closely monitored, with the case manager maintaining frequent contact with both the physician and the client. One of the goals jointly established by the provider and the ISA would be to wean the client over a reasonable period of time without jeopardizing quality care.

Since the ISA does not provide residential services directly, staff work closely with board and care facilities to ensure continuity of care and a positive living arrangement for the individual. The ISA does not have financial responsibility for this residential arrangement, which is paid for by the client's SSI. When a client requires a higher level of residential care but does not meet the criteria for hospitalization, a residential bed in a 24-hour crisis program or in a locked facility is purchased by the ISA.

CLIENT SELECTION AND ENROLLMENT

Clients in the ISA are assigned by DMH based on their cost to the public mental health system over a five-year period. A pool of high utilizers was developed using historical cost data, starting with the highest cost bands, ranging from $30,000 to $80,000 in annual costs. Using identification information and episode information from the county MIS, ISA staff attempted to locate individuals, assess their appropriateness for the program, and to "sell" the program to them.

The most frequent reasons for non-enrollment or disenrollment were a) the inability to locate the assigned client and b) lack of discharge readiness from a state hospital. Disenrollment of a potential client required approval by DMH staff, who could request that the ISA make further attempts to find the individual or to reassess a hospitalized client. If the disenrollment was accepted, DMH assigned a new client to the ISA.

Another reason for disenrollment was client refusal to sign consent to be enrolled in the program. These individuals were pursued vigorously, with mixed results. It was particularly difficult if the individual was involved with another provider who did not want to release the client. Enrolled clients are assumed to be enrolled for the length of the project, if not indefinitely. However, clients can terminate if they refuse the services of the ISA and continue to receive treatment elsewhere or to go without treatment. Intensive casefinding, persuasion, and perseverance are required of case managers in such situations. Ultimately, the client has freedom of choice and can terminate with the ISA without jeopardizing access to other publicly funded services.

THE DEVELOPMENT OF APPROPRIATE SERVICES UNDER CAPITATION

Determining the scope of services to be covered by capitation and establishing realistic capitation rates are important issues to address in negotiating contracts. Persons with SPMI may receive a wide array of services from a variety of social service agencies with many funding streams. In fully capitated systems, all of these funding streams are combined and a capitation rate is established which allows a single point of responsibility to have the resources to coordinate most aspects of services (See chapter by Oss and Mackie). Capitation in LA, however, is mainly limited to mental health services, although financial arrangements can be made to ensure that a client has food, shelter, and clothing.

As a new entity, we have been able to flexibly adapt to the needs of public sector clients, as we had no existing infrastructure or rigid clinical protocols to impede our ability to respond to the new model of service delivery and the changes in the Medi-Cal program. We were able to develop services which were relevant to our population: both culturally sensitive and client-driven. We began by providing services based on the experiences of other programs such as the PACT program in Madison, Wisconsin (Stein & Test, 1985) and Bridges in Chicago (Witcherich & Dincin, 1985). We assumed that intensive case management had to be the primary mode of service, and that home visits and the provision of services in the community were essential in working effectively with our target population.

In negotiating a capitated rate contract, it is important to have language that allows for flexibility regarding the services to be provided. It is essential to avoid being locked into a contract which specifies the amounts of service to be delivered. Flexibility is necessary in developing services that are client-driven rather than in offering clients a predetermined mix of services. The cost of hospitalization must be addressed, because even the most effective interventions cannot prevent the need for this level of care. It has been our experience that a small number of clients will continue to be high utilizers of inpatient facilities, usually as a result of medication noncompliance or drug use. These treatment-resistant individuals can consume the budget of a program if hospital costs are a part of the capitation rate. Some of these costs have been defrayed in this particular ISA by utilizing hospitals which accept fee-for-service Medi-Cal, which, as noted earlier, is not currently billed against the capitation rate. When the private and public Medi-Cal programs are totally consolidated for in-patient services, some method of shared risk between the ISA and the county will have to be negotiated.

It has been our experience that the most effective way to provide coordinated, integrated services within a seamless system is to provide most services directly through the ISA, since the capitated rate is supported through the county general funds and matching federal dollars. Thus, the provision of medication, case management, and psychosocial rehabilitation (out-patient) services was initiated immediately by the ISA.

We originally provided group mental health rehabilitation services at our main clinical site. However, the clients expressed a need to have a place to come on a daily basis which would provide a structured setting and offer support in maintaining community functioning and residential stability. We responded by instituting a day rehabilitation program. Capitation provided us with the flexibility to do this, to respond to the needs of the population, and to add another Medi-Cal reimbursable service to our service mix. Additional benefits to the ISA of providing services directly are the increased ability to coordinate and integrate services, the ease of managing and determining the maximal service configuration for each client, and the opportunity to maximize the involvement of the client and significant others in service planning.

Capitation allows for the development of clinical protocols which are appropriate and relevant to the clients of the ISA. The development of the day rehabilitation program is an example of this. Client-driven services, a major ISA philosophical tenet, is a key to the development of the most effective and least costly clinical protocols. For example, using flexible capitation dollars, we have been able to obtain subsidized housing for some of our clients and have provided independent skills training for them on-site in their apartments, teaching clients how to do money management, household chores, food shopping, menu planning, and cooking.

COMMUNITY INVOLVEMENT

We became involved in the Service Area Advisory Committee as soon as the RFP process began. Community involvement at the grass roots level was imperative to educate the advisory committee about the significance of the ISA as a new community-based delivery, which needed the backing of this community body to ensure that at least one of the ISAs would be located in South Central. Visibility and commitment to improving the area's mental health resources were essential to developing community support for the proposal.

Another avenue for community involvement early in the process was the establishment of a community advisory board for ISA. An advisory board was formed which consisted of the major stakeholders in this new service delivery system: service providers, citizens, consumers, and family members.

INTERNAL TRACKING SYSTEM

The development of an effective client data base has provided the ISA with the capability to generate reports that target management issues, to format information requested by funding source(s), and to capture information relevant for program evaluation and research. The ISA is integrated into the DMH MIS. The MIS is utilized for billing services directly provided by the ISA. It also provides an episode screen. Anyone who accesses that screen can determine all the open episodes for a client who is receiving mental health services in a county funded program. The screen identifies whether the client is enrolled in a managed care ISA and that the clinician must contact the ISA program service coordinator prior to initiating any services. This protects the ISA from being held accountable for unauthorized services provided by other entities.

The internal tracking system is also utilized to run monthly reports of per client costs, which is essential in a capitated program. Management must have timely and accurate information regarding the cost of services directly provided as well as any services purchased from other providers in order to contain costs.

OUTCOMES

In spite of the fact that the ISAs have operated in an environment which has not been user friendly and which has presented problems in tracking costs and coordinating services, the ISAs have had significant and sometimes controversial impact. As pilot programs, they have had to prove that they are cost effective and that they improve the quality of life of the clients they serve. They have come under criticism for aggressive outreach done to enroll clients and for the practice of directly providing services rather than purchasing services when a client has been involved with another agency. Unquestionably, the advent of the ISAs has shaken the system and has imposed itself upon an existing system, which many county and agency staffs had a vested interest in perpetuating. The imposition of the ISAs has increased accountability, the need to justify services provided and the need for culturally competent services.

We have seen dramatic results in our own ISA, by reversing the service utilization patterns from expensive in-patient and emergency services to intensive case management, medication support services, day rehabilitation services, and other out-patient services. *During the first 18 months of operation, in-patient days were decreased by 90% and emergency room visits were reduced by 75%.* Intensive case management services were increased by 95%. Medication support services were increased by 60% and day rehabilitation service were increased by 25% during this same 18 month period.

Survival Tips

Capitated Care Management by Community Psychiatrists

Community psychiatrists (or other providers) can be successful in forming an MCO to provide capitated PSMC services. Locally based capitated ISAs can be effective in improving services to urban clients with SPMI. Successful survival is embodied in the following working principles:

- **Staff investment**
- **Outreach and mobility**
- **Expansion of psychiatric roles**
- **Rehabilitation-oriented programming**
- **Consumer empowerment**
- **Consumer responsiveness**
- **Intensive case management**
- **Cultural relevance**

SURVIVAL TIPS

One of the major points of this chapter is that individual community psychiatrists (or other providers) can be successful in forming an MCO to provide capitated PSMC services. The second major point is that locally based capitated ISAs can be an effective PSMC mechanism for improving services to urban clients with SPMI. Successful survival is embodied in the following working principles:

- **Staff Investment.** This is a grass roots agency that began with the ISA contract. Staff did not bring a lot of "baggage" as to how services "should" be delivered. They had to be creative and innovative in their approaches to incorporate both a managed care philosophy and a strict adherence to quality of life issues. The environment created by the start of a new agency, the use of innovative approaches, and the relationships that exist throughout the agency engender a sense of mutual excitement and hope. Clients and staff are invested in having a successful program and this enhances the growth we see in clients and that they see in themselves.

- **Outreach and Mobility.** Taking services to clients wherever they are in the community, either in the form of home visits or in working with them in the street, has been a major mode of service. All staff, including psychiatrists, make home visits and will even give medication injections, if needed, to clients in the street. Teaching life skills in clients' residential settings has resulted in "in vivo" learning, since they often have difficulty transferring skills from artificial settings.

- **Expansion of psychiatric roles.** In a psychosocial setting, the psychiatrist performs psychosocial assessments, provides medication education and includes the client in the decision-making regarding medications. The psychiatrist works in conjunction with other team members, requires knowledge of community and ethnic/cultural issues, has an all encompassing role which includes case management and social work. Psychiatric interventions take place in natural environments such as the client's residence or in the street. The scope of practice includes money management, skills training, and other psychosocial rehabilitation interventions. This change in the role of the psychiatrist is parallel to the concept of the family physician, in which the individual is followed by one physician, both in the community and in the hospital. The change in the relationship between physician and client results in a decreased focus on disability with an emphasis on productive activity. Instead of talking about disease, conversations between psychiatrist and client are more often about abilities.

- **Rehabilitation-oriented Programming.** The day rehabilitation program provides an environment in which clients feel wanted, needed, and expected, resulting in a bonding process that provides maximum opportunities for symptom stabilization and for rehabilitation. Since all jobs are essential to the smooth operation of the program, clients become contributors rather than recipients of services. This productive activity has the impact of increasing their sense of self-worth and self-esteem.

- **Consumer Empowerment.** The concepts of client-driven services, client empowerment, blurring of staff roles, and a focus on the healthy, functional part of the individual rather than on the illness are all necessary ingredients to successful community integration and rehabilitation.

- **Consumer Responsiveness.** Designing services to meet the needs identified by the clients rather than designing services based on staff preferences ensures client involvement and service relevancy. An example of this is the day rehabilitation program. Based on the expressed need for this more intensive level of care, we developed the day program and have been overwhelmed by the popular response to these services.

- **Intensive Case Management.** Case management services are the "glue" which connects all the elements of the services provided. This results in a coordinated, integrated approach to clients which they have not experienced before. Having all of their mental health needs met by one agency provides them with stability and consistency. "Wrap-around" services prevent clients from getting lost as easily as in more fragmented systems.

- **Cultural Relevance.** Culturally relevant services are essential to making this program a success. It has been important to hire staff from the community of the population being served. Traditions, behaviors appropriate to specific minority groups, belief systems, historical factors, and the relationship between minorities and the dominant society are intertwined into all aspects of program planning and implementation. For example, in the African American community, mentally ill family members are more likely to be living with their families, reflecting a cultural belief in the extended family and in caring for family members unable to live independently. This is integrated into the program by use of home visits which include the client and the family, frequent case management contact with the family, and a high representation of families on the Advisory Council of the ISA. Clients are aware that this is an agency which understands and respects their ethnic and cultural values as well as their psychosocial needs.

REFERENCES

Rothbard, A.B., Hadley, T.R., Schinnar, A.P., Morton, D., & Whitehill, B. (1989). Philadelphia's capitation plan for mental health services. *Hospital and Community Psychiatry, 40*(4), 356.

Stein, L.I., & Test, M.A. (1985). The training in the community living model: a decade of experience. In the New Directions for Mental Health Services series, San Francisco: Jossey Bass.

Weisburd, D. (1986). *A System in Shambles.* Documentary film about the LA Country Mental Health System.

Witcherich, T., & Dincin, J. (1985). The assertive community treatment worker: an emerging role and its implications for professional training. *Hospital and Community Psychiatry, 40*(6), 620–624.

Wright, C., Bronzan, B., & McCorquodale (1988). *The Mental Health Act of 1988.* California Legislation AB3777.

9

Care Management by Public Payers: The VA System

LAURENT LEHMANN

Managed care is not the exclusive province of private MCOs or provider agencies. The Department of Veterans' Affairs (VA) has had decades of experience with managing comprehensive mental health care under a fixed budget. This chapter will describe the ongoing evolution of managed care in VA, offering ideas that may be useful for public mental health care providers and payers.

VA'S MENTAL HEALTH SERVICES

Veterans with serious mental illness constitute a significant portion of the patients served by VA and they are a significant portion of the seriously mentally ill in the nation. Data derived from the 1989 National Health Interview Survey indicate that 405,000–630,000 veterans are accounted to be seriously mentally ill: 14 percent of the total adult seriously mentally ill population in the nation (Rosenheck, 1995). Veterans with mental disorders represent 26.5 percent of all veterans eligible for VA care. While only 10 percent of all veterans use VA health care services annually, 40 percent of seriously mentally ill veterans use VA care.

As with most public mental health systems, VA has a legacy of a core of bed-based inpatient programs, but since the 1960s there have been innovative outpatient programs designed to prevent hospitalization and maintain chronically ill patients in the community. The most recent evolution of these programs is the proliferation of community based communal living programs, with a focus on compensated work therapy, an idea reminiscent of the Fairweather Houses that have served as a model for several of these programs. (Rosenheck, Neale, Milstein, & Frisman, 1995; Friedman, West, & Clark, 1987).

The goal of these VA mental health programs is to provide continuity of care and comprehensive care to the veterans who seek our services, matching the severity and complexity of patients' needs with the type and intensity of services that can best meet these needs. VA's Mental Health and Behavioral Sciences Service incorporates substance abuse services. Comprehensive care includes medical, surgical and dental care as well as mental health services. VA mental health services are not "carved out" from medical services, but rather are integrated with them under a single medical care budget. In addition, VA can provide social and economic supports through VA pensions and other benefits which are available for certain veterans.

VA's budget comes from Congressional appropriations which are planned on a yearly basis: mental health gets $2 billion of the $12 billion VA medical care budget (FY 1994 data). The amount is determined by workload estimates based on the resource allocation methodology existing at the time (see below). Mental health has, at times also been supported by Congressional "add ons" to the budget for specific issues such as the Homeless Chronically Mentally ill (HCMI) and Post-traumatic Stress Disorder (PTSD). These are areas where VA has developed significant and, in the case of PTSD related to military service, unique, expertise. These programs would probably never have occurred if not specially funded by Congress, which was stimulated to action based on reports of VA and non-VA sources of unmet needs. (Kulka, 1988).

VA has, for most of its history, not operated as a managed care organization in the sense that managed care is understood today. Managed care usually implies a health care plan with a fixed population of enrollees, with a fixed set of clinical services available to them, supported by a fixed funding pool (e.g. from premiums paid by enrollees). Often there are utilization controls that direct care towards the least expensive (usually ambulatory) care settings, with the consequence of little or no reimbursement for care outside the boundaries of utilization review criteria.

VA differs from this situation in several ways. The Department of Veterans Affairs provides a range of benefits and services beyond health care for those eligible to receive them. A person who is "service connected" for an injury or disease incurred while on active military duty is not only entitled to medical care, but also receives a pension based on the degree of occupational impairment (as determined by Veterans Benefits Administration [VBA]). Veterans may also be eligible for a variety of other social and economic benefits including assistance with housing and education, support for spouses and children, and even burial expenses.

In terms of health care, VA has been and remains, a "point of service" provider. VA's medical care budget has not been based on a pool of enrollees, some of whom may not require care in a given year, but rather on active users of clinical services, many of whom have severe and multiple disorders, associated with high costs. Before the 1980s, Congressional appropriations covered not only the costs of services as projected, but usually could be counted on to provide end of year supplements to cover cost overruns. There were no clearly identified incentives to cost control, and for the field, keeping a high inpatient average daily census was seen as a good thing.

Access to services was controlled by two elements: clinical judgment and eligibility for care. VA's primary means of identifying its target population is done through eligibility criteria, based primarily on whether a disorder is adjudicated as Service Connected. (Department of Veterans Affairs, 1995). Service connection implies that a disorder was incurred during, or is related to, military service. A disorder may be claimed to be related to military service if it is identified within one year of discharge from active duty. There are a few exceptions to this, one being PTSD which, due to its delayed and recurrent nature, may be Service Connected any number of years after military duty, provided it can be demonstrated that the PTSD symptoms are related to military service (e.g., intrusive recollections of combat). Essentially, a person 100 percent Service Connected is eligible for any and all medical care, inpatient or outpatient; whether related to the Service Connected disability or not, free of charge.

The other criterion for eligibility for VA care is indigence, which is measured by a "means test" (Paralyzed Veterans of America, 1992). In theory, individuals who meet the criteria of service connection or indigence, are eligible for VA care ("mandatory workload"), but there are many variations in practice. Any veteran can get inpatient care provided there is urgent need, but eligibility for outpatient services varies according to regulations based on Federal law. Veterans who are Non-Service Connected and do not meet means test criteria, can only be seen in outpatient care for one year after inpatient discharge, unless it can be documented that outpatient care is preventing rehospitalization: a restriction similar to that experienced by other public sector providers. There are even variations in the kinds of outpatient care Service Connected veterans can receive, based on their degree of Service Connection. The complexities of eligibility promote confusion and discontinuity of care for chronically ill patients. Eligibility reform is a major goal of VA as it tries to reshape itself into a comprehensive primary care provider.

INTRODUCTION OF MANAGED CARE REFORMS

In the 1980s came the increasing perception of national financial crisis and the imperative to control health care costs by improving the management and control of clinical services. The first attempt at this in

VA was the DRG-based Resource Allocation Methodology (RAM) which was operational between 1985 and 1990. Under RAM, facilities competed with each other for a fixed resource pool, as end of year special appropriations dwindled and ultimately disappeared. While lengths of inpatient stay decreased under RAM, medical centers had incentives to provide more services, often extending themselves beyond their resources. This caused budget crises at a number of facilities and concerns about quality of care as limited resources were stretched to an expanding population in need of services.

In late 1990, RAM was replaced by a new system, called Resource Planning and Management (RPM), a prospective, capitation based system designed to better allocate resources based on current and projected workload (Department of Veterans Affairs [VA], 1994a). RPM was designed to estimate future resource needs using risk-adjusted capitation rates to assist in allocation of resources through a negotiation process involving expected number of patients, their case mix and expected costs per patient. RPM has had its problems too. RPM relates its costs to patients through an estimation system called the Cost Distribution Report, rather than through actual patient billing. Also under RPM there has still been a tendency to underreport outpatient costs and overreport inpatient costs, due at least in part to the relatively greater accuracy of the inpatient data gathering system.

In summary, both RAM and RPM have resulted in shortened lengths of inpatient stay in all clinical services, because of relative resource losses for patients retained beyond the DRG "break even" point, but neither system has specifically promoted ambulatory care development. In addition, the fiscal advantages of shorter lengths of stay have caused some facilities that previously provided intermediate or long term psychiatric care (60–90 days or longer) to resist this role, resulting in a "revolving door" effect for some chronic patients which has been noted in other public systems that have experienced similar budgetary constraints.

Under both RAM and RPM, VA facilities were organized into groups that reflected similar range of services and so, presumably, of costs. RPM has also had a problem with "outliers": those facilities whose costs lie above or below the average for their group, particularly for Medical Care Group 8 (MCG 8) which is composed of those 20-odd facilities which provide long term psychiatric care. The reasons for this difficulty are not entirely clear, but the implication is that MCG 8 is not as uniform a grouping as the others. RPM also suffers from being a facility-based resource allocation system, rather than one that is tied directly to actual patient costs. As VA moves more closely towards a "true capitation" system, costs will be more patient-based. This will be facilitated by new data collection systems involving patient encounter forms that will document all inpatient and outpatient clinician contacts. This should also promote incentives towards ambulatory services through improved accounting of these services.

With limitations on the medical care budget, there have been changes in regulations that allow some local initiatives in developing additional funding streams. Chief among these is the promotion of sharing agreements with other public providers, particularly the

Department of Defense, to deliver care to active duty personnel if the workload of eligible veterans allows. There remains, however, a significant limitation on the populations VA can target for sharing agreements, particularly if these should involve services to non-veterans. Another fiscal innovation is the ability to charge veterans for services for which they are not eligible by virtue of Service Connection or indigence. Fees for services and co-payments, which are modest by private sector standards, are collected by a system called Medical Care Cost Recovery (MCCR). In the most recent year for which information is available (FY 1993), MCCR collected $506.5 million (VA, 1994b). What is problematic about this for VA, from a business perspective, is that VA can retain only enough funds to cover its expenses in collections: all other "profits" are turned over to the U.S. Treasury. While these recovered funds contribute to the resource pool of the Federal government, and may be perceived as contributing to funding VA as a whole, it deprives individual VA facilities of a direct incentive for generating more "paying" workload. This is another parallel to non-VA public mental health systems (e.g., Massachusetts) in which revenue savings are sometimes diverted to other jurisdictions.

Plans for moving VA toward a more traditional managed care system include more effective definition of a population of enrollees, not limited to service users. This would broaden the covered population to include more "low risk" patients, hopefully providing more resources for those who need more costly services. While eligibility reform is focused on veterans, it is possible that in the future, coverage might be expanded to include some non-veteran groups, such as veterans' immediate family members or purchasers of specialized services such as mental health or spinal cord injury. Along with these changes, there will be attempts to change existing legislation to allow VA facilities to keep at least some portion of MCCR funds beyond recovery expenses. These funds could be used to improve or expand existing services.

VA MANAGED CARE IN TRANSITION

Entering the 1990s, VA engaged in various forms of self examination to determine how it could improve the efficiency and quality of its clinical services in an era of diminishing resources. There were indications of the directions in which VA mental health wanted to go, including more ambulatory care; more rehabilitation in intermediate and long term care units to promote successful discharge of chronic inpatients and maintain them in the community; and more community based residential care. VA had significant participation in the 1993 White House Health Care Reform Task Force and in 1994, VA developed its own Health Care Reform Task Force, again with the participation of mental health clinicians. Among the goals of this activity was to develop plans for benefits packages in particular areas of VA expertise, including mental health, geriatrics and extended medical care and rehabilitation, as well as ideas about how to better provide and manage the delivery of care (VA, 1994c). It is apparent at this writing that Health Care Reform as envisioned in the Clinton Health Care Plan (H.R. 3600) is "dead" but it is equally clear that Health Care Reform as a concept is vigorously and dynamically alive and VA is reorganizing itself just as the rest of American health care is doing, to ensure its success and survival.

Themes of flexibility and local initiative are at the heart of much of VA's reorganization effort. There will be greater VA participation with the non-VA health care community with the goals of enhancing access to care and continuity of care. Opportunities will exist for the development of ambulatory and community based residential mental health programs. There will be changes in the centralized governance of VA which will result in the National Headquarters (NHQ) housing clinical expertise in the form of program offices which will resemble the current Mental Health and Behavioral Sciences Service more than single discipline services such as Medicine. Given more decentralized authority in program management, it will be necessary for the National Headquarters mental health leadership to ensure that the needs of mentally ill veterans are served and that exemplary mental health programs are not locally dismantled as has happened in some states' public mental health services. Programmatic guidance in the form of practice guidelines and outcome monitoring will be the primary means by which clinical leadership in the NHQ will influence the field.

There is a clear statement of managed care as the basis for VA health care delivery, and primary care will be the mechanism by which care will be delivered. The roles of mental health clinicians in VA's primary care system will be varied. Virtually all current textbooks addressing primary care and mental health do so from the perspective of mental health clinicians providing consultation and/or liaison services to medical/surgical primary care teams (Cadoret & King, 1983; Dubovsky & Weissberg, 1986). Certainly, VA psychiatrists, psychologists and nurse clinicians will serve in these supportive roles: the greater penetration of mental health clinicians into medical primary care teams will improve the identification and treatment of such common disorders as depression and substance abuse which are too often missed in the absence of mental health input in patient care.

What is even more significant is the establishment of mental health clinicians as primary care providers for Mental Health Primary Care Teams, with internists, and medical physician assistants and nurses as support members of the Mental Health Teams. It is a common truth of VA mental health care, and probably of most public mental health systems, that the psychiatrist often functions as the primary care physician for a cohort of seriously mentally patients in his/her care, particularly in inpatient settings, Day Hospitals and Day Treatment Centers. These patients are often those whose illness behaviors make them unpopular and difficult for internists to treat, and who also have great difficulty in developing relationships with any health care providers. The concept of Mental Health Primary Care Teams received the support of VA Chiefs of

Psychiatry and Psychology and VHA leadership in the course of the VA Health Care Reform Task Force activity. While it remains true at the time of this writing that medical politics only acknowledges internal medicine, pediatrics, family practice and obstetrics and gynecology as "The" primary care specialties, it is evident that in practice public psychiatry also has this role and VA will continue to endorse it.

Accepting that VA's mental health primary care presence will include the more traditional consultation/liaison as well as the new Mental Health Primary Care Teams, the question arises as to how these roles will be manifested? The answer is consistent with the diversity of VA practice settings and the spirit of local innovation. VA medical centers range from highly affiliated tertiary care sites, to small, rural general hospitals, as well as about 20 facilities with a major inpatient psychiatric component (50 percent or more of facility beds) formerly called "neuropsychiatric hospitals". The primary care methods that will work for one type of facility will not necessarily fit for another. Even within the same type of facility there may be significant diversity in terms of the skills and numbers of available VA staff and possible community supports. Some facilities have had some form of primary care organization for mental health for years. Others are building Primary Care Mental Health Teams with added internists or family practitioners. Others are developing Mental Health Teams and linking their of their patients to developing medical primary care teams. Some facilities are organizing their primary care teams to cover both inpatient and outpatient care for a particular group of patients. Others are beginning their experiment with primary care in the ambulatory care arena and planning a slower shift into the incorporation of the inpatient units. One approach that is popular in VA Medical Centers that are affiliated with medical schools is to develop teams that are based around patients grouped by diagnosis (e.g., a Mood Disorders Team; a Schizophrenia Team; a PTSD Team).

It is anticipated that clinical services will take shape as product lines to provide a continuum of outpatient and inpatient services to a group of patients with a defined resource base. Local clinical managers will have responsibility for providing quality care for their patient populations as efficiently as possible, with some ability to retain a portion of the profits from efficient operations or from MCCR collections. Gatekeeping functions and the management of access to various levels of care will be assisted by system wide utilization management criteria supported by system wide quality monitors and clinical indicators.

It remains to be seen how this will evolve over time and across VA's national system. It may be assumed that some facilities, particularly those with small mental health services, may resemble HMOs with internist or family practice gatekeepers for mental health referrals. Facilities with more extensive mental health capabilities, such as MCG 8 facilities and highly affiliated tertiary care medical centers can be expected to have more control of mental health services in the hands of mental health clinicians (product line managers).

Much of this reorganization in the delivery of care is quite new and there remain a variety of obstacles and challenges to be met. One of the roles of Mental Health and Behavioral Sciences Service (MH & BSS) in NHQ is to serve as a clearing house for information about the primary care methodologies that different facilities are developing and disseminating them across the system. To facilitate this information transfer there are the existing monthly teleconferences for Chiefs of Psychiatry and Psychology and the meetings and newsletters of the Chiefs' organizations. It can be conjectured that not every facility will develop mental health primary care teams, either because of problems in the mental health groups or their medical colleagues, or their facility leadership. In these cases it will be the role of MH & BSS to identify the issues and assist in resolving them to promote primary care development, particularly if patient care appears to be suffering. How this may be accomplished leads to the consideration of evaluation as a tool in managed care.

PROGRAM EVALUATION

Program evaluation, focusing on resource management and clinical outcomes has been a feature of MH & BSS specially funded programs (HCMI; PTSD; Substance Abuse) since 1986. In each of these cases ongoing studies have identified the resources committed to the programs, in terms of staffing and funding; the demographics of the patient populations using the services; the treatment processes that have been provided to care for these patients, and the outcomes of treatment in terms of symptomatic and socio-economic improvement including patient satisfaction (Fontana, Rosenheck, & Spencer, 1993; Rosenheck, Gallup, Leda, Gorchov, & Errera, 1989). These program evaluations have not only provided Congress, the funding source for these programs, with information on how well their money was being spent, but also has shown MH & BSS where there are problems requiring solution. The use of computerized records and data gathering will enhance the ability to collect relevant program evaluation information in a manner that is minimally intrusive on clinician time. VA's automated data processing capabilities are a strength. It should be noted that any methodologies that VA develops in this area are "public domain" and so are essentially free for other health care entities to explore and use. Any software developed by VA can be accessed through a "Freedom of Information" request directed to VA headquarters in Washington.

For public care providers in a managed care environment, it is particularly important to share information with funding agencies, system users, and advocacy organizations about positive outcomes as well as problems and plans to correct them. This can be done not only by official reports but also through publications and presentations at scientific meetings describing the nature and efficacy of treatment programs. Even more important is the face to face sharing of information with local stakeholder groups, which for VA include affiliated medical schools; Veterans Service Organizations,

---

Survival Tips

Care Management by Public Payers: The VA System

Within a rigid public bureaucracy, a public payer can initiate PSMC.

Significant VA managed care initiatives that may be relevant to other public settings include:

- Decentralization of resource management
- Capitated funding of decentralized service delivery systems
- Shift from facility-based to client-based resource allocation
- Development of objective data-based systemwide methodology for equitable resource allocation
- Fiscal incentives to discourage overuse of hospitalization and to encourage development and utilization of ambulatory options
- Integration of teams of primary care and mental health providers as care managers in clinic settings
- Development of special product lines (e.g., PTSD, SPMI services) that can be marketed to private payers or consumers to enhance revenues
- Centralized quality management through standards of care, preservation of model programs, and outcome evaluation

Disadvantages of public sector systems as care managers must be acknowledged, as illustrated by the VA's slow pace of change, multiple administrative obstacles, and delayed transition to ambulatory care. Systemwide frustration may be reduced by addressing administrative barriers up front, rather than trying to create major service reorganization without major system reorganization.

---

and Congressional staff as well as the more specifically mental health advocacy groups such as the National Alliance for the Mentally Ill (NAMI). By bringing the providers of resources and the system's users into the picture and showing them what is being done and why, what the problems and the possible solutions are, a program can gather support (as well as ideas for problem resolution that may not have been considered by the clinician group). These stakeholders can "buy in" to the program and feel themselves to be in partnership with the providers.

Program evaluation requires the investment of staff resources to carry out the evaluation. One needs to identify what elements of the program are important to monitor and how to get the necessary information. Clinicians must develop these evaluation programs, training themselves in the statistical skills needed to make accurate assessments of the data gathered about programs, or by bringing health systems scientists into the clinical evaluation team. Approaching the question of evaluation, the issue of comparison to standards arises. Mental health in general has far fewer objective standards than other fields of medicine, but this is gradually changing. Whenever mental health standards of care or guidelines are created, it is the business of mental health clinicians to ensure that they have a controlling part in their development. This has been the case with the recently developed Practice Guidelines for Depression created by the American Psychiatric Association and the Clinical Practice Guideline for Depression in Primary Care developed by the Agency for Health Care Policy and Research (American Psychiatric Association, 1993; Agency for Health Care Policy and Research, 1993). Practice guidelines can be expected to evolve over time, for example as new medications result in more effective management of a disorder, but they need clinician direction to ensure that practice is driven by patient needs rather than by purely economic motives.

Controlling costs of health care is a major factor in the development of the managed care movement (Feldman & Fitzpatrick, 1992). This is a significant element in the poor insurance support for mental health care in America: a chronically ill person generates health care costs, and if suffering from a serious mental disorder such as schizophrenia, may not be capable of maintaining employment to pay insurance premiums. This avoidance of the chronically ill or those who need long term care is true for those who suffer from other disorders, but the bias against the mentally ill just digs the hole a little deeper for our patients.

In VA, as noted above, cost controls have primarily come from eligibility controls: with scarce resources, services are limited to "mandatory workload" patients, then to the Service Connected, then to those with the greatest degrees of Service Connection. Length of stay criteria applied through DRGs have also been used. Utilization management in the sense of admissions and intensity of care criteria have not been used in VA until very recently and even then they have been applied to medical surgical services rather than to mental health. Attempts to pilot test existing psychiatric utilization management criteria have suggested that at least one such format, the InterQual 1992 and 1993 criteria, are poor predictors of appropriateness of admission or length of stay (Goldman, Weir, Turner, & Smith 1995). At this point it is clear that VA is going to attempt to apply some form of utilization management criteria at least for acute psychiatric care as part of the effort to match patient care needs with the most efficient type and intensity of treatment. It must be noted that the utilization management pilot project referred to above prominently included several VA psychiatrists and other mental health professionals.

It is not surprising that utilization management criteria developed for private sector use are not immediately applicable to VA use. VA, like other public sector providers, carries certain special mandates and obligations beyond those of the private sector, and these impact the ways in which managed care methodologies can be applied. VA has some unique obligations such as the "Fourth Mission" (beyond clinical care of veterans, and support for research and education in relation to veterans' health care) of support of the Department of Defense in time of war and of Emergency Medical Preparedness in time of national disaster. In terms of disaster relief (e.g., Hurricane Andrew; the Northridge Earthquake), VA is the primary source of medical personnel, including mental health clinicians. The impact of pulling members of primary care teams from the task of caring for their panel of patients to serve in a disaster relief activity is one of the problems that must be addressed in developing VA's primary care system.

A key to ensuring the existence of quality mental health services to seriously and chronically mentally ill veterans will be to ensure an adequate funding base for these services. Among the ways of doing this can be to establish a system wide capitation rate for services to chronically mentally ill veterans based on the existing average rate for the RPM Chronic Mental Illness patient care group. Incentives for the most cost-efficient care will come from serving a known population with fixed resources. The potential exists for savings for more efficient operations being turned back to the mental health product line to enhance or expand services.

The public sector will always have "outliers" in terms of such measures as length of inpatient stay because treatment resistant patients, particularly those who manifest dangerous behaviors, gravitate to our care. For this reason, "risk adjustment" based on the clinical, social and economic realities of our patient population must be taken into account when developing managed care and cost control measures. Again, it is the role of the clinicians to keep our patients' needs foremost in the planning process.

CONCLUSION

VA's experience and plans for the future in terms of managed mental health care can be summarized in five points, which may be relevant to other public sector settings.

1) Establish a resource base for mental health services sufficient to provide high quality care, with decentralized, flexible, risk-based management.

2) Organize mental health services in terms of program or product lines of comprehensive care (e.g., the PTSD product line).

3) Deliver mental health services through interdisciplinary primary care teams.

4) Enhance program monitoring and evaluation to document the resources committed, the processes of care, and the outcomes of care, using electronic communications and computers to optimize evaluation.

5) Collaborate, cooperate and advocate, by sharing your efforts with other community providers and stakeholders.

REFERENCES

Agency for Health Care Policy and Research. (1993). Depression in primary care. *Clinical Practice Guideline Number 5.* Washington, DC: United States Department of Health and Human Services.

American Psychiatry Association. (1993). American Psychiatric Association practice guideline for major depressive disorder in adults. *Supplement to the American Journal of Psychiatry. 150.*

Cadoret, R.J., & King, L.J. (1983). *Psychiatry in primary care.* (2nd ed.). St. Louis: Mosby.

Department of Veterans Affairs. (1995). *Federal benefits for veterans and dependents.* (1995 ed.). Washington, DC: Author.

Department of Veterans Affairs. (1994a). *Resource planning and management handbook.* Washington, DC: Author.

Department of Veterans Affairs. (1994b). *Chief financial officer 1994 annual report.* Washington, DC: Author.

Department of Veterans Affairs. (1994c). *Meeting the challenge of health care reform.* Washington, DC: Author.

Dubovsky, S.L., & Weissberg, M.P. (1986). *Clinical psychiatry in primary care.* (3rd ed.). Baltimore: Williams & Wilkins.

Feldman, J.L., & Fitzpatrick, R.J. (Eds.) (1992). *Managed mental health care: Administrative and clinical issues.* Washington, DC: American Psychiatric Press.

Fontana, A., Rosenheck, R., & Spencer, H. (1993). *The long journey home, III: The third progress report on the Department of Veterans Affairs specialized PTSD programs.* West Haven, CT: Northeast Program Evaluation Center, Department of Veterans Affairs.

Friedman, M.J., West, A.N., & Clark, A. (1987). Integration of VA and CMHC care: Utilization and long-term outcome. *Hospital and Community Psychiatry, 38,* 735–740.

Goldman, R.L., Weir, C.R., Turner, C.W., & Smith, C.B. (1995). Unpublished manuscript.

Kulka, R.A., Schlenger, W.E., Fairbank, J.A., Hough, R.L., & Jordan, B.K. (1988). *Contractual report of findings from the national Vietnam veterans readjustment study.* Research Triangle Park, NC: Research Triangle Institute. (NTIS No. PB90-164203-XAB).

Paralyzed Veterans of America. (1992). *Strategy 2000: The VA responsibility in tomorrow's national health care system.* Washington, DC: Author.

Rosenheck, R. (1995). Unpublished manuscript.

Rosenheck, R., Gallup, P., Leda, C., Gorchov, L., & Errera, P. (1989). *Reaching out across America: The third progress report on the Department of Vet-*

erans Affairs homeless chronically mentally ill veterans program. West Haven, CT: Northeast Program Evaluation Center, Department of Veterans Affairs.

Rosenheck, R., Neale, M., Leaf, P., Milstein, R., & Frisman, L. (1995). Multisite experimental cost study of intensive psychiatric community care. *Schizophrenia Bulletin, 21,* 129–140.

10

Rural Issues in Public Sector Managed Behavioral Healthcare

DENNIS MOHATT

INTRODUCTION

The design of optimal PSMC systems is significantly influenced by the nature of the service area. An earlier chapter described the implementation of a capitated managed care system in an urban area with a predominant ethnic minority population (See chapter by Barbour, Floyd, and Connery). This chapter discussed implementation of PSMC in rural settings.

Due to the lack of rural specific managed care experience and the rapid evolution of managed care strategies, there is little empirical data which informs rural PSMC development. Nonetheless, rural issues which will impact the development of managed care have been clearly illuminated in recent years.

AN OVERVIEW OF RURAL ISSUES

Over one-fourth of the population of the United States resides in non-metropolitan areas, and nearly all states have distinct rural populations. Rural Americans experience incidence and prevalence

119

rates of mental illnesses and substance abuse which are equal to or greater than their urban counterparts (Wagenfeld, Murray, Mohatt, & DeBruyn, 1994).

Rural Americans, however, suffer from chronic shortages of mental health providers and services, which will significantly impact the development of rural managed care options. Over sixty percent of rural areas have been designated as federal Mental Health Professional Shortage Areas (U.S. Congress, Office of Technology Assessment, 1990). As a result, rural residents must travel for substantially longer times to access a mental health provider and are much more likely to see a mental health provider with less advanced training than their urban peers (Schurman, Kramer, & Mitchell, 1985). Rural areas are also less likely to currently offer a full array of behavioral health services. For example, while 95% of urban counties have psychiatric inpatient services, only 13% of rural counties have such services, and outpatient services are available in twice as many urban as rural hospitals (Wagenfeld, Goldsmith, Stiles, & Manderscheid, 1988). Additionally, supportive resources such as public transportation, housing, and vocational, which are vital for promoting independence in persons with serious and persistent mental illnesses are often very limited or unavailable in rural areas (Wagenfeld, Murray, Mohatt, & DeBruyn, 1994).

Rural areas have disproportionate populations of uninsured and underinsured. As a result of rural persons being employed in small business and self-employment settings, they are more likely to be uninsured or have more "catastrophic" insurance coverage, which lacks behavioral health benefits. Only one-fourth of the rural poor qualify for Medicaid, compared to 43% of the poor in urban areas (U.S. Senate, 1988).

The combination of professional shortages and limited array of services, coupled with a thin layer of third party payers, creates a fragile continuum of care for rural residents. The public mental health system is often the only provider in rural areas, serving primarily persons with serious mental illnesses (Wagenfeld, Murray, Mohatt, & DeBruyn, 1994).

The majority of Americans seek, and prefer, treatment in the primary care setting (Regier, Goldberg, & Taube, 1979). This trend holds true in rural settings, where a shortage of primary care providers serves to impede access to care. The problem is further complicated by problems identified with the effectiveness of primary care providers in providing diagnosis and treatment of behavioral health problems. In a recent study of American primary care settings, Schulberg (1991) reported that 80% of psychiatric diagnoses went undetected by primary care providers.

A serious problem also exists in the lack of coordination between rural primary care and mental health providers. Over one-third of primary care providers never refer to mental health providers, while 50% of the referrals made are not completed (Yaeger & Linn, 1990), this trend is mirrored in rural primary care (Kelleher, 1993). Considering the most common form of managed care (public & private) in rural areas is the Primary Care Case Management (PCCM) model (WAMI, 1994), the problems in primary care behavioral health competency create special managed care challenges.

In such a model, the primary care physician assumes the gate-keeping case management responsibilities for a defined population of covered beneficiaries, usually for a nominal fee, while the risk remains with an external organization. Without strong systems of behavioral health treatment and referral protocol, coupled with provider education and support, the risk of inadequate service utilization is high. Furthermore, considering the serious shortage of rural primary care providers, establishing an additional non-treatment role may be perceived negatively by these providers. Finally, the "de facto" mental health system currently operating within the primary care setting may become less responsive to consumers presenting with behavioral health problems if the opportunities for treatment reimbursement are altered, for example through a behavioral health carve-out which limits primary care delivery of such services.

In sum, a range of issues such as professional shortages, fragile service continuums, lack of insurance, geographic distances to care, payer mix, and lack of integration between primary care and mental health creates unique challenges in developing managed care strategies to serve rural areas. These conditions have traditionally resulted in: 1) rural persons going without appropriate care; 2) rural persons accessing care later than desirable resulting in increased cost and duration of care; 3) rural persons being treated at higher (and more costly) levels of care; and 4) rural persons receiving care at greater distance from their home and work, resulting in loss of community ties and difficulty in reintegration (Beeson & Mohatt, 1993). Effective rural managed care strategies must address each of these issues to ensure both cost containment and access.

INNOVATIVE PUBLIC SECTOR SOLUTIONS

Currently more than 33 million Americans receive their health insurance through Medicaid. The cost of Medicaid has increased over 400% since 1980, while Medicaid absorbs an average of 16% of state budgets (WAMI, 1994). The need to control cost is obvious, and managed care is being embraced by the states as the vehicle to cost containment.

Six states have received HCFA waivers to enroll all of their Medicaid consumers into managed care plans: Tennessee, Hawaii, Oregon, Rhode Island, Florida, and Kentucky. It should be noted that Arizona has operated its Medicaid program as a managed care plan for over ten years under a HCFA 1115 waiver, and 42 states are operating Medicaid managed care variations under HCFA 1915b waivers. Of these 42 states, only Rhode Island does not serve a federally defined non-metropolitan rural population. In January 1995, the National Rural Health Advisory Committee (a committee appointed by the Secretary of Health and Human Services to provide input relating to national rural health policy) issued a recommendation to the Secretary of Health and Human Services seeking review of these waivers to specifically address rural impact (author's personal knowl-edge via membership on Advisory Committee). Currently, HCFA review of these waivers does not specifically address rural impact.

The rural issues previously discussed, when not considered in the waiver process, can pose serious barriers to consumer access. For ex-ample, the current 1915b waiver for Nebraska's Medicaid managed care program for mental health and substance abuse contains stand-ards for pre-treatment assessment and supervision of care which may create significant barriers to consumer access to treatment.

These standards, which are part of the waiver, require a pre-treatment assessment of all recipients prior to the provision of outpa-tient care (i.e., psychotherapy, day treatment, etc.) The pre-treatment assessment is essentially a standard psychosocial intake diagnostic process, however the new standards outlined in the waiver require the mental status portion (inclusive of the diagnosis) to be completed by either a physician or licensed psychologist (doctoral level). Fur-thermore, the supervision of care standards require monthly supervi-sion by a supervising professional (physician or psychologist), of all cases where treatment is provided by other mental health providers (e.g., social workers, counselors, psychiatric nurses, etc.) inclusive of a verbal discussion/case presentation. The supervising professional is also required to have face-to-face contact with the consumer at six-month intervals.

Obviously the intent of such standards, albeit influenced by the political process, is to ensure quality of care. However, considering much of Nebraska is rural and has serious shortages of health and mental health professionals (especially physicians and doctoral psy-chologists), these standards could seriously impede consumer access to treatment resources currently available primarily via mid-level providers.

One potential solution involves the development of broadbased provider networks to maximize the efficiency of coordination of uti-lization of limited numbers of providers. Such networks can more easily develop 24 hour telephone availability, schedule provider ac-cess in remote settings, and fund mobile communications and trans-portation systems (e.g., helicopters) to bring providers to the clients.

Another solution involves the application of telemedicine re-sources to the rural areas. This includes the use of uni- and bi-directional communications between the rural site and a site from which assistance, in the form of assessment, consultation, and train-ing can be provided. If such resources are to be used, their value must be recognized by the managed care organization and financial support for their use must be included in the funding for rural ser-vices. Telemedicine may also facilitate utilization of mid-level pro-viders (e.g., physician assistants, nurse practitioners, and masters level counselors) through ready access to on-site audiovisual medi-ated supervision or consultation by senior professionals located in other settings hundreds of miles away.

Even with enhanced technology, however, the evolution of rural Medicaid managed care remains limited by the many rural issues noted above. Such challenges were the focus of the March 1993 conference in Little Rock, Arkansas, sponsored by the Robert Wood Johnson Foundation and Arkansas Department of Public Health: "Health Care Reform in Rural Areas". This conference, which brought together 100 invited participants representing a wealth of rural health care experience, health care policy experts, and staff from both the Clinton administration and congress, focused exclusively upon the examination of the potential fit between rural reality and potential reform strategies.

A clear consensus from that meeting was the viability of cooperative approaches to managed care, rather than managed competition, in rural areas. The development of horizontally or vertically integrated networks was seen as the best fit for a rural response to the health care reform goals of cost containment, enhanced access, and quality improvement (Alpha Center, 1993). Integration, which seeks to achieve these goals through collaboration and cooperation, fits the rural environment. Rather than introducing competition among providers, and potentially disrupting the fragile and limited rural continuum of care, integration seems to be a means to strengthen that continuum by building upon the system's existing resources, and avoiding unnecessary and costly duplication of effort.

VERTICAL INTEGRATION

Vertical integration approaches to managed care seek to network a group of rural healthcare providers, inclusive of primary care and behavioral health to form an integrated service network (Casey, Wellever, & Moscovice, 1994). They seek to develop, via cooperation, a coordinated, consumer focused seamless continuum of care designed to improve access and availability through efficiencies gained by the elimination of redundant services or systems.

A model rural vertically integrated system is the Laurel Health System in Northeastern Pennsylvania. Laurel was founded in 1989 with the merger of five not-for-profit organizations. This network spans the human service gamut inclusive of primary care, nursing homes, senior housing, ambulance service, and hospital.

The continuum of care is focused in Laurel's two major service anchors. The merger linked a primary care and tertiary health system serving a balanced public/private payer mix, with a community health and mental health system which was heavily government subsidized (six federally qualified rural health centers and the community mental health program). To accomplish the merger, however, both major organizations were forced to overcome a history of rivalry dating back to 1972.

Today, however, Laurel is moving forward in its partnership. The move toward managed care has turned its planning focus toward the development of a HMO/PPO option for the local insurance marketplace. Laurel is seen as a model integrated rural health delivery system, successful in its mission to provide the community a seamless system of care inclusive of both traditional health and mental health services.

HORIZONTAL INTEGRATION

The horizontally integrated network brings providers of similar services together to achieve the advantages of economies of scale, and to position organizations to eliminate administrative duplication. Access is enhanced through the redirection of resources formally utilized in redundant administrative functions (e.g., crisis or intake services).

A recent example of such a horizontal integration is the 1994 formation of Northpointe Behavioral Healthcare Systems in Michigan's Upper Peninsula. Northpointe was formed as a proactive response to the evolving managed care environment in public sector mental health. Northpointe was established through the consolidation of two community mental health programs serving three rural counties. The consolidation allowed the CMHCs to centralize executive administration, management information, fiscal management, and human resources for the new entity which employs 300+ and serves more than 3,500 consumers annually.

Neither CMHC alone would have possessed the capital to build the management and information infrastructure necessary for managed care operation. The efficiencies gained through the consolidation have allowed Northpointe to invest its combined capital on managed care readiness efforts. The new entity employs centralized intake and utilization review, tied to an evolving clinical outcome and consumer satisfaction assessment system. (See chapter by Weinstein).

Survival Tips

Rural Issues in Public Sector Managed Care

Develop networks proactively, rather than waiting for networks to be created by MCOs. Emphasize the need for conflict resolution and organizational consultation to overcome old rivalries.

Horizontal networks permit economies of scale, elimination of administrative overlap, and more efficient use of limited resources.

Vertical networks permit better service continuity, with elimination of redundancies and reallocation to fill gaps in the continuum.

Emphasize provision of public mental health services in primary care settings with accessible consultation.

Make use of appropriate technology, especially telemedicine and transportation supports, to overcome the barriers created by sparse population areas and great distances between clients and providers.

Northpointe utilized a portion of Michigan law, known as the Urban Cooperation Act, which allows elements of local government to consolidate to more effectively meet public needs (usually used to form airport and solid waste authorities). This act allows Northpointe to establish for-profit and not-for-profit subsidiaries, and provides the participating county governments legal separation from Northpointe related financial risk.

CONCLUSION

Rural issues create a unique environment for managed care. While managed care in urban settings is characterized by competition, rural managed care will likely take on aspects of cooperation. The formation of both vertically and horizontally integrated networks has been a common response to managed care in rural health care settings. Since managed care seeks to contain costs through effective and efficient clinical management, it is unclear how such a system will address the problems of serious rural underservice.

Integration, which rests upon an ability for collaboration and cooperation, faces many challenges in the rural environment. Historic relationships between providers often may be exclusive of collaboration. Geographic realities of many frontier regions, where the population is widely dispersed and the service continuum extremely limited, may simply not have the resource base which can effectively meet the demands of a managed care approach. Finally, integration poses risks to provider autonomy. Through collaboration the partners must agree to share authority, accountability, risk, as well as benefit or loss. In a managed care environment, it is essential to ensure beneficiaries are linked with both the most appropriate level of care and provider of care. For an integrated network to succeed, the partners must be capable of addressing a myriad of issues arising out of such shared responsibility for utilization and outcome. As with any group process, the key to success (cohesiveness) will be the member's ability to resolve conflict.

REFERENCES

Alpha Center. (1993). *Healthcare reform in rural areas: A report from the invitational conference sponsored by the Robert Wood Johnson Foundation and Arkansas Department of Health.* Washington, DC: The Alpha Center.

Beeson, P.G., & Mohatt, D.F. (1993). Rural mental health and national healthcare reform. Arlington, VA: National Association of State Mental Health Program Directors.

Casey, M., Wellever, A., & Moscovice, I. (1994). Public policy issues and rural health network development. Minneapolis, MN: University of Minnesota Rural Health Research Center. (Working Paper Series).

Kelleher, K. (1993). Rural mental health and primary care. Lincoln, NE: Paper presented at the National Association for Rural Mental Health Annual Conference.

Regier, D.A., Goldberg, I.D., & Taube, C.A. (1979). The de facto U.S. mental health services system. *Archives of General Psychiatry, 35,* 685–693.

Schulberg, H. (1991). Mental disorders in the primary care setting: Research priorities for the 1990s. *General Hospital Psychiatry, 13,* 156–234.

Schurman, R.A., Kramer, R.D., & Mitchell, J.B. (1985). The hidden mental health network. *Archives of General Psychiatry, 42,* 89–94.

U.S. Congress, Office of Technology Assessment. (1990). *Health care in rural America* (OTA:H:434). Washington, DC: U.S. Government Printing Office.

U.S. Senate. (1988). *Report of the Special Committee on Aging.* Washington, DC: U.S. Government Printing Office.

Wagenfeld, M.O., Goldsmith, H.F., Stiles, D., & Manderscheid, R.W. (Eds.). (1988). Inpatient mental health services in metropolitan and non-metropolitan counties. *Journal of Rural Community Psychology, 9*(2).

Wagenfeld, M.O., Murray, J.D., Mohatt, D.F., & DeBruyn, J. (Eds.). (1994). *Mental health and rural America: An overview and annotated bibliography 1978–1993.* Washington, DC: U.S. Government Printing Office.

WAMI Rural Health Research Center. (Winter 1994). Medicaid managed care coming to rural America. *Rural Health News, 1*(1), 1.

Yaeger, J., & Linn, L. (1990). Studies in the screening and feedback of depression and anxiety in primary care outpatient populations. In C. Attkinson & J. Zicj (Eds.) *Depression in primary care: Screening and detection* (pp. 117–138). New York: Routledge.

Section III

Program Management Issues: Introduction

CHARLES RAY, MONICA OSS and LEE ANN SLAYTON

The readiness of CMHCs (now termed community behavioral health provider organizations- CBHPOs) to adapt to the implications of the PSMC revolution has become one of the most compelling issues facing CBHPOs in the coming decade.

Ironically, the movement toward public sector managed health and behavioral health incorporates many of the original concepts of the CMHC movement: development of a comprehensive, integrated and coordinated system of mental healthcare, provided in the least restrictive environment.

During the past decade, the evolution of the CMHC movement has led to great variability among CMHCS. Many have expanded their array of services, branched into addiction treatment services, and actively sought private-sector dollars and clients to enhance their payer mix. Others have formed strategic alliances with other public providers, and with community-based not-for-profit organizations. Many have abandoned the concept of "catchment area" to compete regionally or state-wide for certain contracts. To reflect these changes, we are now referring to them as community behavioral health provider organizations (CBHPOs). Ironically, the CBHPOs that pioneered many of the innovative, resource-sensitive, and clinically effective programs (such as partial hospitalization, psychosocial rehabilitation, home healthcare, and case management) now find that these have been adopted by private-sector providers who compete with CBHPOs for behavioral health benefit dollars not only in the private sector, but now in the public sector as well.

Only a few years ago, there appeared to be an assumption that the traditional public sector market of CBHPOs was largely exempt from competition and managed care trends. Now, as an expanding percentage of individuals are covered by public or private sector managed care, CBHPOs must increasingly compete with private sector providers for public and private dollars disbursed by private managed care organizations who have large public sector contracts. Consequently, for several years, active discussion has taken place about the roles and challenges facing CBHPOs attempting to participate in managed care. Such discussions focus on revenue diversification strategies, extension of core competencies into new markets, and protection of the social mission through the development of contemporary business-focused management styles.

What does this mean for the current generation of CBHPOs? The current trends pose a significant threat. Over the past few decades, CBHPOs have become relatively conservative organizations, operating on the assumption that their funding would be relatively stable, and would change relatively slowly. Their governing boards have typically been involved in stewardship issues, accounting for funds and quality of service. Now, these volunteer boards must make complex policy decisions that balance their social missions with contemporary business practices. They need to consider access and availability of care, efficiency and productivity, financial management, their local community role, and recruiting and retaining the staff required to operate increasingly complex systems. Most nonprofit boards have not traditionally been involved in such issues and are understandably likely to be overwhelmed by such demands.

These same challenges face CBHPO managers as well. Traditionally, CBHPO managers have been responsible for managing a fixed budget and providing services within it. They did not need to generate additional revenue or provide sophisticated marketing plans, as the public sector defined both the patient or consumer and the rate of reimbursement. Managers were not expected to have sophisticated knowledge of different markets or payers, or of ways to provide services according to the demands of different market segments and/or patient relationships.

In the new PSMC environment, CBHPO managers need to acquire a new set of executive skills and become much more sophisticated about finance, marketing, human resources, and managing effective operations. The traditional clinical manager is poorly prepared for these dramatic systems changes.

As states across the country move toward privatizing portions of the public mental health system, survival has become a new challenge for CBHPOs. States may continue the traditional public systems in some modified form using CBHPOs and other providers, or the system may be open to intense competition between private groups, CBHPOs, and others. The uncertainties have led many traditional providers to wonder how they can survive in either type of system.

Survival Tips
Developing Managed Care Readiness • CBHPOs no longer have a public funding stream protected from competition. Therefore, CBHPO leadership must develop management skills suitable for a competitive privatized market. • Management skills include expertise in finance, MIS, marketing, human resources, and maximization of efficiency. • Do not focus on cost containment and cutting; rather, utilize resources to maximize creativity, develop new products, and enhance productivity. • Sophisticated fiscal and clinical information systems are essential. • Non-profit community boards require significant training and support to keep up with the pace of change and to be helpful in the process. • Develop one or more of the following survival strategies consistent with the organization's overall mission: revenue diversification, specialized program development and marketing, development as a MCO capable of managing risk-based contracts (See chapter by Oss and Mackie). • Promote mergers, affiliations, or networking (See chapter by Weinstein). • Develop competency in utilization and quality management (See chapters by McFarland, Minkoff, Roman, & Morrison, and Berlant, Anderson, Carbone, & Jeffrey).

This section emphasizes some of the specific skills or systems that agency managers must develop to survive the challenge of PSMC. One set of skills involves "market positioning" — maintaining the status quo versus promoting mergers or affiliations versus developing new managed care oriented "product lines" — and contracting for services using new risk-based methodologies, such as capitation. A second set of skills involves the process of network development, as exemplified by the formation of Behavioral Health Networks (BHNs) in Vermont, New Hampshire, and Maine. The third set of skills reflects the need for CBHPOs to develop managed care competencies, which in effect make them "mini managed care clinical organizations". These skills are necessary to be credible to PSMC payers, to successfully manage risk-based payment methodologies, and, most important, to continue to assure quality service provision and are discussed in the chapter on utilization management. Survival tips in each chapter emphasize concrete administrative strategies that promote readiness and facilitate the development of the skills and systems noted above.

CBHPOs are the heirs to a rich tradition of coordinated and comprehensive services to achieve appropriate clinical outcomes in the least restrictive settings. The early CBHPO focus on prevention, coordination of services, continuity of care, and partial and residential services, as well as psychosocial and case management methodologies, underlies contemporary PSMC programs. If CBHPOs individually and collectively can meet the challenge of managed care readiness, they will not only survive, they will thrive in the era of PSMC.

11

Contracting Issues

MONICA OSS and J. JAY MACKIE

PREPARATION FOR PSMC CONTRACTING

A major challenge for public sector mental healthcare organizations is to learn how to successfully develop and compete for contracts. The external environment is beyond the control of public providers. However, regardless of the individual decisions about managed mental health models made by individual states, all of the models favor mental health delivery systems that can both provide care for the traditional public sector client and accept financial risk for the population like an insurer would.

With this strategic goal in mind, public mental health providers can prepare for PSMC contracting by developing some basic managerial and operating skills. This basic skill set requires the following administrative infrastructure, which is described in several other chapters:

- Cost accounting system that accurately determines provider costs per unit of care, per course of treatment, and per patient
- Competitive cost analysis in local marketplace
- Financial systems to manage risk-sharing or risk-based contracts
- 24-hour, centralized patient intake and tracking system
- Internal prospective utilization review capability
- Quality measurements systems

- Integrated (financial/clinical) management information system
- Centralized billing capability

In addition to this management infrastructure, providers should start to develop or affiliate with the continuum of care that is required in managed mental health systems. The continuum of care should be multi-modal (integrated across all levels of care) and multi-specialty (serving all required populations: mental health, chemical dependency, MR/DD, children services, etc.). This multi-modal and multi-specialty continuum would also have to meet the geographic coverage requirements of the contracting model, which could be local in the case of an HMO, and regional or state-wide in most state models.

The elements that should be evaluated in developing a multi-modal continuum of care include:

- 24-hour emergency assessment and crisis intervention
- Hospital diversion programming (23-hour observation beds, in-home crisis stabilization, etc.)
- Outpatient psychotherapy and counseling services — both individual and group
- Medication evaluation and management programs
- Continuity of care — both relapse prevention for chemically dependent patients and assertive community-based treatment and case management models for mentally ill patients
- Intensive non-residential treatment programs — partial hospitalization, structured outpatient treatment programs
- Acute inpatient capability
- Non-acute residential/group home/halfway house availability

In addition, a competitive continuum of care should have the following characteristics:

- A multi-disciplinary professional staff
- Adequate geographic coverage for both adults and for specialized children services
- Clinical staff with credentials/training in chemical dependency treatment
- A proportionate mix of male and female staff
- Clinical programming that is specific to clients from all socio-economic and cultural backgrounds
- Foreign language fluency appropriate to a geographical area
- Staff with a working familiarity with community resources.

Development of these integrated delivery systems requires substantial capital. This need for capital is driving an unprecedented consolidation among traditional public providers, in the form of mergers, strategic alliances, and joint ventures. These new alliances of public providers have, in their short history, been quite successful in securing and successfully managing public managed mental health contracts. Their success in competing with the large MCOs is spurring price competition for public contracts. It is this price competition that is causing the large MCOs to embark on a strategy of backward integration, i.e., the acquisition or development of provider delivery system capabilities. In other words, at the same time that public mental health providers are organizing to accept risk and assume some "insurance" functions, MCOs are becoming providers of care. The most prominent example of this backward integration is the merger of Green Spring Health Services with Charter Medical Corporation into the new organization, Magellan. It appears that the public mental health landscape will be dominated by large integrated mental health delivery systems that can both provide treatment services and insure mental health benefits. These large systems, capitated by payers, will replace the current dichotomy between "provider" and "insurer". In addition, it is likely that these larger systems will be equally successful in the privately-financed and publicly-financed health care markets and may replace the current two-tiered public/private mental health delivery system.

What does this mean for planning for contracting? Planning for effective inclusion in managed care contracts requires attention to the five following important strategies: 1) product development, 2) market positioning, 3) accurate cost accounting and rational pricing, 4) cost reduction, and 5) influencing public policy. These will be described in more detail in the remainder of this chapter.

PRODUCT DEVELOPMENT

This strategic area is covered in chapters 19–24 and involves the development of the kinds of services that would be more attractive to payers. These include time-sensitive psychotherapy services, alternatives to acute hospitalization, integration of various previously distinct service areas (e.g., psychiatric and addiction services or psychiatric services in primary care facilities), and services to special population groups, such as children and the elderly. The principles associated with success with this strategy are to maintain a focus on value-based service development, attention to quality, and the use of networking to complement missing skills or services.

Providers should present their program strengths and sell "value" as opposed to "price". Analyze what is different and what is better, when compared to competitors. Those differences should be stressed in promotional materials, presentations, and proposals, in terms that are relevant to consumers, MCOs, other providers, or employers. This "value based" positioning is essential in competing against less expensive programs or services.

MARKET POSITIONING

There appear to be a number of market niches available to provider organizations in the evolving mental health field. However, these niches look very different in size, structure, and management than public mental health organizations of even a decade ago. In our work with provider organizations, we often see five types of strategic market positioning:

1. Become (part of) a large integrated mental health delivery system (with contractual relationships other than fee-for-service). A growing number of mental health providers are "affiliating" to create integrated delivery systems that can partner with or compete with specialty managed mental health programs.

2. Develop a niche as the low-cost/high-value provider of a particular service in a particular geographic area through fee-for-service contracts with managed mental health and integrated mental health delivery systems. The challenge with this market place position is both that fee-for-service contract rates are falling (or at least not keeping pace with inflation) and that the managed mental health programs are developing their own delivery system capability.

3. Provide a very specific treatment service, with a large geographic market area. For some organizations, specialization is a possible market strategy. Selected populations — the hearing-impaired, individuals with severe medical and mental problems, the HIV/AIDS patient population, pregnant women, foster children, etc. — represent market niches that can draw patient referrals across a large geographic area and a large number of health plans.

4. Position the practice or program as a specialized provider of a high-value privately-paid service (in terms of quality/cost ratio). For some services, individuals and employers will be willing to pay outside of their selected health benefit plans.

5. Offer a specialized mental health service for a payer outside of the health care system. Some mental health provider organizations are moving outside of the health care payment system, applying their expertise to develop programs for workers compensation system, juvenile justice, child welfare, education, or other payer sources.

ACCURATE COST ACCOUNTING AND RATIONAL PRICING

In markets with evolving public mental health programs, one of the most common problems faced by traditional public mental health providers is that of price competition. For many providers, state and local funds have provided a financial safety net when fee-for-service income was inadequate. At the same time, state and local regulation adds a layer of administrative overhead that often causes the plans to be non-competitive on a price basis. The rapid consolidation of control of mental health and chemical dependency funds among the leading managed mental health programs is reducing fee-for-service reimbursement options. While the number of inpatient and residential mental health and chemical dependency treatment beds is dropping, the all-inclusive per diems paid for those services are dropping even more quickly. The number of partial and day treatment programs is rising rapidly, but patient acuity is increasing and reimbursement is declining. The number of private providers offering services for patients traditionally served by public mental health programs is rising.

Regardless of quality, content, or cost of a provider's programs, the provider must have accurate information concerning its costs and a rational pricing strategy in order to negotiate contracts effectively and safely. Public providers beginning the process of contracting with MCOs often experience themselves in an unequal negotiating position. The MCO is a powerful purchaser of services, may feel little obligation to maintain continuity of service provider, and may have virtual monopolistic market control to drive down price. To "level the playing field", public providers need to have accurate data on their services, modern management information systems for analyzing such data on a real-time basis, and competent fiscal officers to assist with the budgeting and pricing proposals. In addition to having these skills and technical supports, they must attend to bringing down their costs.

COST REDUCTION AND EFFICIENCY ENHANCEMENT

For most public mental health programs, there are only a few options for competing in a low-cost market.

Lower direct costs. Analyze direst service costs in order to discover what efficiencies are possible. Only by understanding costs per unit of care, per patient, or per course of treatment will the provider be in a position to develop an effective management and marketing strategy. For some organizations, increasing clinical staff productivity is an issue, while for others, decreasing no-show rates is essential. In some instances, decreasing clinical staff cash compensation or non-cash compensation is required.

Lower indirect costs. Analyze indirect costs, such as the costs of overhead in terms of administration, regulatory compliance, and other factors. Again, reorganization of existing management staff to reduce layers of management, increasing administrative efficiency through automation, and closing clinical programs with high administrative and regulatory requirements may have to be considered.

Propose changing the pricing structure. For provider organizations whose payment is currently limited to fee-for-service arrangements, developing per case, per episode, performance-based, or capitation pricing agreements may eliminate competition on a unit-price basis.

Change the financial relationship to the providers in the system. Payment for clinician services can range from employment agreements, to retainers, to fee-for-service billing arrangements, to subcapitation. As the program's payment arrangements evolve, the financial relationships with clinicians may need to change to reflect the same financial incentives.

Do competitive research and determine what competitors are doing to lower their costs and prices. Understanding the delivery system of low-cost provider organizations in the marketplace is essential to developing a competitive strategy. With that knowledge, provider organizations can decide whether to adopt the same practices (to achieve the same financial result) or use the information to position their services as "superior" in the marketplace.

As changes continue in the mental health field, price pressure will continue until the supply of programs and professionals roughly matches the funds, both third-party and private pay, that are available to pay for services. The challenge for mental health organizations is to develop a strategy to cope with this period in health care system development.

PUBLIC POLICY INFLUENCE

Current providers must also influence public policies in order to balance the need to compete for contracts in the new managed care environment with the traditional mission of serving their communities. Key policy issues are highlighted below:

Adequate implementation time & technical assistance. As public mental health systems become "deregulated", the issue of transition and implementation strategies arises. Policies related to implementation must allow for a realistic transition phase.

Regulatory reform. These sweeping changes in financing will require significant regulatory reform. As care management and care provision functions blend in the same organization, a review of malpractice regulations and the relative responsibility of individual providers and organized systems of care will be required. As public and private systems merge, existing (and usually quite complex) regulation of public and private providers will need to be reexamined. Issues such as reporting, accreditation, and licensure will likely change. One major change that will be required will be the shift from the traditional reliance on inspection and auditing of clinical records to quality improvement focused requirements for organizations to develop and describe their quality assurance and utilization management processes.

Obligations to serve the uninsured. A potential dilemma for public sector providers taking on PSMC contracts is that the contracts may not explicitly include services for some persons who have traditionally depended on public providers. In the past, CMHCs and other private non-profit organizations served as the mental health "safety net". As new health care financing plans emerge, we are removing the program-funded safety net and replacing it with a service system that is both eligibility-driven and often capitated. As a nation, we continue to have 18–20% of the non-elderly population without any health or mental health coverage and an additional segment of the population underinsured for mental health by virtue of the lack of parity within existing health plans. The effects of lack of insurance and underinsurance for mental health needs will become more apparent. In the long-term, if the merger of systems, public and private, and the systematic transformation of the current public mental health system is to be considered a success, it should result in employers offering parity in mental health benefits and policymakers mandating parity and universal coverage. However, in the interim, this lack of safety net poses extreme ethical and financial dilemmas for providers of mental health services, especially those whose traditional mission has been to serve those most in need.

During this period, as financing is limited to specific services for defined populations in an environment where private and public health plans do not offer equitable coverage, the demand for "charitable" services will continue to increase. For all provider organizations, both public and private, the strategic ethical questions are how to address the compelling pressure of uncovered clients who have genuine service needs, how to generate enough revenue from managed care contracts to subsidize uncompensated care, and how to allocate or ration services among the people requesting uncompensated care. Providers need to articulate these concerns in the public policy arena, so that they do not get penalized financially for continuing to serve the needs of the most disadvantaged clients.

Survival Tips

Contracting Issues

- **Develop basic administrative infrastructure for PSMC contracting.**
- **Develop or maintain elements of a multimodal service continuum.**
- **Consider the five important contracting strategies:**

  1. Product development

  2. Market positioning

  3. Accurate cost accounting and rational pricing

  4. Cost reduction

  5. Influencing public policy

12

Developing Community Based Provider Networks

MATTHEW WEINSTEIN

INTRODUCTION

In response to increasing Medicaid managed care initiatives, community mental health centers (CMHC), traditionally the leading providers of services for medical assistance and indigent clients, have begun to organize networks to protect their market position. CMHCs in Tennessee, Maine, New Hampshire, Vermont, New Jersey and Oregon have formed consortia for coordinating services in response to statewide health care reforms. Florida also formed an Independent Provider Association with more than 50 centers with the express purpose of providing services to both commercially and publicly insured clients both regionally and statewide. The purpose of this chapter is to provide some guidance in forming a network of community mental health and public agency providers intending to deliver services in the public sector.

ORGANIZATION

Mission. The first element of forming any network of providers is to clarify the mission of the organization. It is important that all of the founding members as well as new participants can articulate in clear terms the purpose of the network. The leadership structure of the network should promote, clarify and enforce the mission of the organization. In the early stages of development it is also important to emphatically communicate the considerations, deliberations and decisions of the organization. Suggested items to include in the mission are as follows:

1. Engage in ethical business practices.

2. Deliver clinically competent services.

3. Establish economically competitive pricing.

4. Promote the use of least restrictive levels of care.

5. Pool member resources to more efficiently manage the costs of providing care.

6. Share responsibility within the membership for directing the activities of the network.

7. Create optimal geographic access to clients.

8. Aggressively pursue contracts and market opportunities.

Governance. Governing structures should promote representation from the membership. Rotation of board and committee members with varying terms allows for balanced participation and continuity. For example, board members could be elected for three year terms with one third replacement each year.

Determining which legal structure is most appropriate and the selection of an attorney should be delayed until broader management issues (discussed below) have been addressed. Rushing to form a new corporation will not address the threatening tone of the marketplace. Premature formation of a corporation can be costly, as future management decisions may require bylaw revisions, membership agreements, and tax and antitrust considerations not contemplated from the onset. Thus, it is strongly recommended that the formation be done at the completion of planning and development activities.

The founding parties, which usually constitute the initial board, are provider organizations that put in seed money and want to maintain authority within the organization. It is important to remember that future agencies that bring value to the network may want to have an equal footing with the founders. Consequently, many networks differentiate levels of members, e.g., Class A members have voting rights, sit on the Board and have greater financial responsibility to the organization and Class B members deliver clinical services but may not wish to be at risk for additional financial commitment. Provision should be made to add new members who have demonstrated competency and managed care market penetration to join the organization with an equal footing regardless of the timing of their membership. It is further recommended that specific planning taskforces be created as listed below.

PLANNING

It is recommended that the following specific planning taskforces be created:

- **Organizational taskforce.** The primary management goals of the organizational taskforce are to provide leadership, solve problems, educate and encourage participation and conflict resolution. This group should handle matters relating to legal formation of the network, board construction, and internal communications and may act as an interim board until all legal formation processes have been completed. In addition, the organizational taskforce acts as a clearing house for recommendations, questions and activities of the other taskforces. The person selected to chair this group must be prepared to provide a hands-on leadership to overcome many of the natural resistances typically found in participants in new ventures.

- **Finance taskforce.** The finance taskforce is charged with developing start-up and operating budgets relying upon the work of other taskforces to determine which operating systems will be selected. The finance taskforce also must evaluate reimbursement options (e.g., fee for service, case rate and capitation) which should be shared with members as their unit costs for providing services will influence pricing strategies. Finally, the finance taskforce needs to be charged with determining what capitalization may be necessary for capitation contracts. Cash reserves may be required by private third party payers or state insurance commissions to prove viability to take financial risk.

- **Clinical operations taskforce.** The first priority of the clinical operations taskforce initially is to design a single point of access clinical triage service. A centralized system for telephonic evaluation, assessment, disposition and scheduling is critical for delivering immediate access for clients and demonstrating network viability. The clinical operations taskforce must also develop a utilization management program which begins by defining criteria for different levels of care, the onset of treatment, continued care, transfer of cases between levels of care and termination of treatment. Utilization review criteria must be clearly defined; criteria for case review may include the following:

1. Cases in treatment too long

2. Cases terminated too quickly

3. Cases terminated prior to the conclusion of therapy

4. Reported critical incidents or complaints

The clinical operations taskforce also needs to address outcome evaluation by selecting client satisfaction surveys and outcome measures to assess clinical efficacy.

- **Provider relations taskforce.** The provider relations taskforce is responsible for determining the criteria for membership within the network. Applications must be devised for both institutional and individual providers. A written credentialling process must include standards for granting provider status, grievance procedures, and standards for terminating provider status. Subsequently, legal documents relating to provider agreements need to be drafted which define the terms under which institutions and individual providers will deliver clinical services on behalf of the network. Some basic elements of these agreements include providers' indemnification, specific malpractice insurance requirements, payment rates, record keeping specifications, data reporting, scheduling access and client satisfaction/outcome participation standards. The provider relations taskforce must delineate membership to ensure geographic, multi-disciplinary, multi-specialty and vertical level of care coverages beyond traditional inpatient, partial hospitalization and outpatient services. Examples of specialized alternative services which may be considered are residential, group home, in-home, crisis partial and ambulatory detoxification. The provider relations taskforce must fill in any gaps that might exist. Lastly, the provider relations taskforce develops communication and education events for the members to generate provider relations development and recruitment opportunities.

- **Management information systems taskforce.** The management information systems (MIS) taskforce has a difficult challenge to integrate data from member agencies. Examples of data requirements include the following:

1. Initial Encounters (all calls to the single point of access)

2. Service Utilization Data

    a. Volume of service per episode of treatment

    b. Total cost of care per episode of treatment

    c. Intensity of service for longterm clients

3. Provider Profile Statistics

    a. Number of visits by provider per episode of treatment

    b. Cost of care by provider per episode of treatment

    c. Client satisfaction data by provider

    d. Client outcomes data by provider

Additional data bases which may need to be developed include certification and recertification of authorizations for care, treatment terminations, credentialling, billing and claiming. The primary challenge is to develop a consensus among the members on how to integrate their current information systems with the network requirements and then develop an implementation plan that is financially feasible. An approach that facilitates merging electronically diverse data can be to use an interface software that reconfigures and downloads a variety of electronic data into a centralized computer that processes information, organizes statistics and creates reports. When researching software it is important to place high priority on integrated systems which allow data from different functions to be drawn into comparative reports and statistical analyses. Integrated applications provide the opportunity for eliminating separate software and service agreements. Lastly, MIS has to be viewed as a long term progressive activity. It is impossible to begin integrating providers and technologies without a careful implementation plan that brings people on-line sequentially and brings systems within the MIS on-line incrementally. A gradual, medium to long range plan which starts with the selection of an ideal system and allows members to come on-line sequentially seems to satisfy most of the reluctant participants.

- **Marketing taskforce.** The marketing taskforce is initially charged with the responsibility of developing a system for contacting potential clients for the network and determining their needs. This market research process will assist in driving the clinical and management service program decisions. In addition, it will help educate and orient the membership to a customer driven service model. Each of the potential customers should have an individualized marketing approach. Any contacts that are to be made with potential customers should be fully integrated and accountable into a detailed marketing plan which takes advantage of historical relationships that may exist with the network members but also shifts the emphasis from purchasing services from individual members to now purchasing services from the network in an integrated fashion. Examples of customers include Managed Care Organizations (MCO), Health Maintenance Organizations (HMO), Preferred Provider Organizations (PPO), primary care physicians, and multi-specialty medical group practices. A listing of all potential customers should be made with detailed information including the following: name of organization; type of organization; contact person; telephone number; address; number of covered lives; preferred method of reimbursement (fee for service, case rate, capitation); and, current preferred providers.

MEMBERSHIP

Big networks seem like a great idea, but the market demand is for a well-managed network. The mission of building a managed care competent network may conflict with a strategy relying upon inclusion for all community mental health centers and service agencies in the state or region. In addition to the issue of potential geographic overlap and excess services, the primary problem with the strategy of inclusion is that it does not qualify members with criteria that are consistent with the mission. If certain members have high costs and inefficiencies, they become a liability when pricing services and bidding on competitive contracts. Similarly, if certain members cannot assure ease of access and schedule initial appointments quickly, they will jeopardize the clinical reputation of the network. It is critical not to downplay or disregard the importance of these standards when evaluating potential members.

Shared values. Criteria that are basic but essential to the success of any managed care network require all members to embrace without compromise ethical conduct, clinical competence, economically competitive pricing, pooling of resources and shared control of the management. A principal element that drives the decision to treat clients in an ethical manner demands that only necessary and medically appropriate treatment will be delivered to clients. This applies to the frequency and volume of services, as well as to the level of care (i.e., utilization of the least restrictive and least expensive modalities and environments). A second ethical consideration involves promoting consumer independence. As much as possible, treatment should consistently encourage the development of independent skills, rather than the reliance on ongoing psychotherapy, even where the individual suffers from a longterm illness which requires ongoing medication and support. There are historical styles of psychotherapy which may be counterproductive in the current managed care environment. When treating clients who do not have serious mental illness, it is incumbent upon the clinician to introduce the goals associated with terminating treatment in the very first session. The symptoms, prognosis, treatment options, and expected outcome are generally discussed at the conclusion of the diagnostic process by most medical practitioners and this model should be applied consistently to behavioral health care as well. For persons with SPMI, this concept can be translated into helping the consumer achieve the goal of best possible functioning with least necessary utilization of mental health services.

Clinical quality. It is important that the clinical work performed in the network adhere to competitively high quality standards. The network must develop formal Continuous Quality Improvement (CQI) systems to measure key areas of performance and to ensure that each member program participates sufficiently in the CQI process. In addition to consistent case management methodologies and credentialling standards which rely upon focused evaluation of providers, there must be uniform support for outcome studies and client satisfaction tools. It is strongly recommended that methodologies be implemented that are efficient, useful, and mission oriented. Many of the tools today are extremely long and research oriented and it is not clear that this provides added value. The time required to complete the questionnaires should be as brief as possible, as time efficiency is an important challenge for managed care competent systems. The network should review statistics and take action with regard to positive and negative results. One proof of a network's viability is that it manages its own providers in an accountable fashion. Integration of data from credentialling, outcome studies, and client satisfaction surveys into a shared database for purposes of providing periodic reports to providers and to management is critical for the creditability of the process (See chapters by Berlant et al. and Essock and Goldman).

Economic criteria. It is critical that all members of the network support the philosophical mission of economic performance. Providers themselves must embrace the development of a low cost clinically effective service. This incorporates competitive pricing, and assures the least restrictive level of care. From the clinical point of view, a solution focused, time sensitive treatment approach to client care is essential (See chapter by Ludwig and Moltz). It is important to note that outlier cases cannot be resolved in short term treatment or time effective therapy. However, it is essential to understand that the core of treatment can adapt these practices and that longer term therapy certainly can be given consideration when criteria are met. The goal is to have the number of outlier cases be a small percentage of the total clinical activity. Managed care has provided opportunities to redesign treatment techniques which allow for creative use of client time and therapeutic intervention. The last element of economic consideration involves the support of new programs and alternative delivery systems which might include: in home care, intensive outpatient treatment, crisis intervention/diversion programs and community-based support groups. Many of the 1915(b) and 1115(b) Medicaid waivers that have been granted to states delineate these clinical settings as desirable alternatives to historically limited Medicaid benefit designs. Any creative programming must be cost effective, expedite treatment and promote positive clinical outcomes.

Capacity to "partner". The organizational dynamics of a network require that providers share the business and clinical goals and objectives as well as the leadership and direction of the organization. To that end each of the founding members needs to accept that there will be a horizontal (or team) management which replaces the traditional vertical model of hierarchy. The capacity to partner also involves clinicians supporting an improved process to transition clients from one service to another anticipating the next program or level of service. In order to motivate the transfer of clients, the economic incentives for the system must also be aligned. Any financial disadvantage of losing a case must be replaced by incentives for having high degrees of clinical outcome at each level of care. Lastly, a willingness to pool resources to reduce operating costs and finance new systems for the network is an absolute requirement. It is one thing for people to agree on policy, but it is a far greater commitment for them to agree on financial contribution, economic sharing, joint billing systems, contracting methods, and pricing strategies.

Promote affiliate relationships. One of the major shifts in relationships between providers is that competing for market share has shifted from "going it alone" to creating networks, joint ventures, and mergers. A clear benefit of these unions is that diverse markets can now be served by a broader group of providers who integrate broadly based programs and services. For example, the public sector has had a strong emphasis in child services, services to persons with SPMI, crisis services, and drug and alcohol programs and the private sector has had traditional emphasis in free standing inpatient programs and multi-disciplinary private mental health practices. Networks can blend these systems into fewer isolated product lines. Alliances can also be promoted with primary care providers who control distribution of specialty services within HMOs and PPOs and multi-specialty medical practices who frequently need behavioral health care providers to supplement their practices. Finally, general hospitals with or without psychiatric inpatient services can be greatly enhanced by joining integrated delivery systems multi-level behavioral health care providers.

Other important potential affiliates are managed care programs such as managed care companies, HMOs, PPOs and EAPs who may seek opportunities to integrate and protect their market through affiliation with managed care friendly and competent provider networks. Many agencies naively believe that partnering with a managed care organization will eliminate their need to build a new infrastructure. In fact, managed care organizations prefer to have the provider networks come to them fully prepared and qualified to do business with their own systems in place.

INFRASTRUCTURE

The tangible systems developed and operated by the network provide an infrastructure which carries out the administrative and clinical operating system requirements. These systems must be efficiently organized and operated.

Single point of access. The clinical protocols and the credentials of the staff performing single point of access are carefully examined by many third party payers and the standards that any network must meet should be determined by regional market demand. Clinical protocols are available in sample procedure manuals and computer software which can be easily adapted for network use. The clinical resources of the network must be immediately available so each agency must create reception procedures which allow referral to be easily facilitated. In advanced systems, access to scheduling, electronically or manually, is also available.

Twenty-four hour medical and emergency coverage. The network must develop an on-call rotating system for physician coverage which should be in writing and scheduled in advance. Statistics as well as incidents occurring from lapses in on-call responsiveness and client disposition must also be maintained in order to provide a method to review and enhance system performance.

Standardized quality assurance reports. Monthly statistical reports must be developed for analysis and feedback. Incident reporting must be comprehensive to document any unusual or negative events surrounding treatment and/or involuntary terminations. It is critical that terminations are recorded in a timely fashion as statistical analyses of cost per case, number of visits per case and provider profiles for cost per case will not have a uniform statistical base. Client grievance procedures should also be standardized so that follow-up and problem resolution can be uniformly administered.

Outcomes and client satisfaction. It is strongly recommended that all members of the network be required to participate in unified outcome and client satisfaction studies and the database produce monthly statistics which are circulated to all members which indicate current levels of performance. There are a broad variety of products on the market from which to choose.

Case management, treatment and credentialling protocols. Standardized methodologies with written policy and procedures should be agreed upon within the network for case management, treatment protocols and credentialling. Many third party payers will want to audit these documents to verify consistency among the network providers. The network should develop a unified credentialling process including primary source verification (NCQA standard), documentation requirements, clinical experience, educational background checks, as well as the provider/institutional applications. Provider networks have a tendency to include or exclude members based solely upon community reputation, professional relationship and/or political agenda. Adhering to strict credentialling protocol will not only limit potential liability but also insure that higher clinical standards are being set by the network.

Medical records. A network goal should be to establish a standardized medical record format. The elements of the record which should initially be uniform would include the initial assessment, the initial evaluation, the face sheet, the treatment plan, progress notes, after care plan and discharge summary. One of the potential benefits of forming a network is to standardize records and streamline them to eliminate excessive documentation, duplication, and extraneous materials and content. In considering electronic medical record systems, a number of products are now available which have been specifically designed for behavioral health care and not only include the elements described herein but also may have simplified case documentation.

FINANCIAL REIMBURSEMENT FLEXIBILITY

The evolution of financial relationships between providers and third party payers has shifted from a standard fee-for-service or negotiated rates to newer methodologies which have the providers, individually or through a network, share some of the risk. Case rates which evolved from the Medicare Diagnostic Related Groups (DRG) were the first steps in shared risk with providers. By paying a flat rate for the entire episode of illness, providers have the incentive to conclude therapy in a shorter number of sessions. This established a reversal of financial incentives which promote creative techniques of time effective and problem resolution therapy that rewards rapidly concluding treatment. Case rates are growing in popularity and networks must be careful and cautious in negotiating these rates as comparisons to fee for service must assure that the average number of visits per incident of illness divided into the case rate provides for adequate reimbursement per unit of service.

As case rate is a calculation of the average cost per incident of illness, capitation is a calculation of the total cost of care over an entire population. When a network considers bidding on a capitated contract, it is important to consider historical utilization data on the targeted population. Many times this information is not available or the competition for providing services pushes the pricing strategy to a position that allows very little margin for error or risk. The complexities and variables are so extreme from population to population that careful actuarial considerations must be balanced against the network's willingness to take risk. In any event, providers will more often be expected to accept capitation as a method of reimbursement. Some industry projections conclude that 50% of all reimbursement dollars will be capitated within the next 10 years. Those providers developing the infrastructure and risk taking capability will certainly be at an advantage in maintaining and increasing their market share in the future.

MANAGEMENT INFORMATION SYSTEMS

Elements within the system can include the following: referral tracking, inquiry response, intake, client registration, benefits eligibility, assessment, disposition, referral, scheduling, certification, recertification, treatment termination, outcomes and client satisfaction. In medical record based data systems, additional medical record components may include the initial evaluation, treatment plans, progress notes, after care plan and discharge summary. The financial Management Information Systems would be similar to those historically available in that they would include billing, general ledger, accounts receivable, accounts payable and payroll capability.

Other MIS functions may include a credentialling module with statistical information from the medical record and the financial database such as the number of visits/cost per incident of illness by clinician/agency. An enhancement that is required in capitation contracts is a claims processing system that would allow the network to pay providers for services rendered. Networks should consider contracting for expert advice on software and hardware specifications as well as implementation strategies.

EXAMPLE OF CREATIVE RESPONSE: VERMONT'S BEHAVIORAL HEALTH NETWORK

Vermont's community mental health system has, until recently, been spared the difficulty of adapting to the requirements and restrictions of managed care. Over the past few years, however, a number of national corporations' Vermont subsidiaries have contracted with managed care companies. The state has signed with American Biodyne to manage its employees' mental health and substance abuse benefits. As a result, the community-based providers are currently witnessing an erosion of unrestricted third-party dollars in their outpatient programs as more indemnity insurance plans become "managed". The continuation of this trend has forced the CBHPOs, which wish to hold on to their outpatient business, to accept the inevitability of managed care and find ways to make it work for them.

Consequently, the Vermont CBHPOs organized and incorporated as a Behavioral Health Network (BHN), and were able to capitalize on their strengths as a "network" by negotiating collectively for their first major managed care contract. In 1991, American Biodyne and the Vermont Council of Community Mental Health Services worked together to come up with a general agreement that would guide individual negotiations between Biodyne and each CBHPO. This approach reduced administrative time for both parties, while giving the providers greater clout than if each organization had contracted independently. A major concession granted by Biodyne was the recognition of the organizations as the actual providers, who in turn were given the authority to credential and approve the staff as they deemed appropriate to provide managed care services. Biodyne required tangible evidence that the providers were up to this task and requested state certification for the CBHPOs participating in the contract. Another success for the organizations was the rewording of what was identified as an "appropriate service" from "medically necessary" to "clinically necessary". As a result, standards of care other than a physician's (such as a psychologist's, a nurse's, or a social worker's) could be used to determine acceptable levels of treatment in a given case. This was a relevant factor in rural Vermont.

Currently, as the prospect of PSMC looms on the horizon in Vermont, BHN has formed a joint venture with another managed care company, Options, to compete for control of the PSMC dollars; Biodyne has become their major competitor. The ultimate implications of these types of partnerships for traditional public sector nonprofits remain unclear; nonetheless certain trends seen to be emerging. First, the concept of partnership with a managed care company is still a new one, and both sides are still learning more about each other's corporate cultures. In particular, the strategy of "choosing sides" with one payer or provider group to compete against other payers or providers may run counter to CBHPOs' natural inclination to design inclusive systems which are highly collaborative. Also, managed care remains unfamiliar to some community-based providers whose revenues have historically been more dependent on government subsidy than on individual consumer choice. Finally, the providers themselves are undergoing major internal organizational and operational changes in order to remain viable within the increasingly competitive healthcare environment.

Outside of Vermont, a major impact of the development of BHN has been the expansion of similar networks in other states (e.g., Maine, New Hampshire). Even where no formal managed care partnership exists, state provider associations have played a role in designing and evaluating the PSMC system, and in providing support for CBHPO members to become more managed-care ready. For the most part, however, these networks have not figured out how to exercise their potential power most effectively; this remains a major challenge.

Survival Tips
Developing Community Based Provider Networks Develop a clear, consensual mission. Develop the clinical and management structure prior to incorporation. Create categories of membership. Initiate specific planning taskforces dealing with organization, finance, clinical operations, provider relations, MIS, and marketing. Create network-wide clinical programs that are visible and relevant, e.g. 24-hour mobile crisis services, centralized triage, utilization management. Be selective in adding members. Promote the shared values and vision derived from the mission statement. Develop an effective clinical and management network infrastructure. Emphasize: ethical business practices, use of least restrictive care, pooling of resources, economically competitive pricing, collective governance with clear structure, optimizing access, and facilitation of new membership to promote expansion.

CONCLUSION

The market pressures of assembling well managed and integrated delivery systems are omnipresent. The uncompromising principles in developing a viable organization require integrity in ethical conduct, clinical competence, economic competitiveness, shared financial and operating systems and a genuine dedication to partnership oriented management. Building in successful network requires customer driven clinical programming, access, infrastructure development, electronic data and reporting systems, financial pooling and risk taking, and an aggressive competitive marketing plan. The ongoing organization and management of these activities require a new dimension of leadership, sharing and communication that can reshape our industry with long term economic benefits to deliver more services to more people at a better price.

13

Utilization Management

PART I: UTILIZATION MANAGEMENT TECHNIQUES
BENTSON McFARLAND and KENNETH MINKOFF
PART II: UTILIZATION GUIDELINES, PRACTICE
STANDARDS, and TRAINING INITIATIVES
BRENDA ROMAN and ANN MORRISON

OVERVIEW

Utilization management is a major focus of both private and public sector managed care. It can be defined as "the attempt to control cost and improve outcome by managing the utilization of services by clients and the provision of services by clinicians in programs" (Glazer, 1992a).

Utilization management can be both external, performed by a utilization review company or managed care organization external to the provider, or internal, performed by the provider itself. Utilization management can also occur on the system level (e.g., a statewide managed care effort), the program or agency level, the service level (e.g., inpatient treatment) or the individual provider level. Part I focuses on techniques of utilization management and Part II describes ways that providers can adapt to the utilization process and how to effectively relate to utilization reviewers.

PART I: TECHNIQUES OF UTILIZATION MANAGEMENT

There are a variety of techniques for utilization management in public sector managed care (PSMC) that can be applied internally or externally and at different levels of focus. These are provider selection, service limitation, continuum development, and financial incentives and risk sharing, which are described in the next sections.

PROVIDER SELECTION

Provider selection serves the function of utilization management in three major ways. First, network development limits the numbers of various types of services (e.g., inpatient beds) or providers (e.g., psychiatrists) to reduce pressure for increased utilization resulting from oversupply. Second, credentialling selects providers using criteria that include demonstrated capacity to manage utilization successfully (through providing historical data on average length of stay or average number of outpatient visits per treatment episode) and to work collaboratively with utilization reviewers. Third, profiling reviews providers' current utilization patterns and uses that data both as corrective feedback and to influence referral patterns. Profiling may also incorporate client outcomes and satisfaction data. In some private networks, profiling results in a small fraction of "low utilization" providers receiving the bulk of outpatient referrals (Hymowitz and Pollock, 1995). Clearly this type of strategy must be used much more cautiously in public settings that serve persons with SPMI.

SERVICE LIMITATION

External managed care or utilization review companies exert their influence on utilization through their power to authorize payment for services provided. Internal utilization management may function as the proactive mechanism to ensure that planned services fit defined authorization limits so that struggles over external authorization occur less frequently. Internal utilization management may also be empowered, especially in capitated systems, to deny credit (e.g., for productivity or for internal payment) to clinicians or programs that provide unauthorized services. Service limitation usually involves processes of utilization review, which in turn may include one or more of the following components: prior authorization, concurrent review, and retrospective review or audit.

Service limitation occurs administratively through *benefit limitations* and clinically through *medical necessity determinations* (utilization review). Benefit limitations are payment limits that are built into the payer's or MCO's authorized benefit structure, independent of clinical status. Examples of this are per episode limits, calendar limits, or lifetime limits on outpatient visits, inpatient days, or expenditures. Some MCOs or insurers have individualized case management (ICM) programs which permit flexibility of benefit limitations for selected high utilization or at-risk clients. Another form of benefit limitation may involve restriction of coverage of certain "untreatable diagnoses" (e.g., conduct disorder), specific level of care (e.g., day treatment), types of care (residential), types of care giver (e.g., unlicensed), or patterns of care (e.g., chronic custodial care) (Glazer, 1992b).

Medical necessity determinations classically involve assessment of whether the intensity of service (IS) provided matches the severity of illness (SI) (Jacobs & Camprey, 1991), and whether the proposed treatments meet effectiveness and efficiency criteria for treating the patient's condition. This process involves evaluation of the following criteria:

1. *Illness Criteria*

First the client must have a DSM-IV defined illness that is the focus of treatment. V-Codes (e.g., family conflict) are usually excluded. As PSMC spreads, the focus on "illness" may be problematic for some CMHCs who would have prided themselves on avoiding the medical model in developing a more egalitarian, non-stigmatizing, or rehabilitative approach to service delivery. This can be particularly true in agencies which specialize in using family systems approaches to treating children.

2. *Medical Care Criteria*

The services provided must be defined as medical care, thus, services regarded as "social" (e.g., club houses), "residential" (e.g., halfway houses), or "recreational" (e.g., activity programs) are likely to be excluded from reimbursement even though they may be necessary components of care for a person with SPMI. The boundary for what is considered medically reimbursable care is not clear-cut. In different states, payers and systems draw the line differently. Many non-medical CMHCs or professionals prefer the term clinically necessary. Although this was actually adopted in one state, it is not in general use. Regardless of the term used, systems moving towards PSMC must be clear about how non-medical but necessary care, like housing, will continue to be funded.

3. *Necessity Criteria*

The determination of how much of what kind of care is necessary is probably the issue associated with most controversy in any type of managed mental health care. Necessary treatment is defined as effective treatment in the most efficient manner possible which is required to alleviate symptoms, improve significant role functioning, maintain safety, and prevent deterioration. Desirable treatment, on the other hand, is something which may be beneficial but is not required for alleviation of symptoms or to prevent deterioration of functioning. Patients requesting therapy for "personal growth" or patients who wish to be hospitalized for a "rest" from family pressures are clearly seeking desirable but not necessary services. The issue becomes more complex when it is not the type but the amount of service that is at issue: a patient who would benefit from twice-weekly therapy but only needs once per week treatment or who would appreciate the support of an additional week of day hospital but does not really need it. In these instances, the distinction between necessary and desirable can challenge clinical judgment and create problems in the provider's relationship to both the payer or the utilization manager and the client. One of the most significant challenges facing PSMC, MCOs, and providers is the development of clear, objective, operational, and workable criteria for distinguishing necessity from desirability (Cigna, 1991). This will be discussed in more detail below.

4. *Effectiveness Criteria*

An effective intervention is an accepted treatment for the defined condition that is likely to result in improvement of target symptoms, attainment of defined goals or prevention of deterioration.

In order to document meeting effectiveness criteria for internal or external utilization reviewers, clinicians must be prepared to develop and discuss a treatment plan which describes in measurable, behavioral terms how the effectiveness of that plan's outcome will be determined and how transition to the next phase of treatment will be accomplished.

Challenges in identifying effectiveness criteria in public sector settings relate to the following issues:

- How to develop targeted, focused interventions for clients with chronic non-psychotic conditions (e.g., conduct or character disorders) which may be ultimately incurable and for which at-risk utilization management entities might be under incentives or pressure to deny any service that is futile (Flynn, 1994; McFarland and George, 1995).

- How to justify continuing services for stable clients with SPMI for whom no short-term improvement in functioning is anticipated (Gerson, 1994; Flynn, 1994).

- How to distinguish reimbursable treatment programs (e.g., day treatment and residential treatment) from support programs (e.g., social clubs and half-way houses).

- How to determine when hospitalization of individuals with SPMI or individuals who are chronically at risk of harming others (e.g., habitual sex offenders) stops being active treatment at hospital level of care and becomes merely custodial or protective.

In each instance, the solution to the challenge involves being able to develop treatment plans which identify attainable and necessary goals with specific and time-limited interventions. For example, a clinician treating an adolescent with conduct disorder involving aggressiveness at home requests ten sessions of individual psychotherapy to "develop trust, build self-esteem, and improve behavior". The request is likely to be denied with the comment that the treatment is unfocused and probably ineffective.

A second clinician with a similar case requests six individual sessions to "identify family and interpersonal situations which lead to anger and aggressiveness, and to develop and practice alternative methods of anger management." Four additional family sessions are requested to "observe how those situations emerge in vivo, to engage the family in supporting alternative strategies, and rehearsing their implementation". This plan is more specific and focused and is more likely to be approved even though it is requesting more costly services.

5. *Efficiency Criteria*

Efficiency is defined as *the least intensive and least expensive service plan that is sufficiently intensive to address the patient's needs.* In short, there must be a fit between intensity of service criteria and severity of illness criteria for each intervention. Efficiency generally involves the application of level of care criteria (often daily) to determine appropriateness of service intensity (hospital vs. crisis residential vs. day hospital) during acute episodes and application of *population based utilization standards* to determine normative expectations for ongoing service in patients who may need continuing care. Those will be discussed in more depth later in this chapter.

CONTINUUM DEVELOPMENT

In order to ensure the most efficient service utilization, managed care entities have encouraged providers through reimbursement incentives to create a comprehensive range of services with varying intensity and costs to accommodate clients with a range of diagnoses in the most appropriate settings. This prevents overutilization of more expensive levels of care that result from unavailability of suitable lesser levels of care. Sample service types are listed in Table 1. Integrated psychiatric and addiction programs are listed in Table 2.

Case management supplies the continuity aspect of the continuum and may be provided as a distinct clinically reimbursable service, as an integrated component of the utilization management function, or both. Case managers provide clinical continuity for patients moving through the system, as well as monitoring the appropriateness of utilization. High risk clients, frequent recidivists, or system "misfits" (e.g., dual diagnosis clients) may be assigned to an intensive or assertive case management team which provides mobile outreach and more aggressive follow-up. Such teams are well documented in their ability to reduce hospitalization and to improve outcome (Burns & Santos, 1995; Kane, 1995). Assertive case management is a costly service that can be provided at different levels of intensity and cost as

TABLE 1: Sample Service Types

Adult & Child Psychiatry	Adult Addiction
Hospital: Locked	Observation Bed
Hospital: Unlocked	Hospital Level IV Detox
Observation Bed	Hospital Level III Detox: Dual Dx
Crisis Residential: Medically Managed	Hospital Level III Detox: Not Dual Dx
Acute Respite: Staff Support/ Foster Care	Residential Rehab (Level IIB)
Partial Hospitalization	Ambulatory Detox: In Sober House
Intensive Outpatient Group	Ambulatory Detox: At Home
Mobile Family & Systems Crisis Stabilization	Partial Hospitalization: Day
Intensive Case Management	Partial Hospitalization: Evening
Crisis Intervention	Intensive Outpatient Group Program
Individual, Group, or Family Treatment	Intensive Case Management
	Crisis Intervention
	Individual, Group, or Family Treatment

TABLE 2: Integrated Psychiatric and Addiction Continuum

Integrated Psychiatric and Addiction or Dual Diagnosis Inpatient Services: Locked

Integrated Psychiatric and Addiction or Dual Diagnosis Inpatient Services: Unlocked

Integrated or Dual Diagnosis Crisis Residential

Dual Diagnosis Detox

Integrated Dual Diagnosis Partial Hospitalization

Integrated Psychiatric and Addiction Crisis Triage

Integrated Psychiatric and Addiction Outpatient

clients improve. The efficiency of such utilization itself needs to be carefully managed.

FINANCIAL INCENTIVES AND RISK SHARING

Because fee-for-service practice creates incentives for over-provision of services, MCOs may create risk sharing arrangements with providers such as capitated payments or case rates. These mechanisms encourage more innovative and efficient treatment approaches, but also risk encouraging under-treatment or limitation of access. Either strategy shifts the burden of utilization micromanagement from external (MCO) to internal (provider). Capitated providers have more flexibility and authority to design their own benefit packages, but must also develop an effective mechanism for utilization management and a methodology for quality and outcome assessment which protects against under-treatment.

Internal utilization management risk-sharing strategies in capitation include:

1. Salary Model

Hire salaried clinicians (no fee-for-service incentive) with fixed caseload and intake requirements. This provides an incentive for efficient utilization but may risk under-treatment of clients with SPMI. Caseload requirements can be adjusted based on severity and chronicity of clients.

2. IPA Model

Develop clinician panels which are collectively capitated, in which individual clinicians are paid on a fee-for-service basis but must meet regularly to monitor each other's utilization (Pomerantz, Liptzin, Carter & Pearlman, 1994). Within this system each clinician is financially motivated to deliver services, but also motivated to discourage fellow panel members from providing excessive care. This approach can lead to standardization of practice patterns among the panel members (Pomerantz, 1995).

PART II: UTILIZATION GUIDELINES, PRACTICE STANDARDS, AND TRAINING INITIATIVES

Providers and payers operating in the PSMC environment need to develop creative and proactive survival strategies to enhance the ability of clinicians and programs to function in this new environment and to facilitate the provision of quality services while minimizing financial liability and reducing payer/provider conflict. This is particularly true for public sector providers who wish to assume MCO functions or to take on capitated contracts.

Survival strategies involve two major elements:

1. Development of clear guidelines, standards, or criteria to guide utilization determinations throughout the service continuum, e.g., level of care criteria, population based utilization guidelines, and practice standards

2. Training staff in required utilization management skills, e.g., making level of care determinations, treatment planning, and relating to internal and external utilization reviewers

SERVICE UTILIZATION GUIDELINES

Managed mental health care service utilization guidelines are required in two major areas. Efficient provision of acute care services requires "level of care" criteria that permit the monitoring of intensity of service requirements on a daily basis as the severity of illness changes. Planning or monitoring utilization of outpatient services by public patients involves a population based utilization guideline that defines expected service requirements for various client categories. Each of these will be discussed below.

1. Level of Care Criteria

In the most current and creative managed care systems, the concept of a linear continuum of levels of care is being replaced by the concept of a multidimensional service matrix (McGee & Mee Lee, unpublished manuscript), in which acute service programs are viewed as being comprised of three relatively distinct dimensions of intensity. These are the level of residential or social support, the level of treatment program intensity, and the level of case management or care management intensity.

The residential support dimension ranges from involuntary hospital settings with twenty-four hour nursing care to acute residential settings with twenty-four hour staffing and eight hours or less of on-site nursing, to group residential settings with less than twenty-four hour staffing, to supported group or individual housing, to independent group living (e.g., sober house), to family support or foster care, to independent living.

Treatment program intensity ranges from a full day of programming (in any setting) to a part day daily, to a few times per week, to group or individual two to three times per week, to weekly therapy or less. Frequency of psychiatrist contact can be another variable within this range.

Level of case management intensity may also be independent of treatment intensity or residential support. Some patients may be seen infrequently or seen daily for brief check-ins but receive intensive outreach monitoring and case coordination. Others may be seen all day long (as in a clubhouse) but receive little individual case management. Thus, for example, high residential support may have low treatment program intensity (e.g., a locked observation unit with high levels of nursing monitoring, no group or individual treatment, but with intensive case management), and low residential support may have high treatment intensity (e.g., independent living plus seven day intensive addiction day programming with only moderate case management).

Using these three dimensions, one can create an array of service mixes with behavioral criteria that define the service and the severity of illness that matches each intensity of service combination. Other variables that affect the service array include age, diagnosis, and acuity. Utilizing the program types listed in Tables 1 and 2, level of care matrices have been constructed in PSMC settings. This concept is being used by the American Association of Community Psychiatrists to develop model level of care criteria for implementation in PSMC settings.

2. *Population Based Utilization Criteria*

Population based utilization management involves attempting to predict patterns of service utilization over time for average or typical clients in a defined cohort. This is characterized by a particular set of diagnostic, demographic, acuity, severity, and disability variables. This methodology may be used to create strategies of utilization management for ongoing cases, especially for intermediate residential or day programs or outpatient programs. The goal is to limit intensive case specific utilization review to identified outliers and to provide standards for quality assurance. Population based utilization criteria can also be used to determine tiered case rates or capitation rates, by which a large regional or statewide MCO can reimburse providers based on the case composition of the clients who are served.

George, McFarland, Angell and Pollack (1995) have developed a set of population based utilization criteria guidelines for application as a quality assurance process to promote adequate services to clients in the Oregon Health Plan. These guidelines were developed for adult and child patients with a range of disorders (55 diagnostic groups), whose conditions are of sufficient severity to warrant treatment from a mental health professional rather than being managed only by the primary care provider. The guidelines assume that within each cohort a defined percent of patients would comprise an "average" group, an "outlier" group, and an "extreme outlier" group with regard to service utilization. The guidelines for schizophrenia are illustrated in Table 3.

Another version of population based utilization criteria was developed in King County (Seattle, Washington) in a PSMC system relying on tiered annual case rate payments to providers for treating clients with different levels of ongoing outpatient service needs.

TABLE 3: Population-Based Utilization Guideline Example Showing Annual Averages for Service Delivery

Condition	Schizophrenic disorders					
DSM-IV codes	295.00 through 295.99					
Age group	Children and Adults					
	Average Patient		Outlier Patient		Extreme Outlier	
Services	% pts	Units	% pts	Units	% pts	Units
Individual, including med mgmt. (hours)	75	15	20	20	5	30
Group (hours)	75	26	20	26	5	26
Consultation (hours)	75	6	20	6	5	6
Case mgmt. (hours)	75	12	20	26	5	36
Skills trng. (hours)	55	48	40	150	5	336
Day treatment (days)			20	180	5	180
Residential (days)			20	365	5	235
Acute hospital (days)			20	8	5	8
Long term hsp (days)					5	120
Medication evaluation	All patients need a medication evaluation					
Psychological testing	Rare: Individualized assessment of need					
Electroconvulsive trmnt	Rare: Individualized assessment of need					

The King County criteria define the following outpatient categories for older adults, adults, and children:

Tier	Description
1A	Brief Intervention
1B	Aftercare
2A	Brief Intensive
2B	Extended or Maintenance Treatment
3A	Rehabilitation
3B	Exceptional Care

PRACTICE STANDARDS

Development of practice standards or practice guidelines involves creating program based or system based criteria for what constitutes an appropriate treatment intervention for a particular type of client. On a broad scale, practice guidelines are a quality management tool to help individual practitioners adhere to a standard of care. On a narrower scale, however, programs can develop practice guidelines to help address thorny utilization questions:

- When should people with schizophrenia have individual therapy? What determines the length of session, frequency of visits, and length of treatment?

- At what point should depression clients seeking or receiving psychotherapy be referred for medication evaluation?

- What are the indications for long-term versus short-term psychotherapy, for weekly versus biweekly versus monthly therapy? (See chapter by Ludwig and Moltz)

CLINICIAN TRAINING INITIATIVES

1. Level of Care Determinations

All clinicians connected with acute services need to develop proficiency in level of care determination and application of both program based and payer based utilization criteria. This training is so crucial to managed care survival that we believe it should be considered a core competency for all provider or clinical staff, including physicians, and not just utilization review staff. Providers should develop a level of care competency assessment tool based on the criteria and then require that clinicians attain and maintain a basic score in that tool. Training needs to be provided and updated at least annually. Sample assessment items may include rating clinical examples and justifying the ratings as well as items reflecting basic knowledge of the criteria.

2. Treatment Planning

Behaviorally focused, goal-oriented interventions and specific treatment programming in acute care and outpatient settings are also essential for PSMC survival and also should be considered a core competency. While it is beyond the scope of this chapter to discuss treatment planning in detail, it is important to point out that an agency's treatment planning may satisfy institutional certification criteria (e.g., JCAHO) but still not be adequate for managed care. PSMC treatment plans must behaviorally define the outcome which will allow the patient to move to the next level of service intensity and the specific interventions which will achieve that outcome.

For example, in a continuum of care within a hospital and a step-down residential program, the outcome for a suicidal patient to move from hospitalization to residential treatment may be defined not mainly by a reduction in suicidality but by an increased ability of the patient to take initiative to seek out staff support when suicidal feelings occur. Targeted interventions to develop and monitor such behavioral signs are a crucial component of the treatment plan.

Similar issues apply in this case example regarding a recidivist alcoholic. The plan must address what will be different in the current treatment episode.

> Mr. T has a history of severe alcohol dependence with delirium tremens, seizures and blackouts. After a several-day drinking binge, Mr. T started threatening suicide, so the family called police to escort him to the emergency room. After being detoxified, Mr. T pleaded that he's "changed and committed to sobriety." His addictionologist recommended an inpatient rehabilitation program, and called the insurance company for approval. Since this was Mr. T's twelfth admission in the past year with an inpatient rehabilitation stay of thirty days six months ago, that yielded only four hours of sobriety after discharge, the physician reviewer required a treatment plan detailing the ways this would increase the likelihood of a period of sobriety following discharge. The treating physician became very frustrated by such questions and hung up. The physician reviewer approved five days necessary to complete detoxification, but could not find significant documentation to support any increase in likelihood in this patient's motivation or commitment to sobriety, thus denied inpatient rehabilitation.

In the above case, the addictionologist could likely have succeeded in obtaining approval if a new treatment plan had been pursued, as this patient has little hope of sobriety without a significant change. If, for example, the plan had been for the patient to attend day treatment and to demonstrate commitment to going to a halfway house, approval would have likely occurred.

Similarly, physician reviewers will be unlikely to approve any addiction services beyond detoxification if family or other support networks are not involved in the treatment plan. In some cases the patient's support system is so toxic that one must "start all over." Concurrently, a plan utilizing the twelve-step program to begin creating a new support system with involvement of sponsors whenever possible will usually increase the likelihood of approval of this service being provided. However, informing the reviewer that "step three has been completed" will do little to support further intensive services without information as to how this will impact the patient's further success at sobriety. Providing specifics about emotional or behavioral disturbances and the recovery environment, along with specific plans to address deficits in these areas, will also increase the likelihood of approval.

Competency in treatment planning can be developed and maintained by training all staff, including physicians, in writing treatment plans and subjecting the plans to audit. All staff should be required to demonstrate the ability to write three to five acceptable treatment plans, either for their own patients or for sample patients.

3. *Relating to Utilization Reviewers: Program Level*

In addition to the specific skills described above, learning how to relate to utilization reviewers, both at the program level and the clinician level, can greatly enhance PSMC adaptation. At the program level, the following guidelines are useful:

a. *Establish an individual or department responsible for coordinating relationships with managed care reviewers.* In acute care settings these individuals may perform the reviews themselves. In outpatient settings they may coordinate contacts between clinicians and reviewers. Most public sector programs, in which there is less familiarity with concurrent external utilization management, have not developed requisite systems for facilitating communication. Reviews go poorly if the reviewers must relate to multiple or inconsistent clinicians with whom they have no ongoing relationship or trust.

b. *Utilize scales or instruments to help clinicians report clinical data more objectively.* Examples include the Brief Psychiatric Rating Scale (BPRS), Beck Depression Scale, and detoxification severity scales (Overall & Gorham, 1962, Cigna, 1991).

c. *Develop patient registration and tracking procedures that proactively gather timely and accurate insurance information and keep track of prior authorization requirements.* Investment in an appropriate and effective MIS system will pay for itself. Public hospitals and clinics are particularly at risk of approaching third party payment in a leisurely, cavalier, or arrogant manner, thus setting up future difficulties with reviewers, who want data that substantiates the claims.

d. *Promote the development of a service intensity continuum and insure that the levels of care provided are at the appropriate intensity for the levels of care requested and that they are documented accordingly.* Many inpatient programs treating patients with SPMI have difficulty distinguishing acute hospital level of care from chronic or custodial care.

    In order to meet the intensity of service criteria of utilization review for acute care, it is expected that patients will be seen by a physician daily (even if the hospitalization is expected to last six weeks), that medication adjustments will be made and considered in a timely fashion, that discharge planning will begin at the start of the hospitalization (even if the hospitalization is expected to last many weeks), that the full range of psychiatric treatments (including ECT, clozapine, family therapy, individual therapy, and psychosocial rehabilitation) will be considered for patients when appropriate and not simply if it is offered within the facility. In addition, if there are "systems issues" impeding care, such as a family disengaging from a patient, a need to obtain court orders, a lengthy screening process for access to special services, or agency turf battles, these should be documented thoroughly to explain what is being done to address these impediments. Medical necessity may still be approved if it appears that the psychiatrist and the treating team are actively trying to solve systems problems which could contribute to a patient quickly relapsing. Conversely, a passive approach to these types of problems may result in denial.

> Timmy, a minor, was admitted to a public hospital for increasing behavior problems at his foster home. The attending physician strongly suspected psychosis, but after three weeks in the hospital had not initiated any medications, as "the father was unable to come in due to work conflicts." The physician stated the treatment plan definitely included medications but had done little to get the necessary informed consent and could not offer a plan as to how this would be accomplished in a timely fashion. Since the patient remained without behavioral problems in the hospital and no medication was initiated after three weeks, despite this being a discharge criterion, the case was denied further authorization for lack of intensity of services.

In this instance, availability of alternative levels of care (e.g., residential, partial hospitalization or intensive outpatient) might assist the facility in continuing the treatment, because the physicians and other staff would be more familiar with criteria for various levels of service and would therefore be more likely to provide appropriately intense service at each level and would be able to request transition to a lower level of care when the patient could move along.

For example, for approval in a partial program or a crisis stabilization, the patient must exhibit a moderate deterioration of functioning, and the clinician must provide a rationale which best describes why treatment in a less intensive outpatient setting would be ineffective, unsafe, or likely result in inpatient care.

> Mr. D had a long history of schizophrenia with fair control of positive symptoms on traditional antipsychotics, though delusions persisted. Clozapine had been discussed as an option. However, both the psychiatrist and the patient were extremely reluctant to change the medication on an outpatient basis due to a history of rapid decompensation and violence when the patient was plagued by hallucinations and delusions. Additionally, the patient did not want to be hospitalized for any medication changes as "I've been out five years and don't ever want to go back." The psychiatrist discussed her concerns with the insurance reviewer and ultimately two weeks were approved in a partial hospital program with the goals to try clozapine under close supervision.

e. *Develop a policy of proactive utilization management.* Staff should be encouraged always to move patients to the right level of care, even if it means a loss of a higher level of reimbursement, though not if it means no reimbursement due to lack of coverage. Clinicians who are taught to "game" the system lose respect for the integrity of the process and also lose the trust of reviewers, which in the long run is more costly.

f. *Create a procedure to facilitate appeals.* Programs should instruct clinicians never to discharge a patient or alter a treatment plan solely because of lack of authorization of reimbursement. If the clinician genuinely believes a necessary service, as opposed to one that is merely more desirable but less efficient, is being denied, then the necessary treatment should be provided and an appeal initiated. There should ideally be an internal utilization management consultant or team of experts to review those cases and to determine if an appeal is really warranted. If so, the utilization management consultant or team could help to process the appeal or help the clinician to negotiate an alternative strategy.

4. *Relating to Utilization Reviewers: Clinician Level*

At the clinician level, training needs to focus on helping clinicians develop a set of basic attitudes and skills to facilitate communications with reviewers.

a. *Address attitudes towards managed care.* In spite of the fact that many managed care principles (e.g., crisis intervention or brief focal treatment) were originally developed in military psychiatry and later adopted by the CMHC movement (Hausman & Rioch, 1967), public sector providers often have strong negative attitudes towards managed care. These attitudes interfere with their willingness and ability to participate effectively in utilization management. Public psychiatrists have always functioned in a highly regulated "managed benefit" environment, integrating stewardship of a defined population with a commitment to fiduciary responsibility, through a process of "group self-management" (Sabin, 1994). Nonetheless, obstacles to acceptance of managed care arise because of resentment of micromanagement techniques of utilization review and because of the inability to communicate to reviewers that the agency shares a commitment to group self-management and fiscally responsible practice.

Clinical staff need specific training to address their negative attitudes. This can be accomplished through facilitated group process experiences to discuss feelings and through specific education regarding the commonalities between PSMC and CMH ideology (See chapter by Minkoff). If managed care reviewers are perceived as sharing a common vision, they can be more easily approached as potential collaborators to help clinicians prepare to do reviews.

b. *Help clinicians prepare to do reviews.* Communicating effectively with managed care reviewers is a particular skill which requires preparation and practice. Clinicians should do the following to prepare for a review.

- Review the chart and have it available.

- Have a specific treatment plan in mind and be able to justify levels of care requested. Describe symptoms specifically and objectively.

- Anticipate the reviewers' questions (e.g., family involvement, primary care provider (PCP) involvement, and anticipated time frame, etc.).

- Review the plan with other team members and any utilization review experts on the staff.

- Prepare a backup plan if the original request for authorization is denied.

- Try to view the case from the reviewer's perspective and form an alliance with the reviewer. If you have a weak argument, acknowledge that you are aware of it and explain the problems or mitigating circumstances.

- Reviewers appreciate thoughtful psychiatric care. Share your thought process. Be willing to accept reviewers' suggestions or consultation.

Survival Tips

Utilization Management

Techniques of Utilization Management:

- **Provider selection through network development, credentialling, and provider profiling.**

- **Service limitation through benefit limitations and clinically through medical necessity determinations (utilization review).**

- **Continuum development creating a comprehensive range of services with varying intensity and costs to accommodate clients with a range of diagnoses in the most appropriate settings.**

- **Financial incentives and risk sharing to shift the burden of utilization micromanagement from external (MCO) to internal (provider).**

Utilization Guidelines, Practice Standards, and Training Initiatives:

- **Service utilization guidelines through level of care criteria and population based utilization criteria.**

- **Practice standards creating program based or system based criteria for what constitutes an appropriate treatment intervention for a particular type of client.**

- **Clinician training initiatives in the following areas:**

  1. Level of care determinations

  2. Treatment Planning

  3. Relating to Utilization Reviewers

- Do not lose your temper. Focus on attaining the next level of care, not total symptom resolution. Justify the full twenty-four hour intensity of services, if requesting hospitalization as opposed to acute residential care.

- Be willing to appeal to the next level if necessary, but do so in a collaborative manner.

CONCLUSION

Utilization management is a central mission and strategic thrust of managed care. This chapter has described an overview of external and internal utilization management, including principles, definitions, and techniques. Survival strategies in PSMC settings involve proactive service continuum development, implementation of service utilization guidelines (level of care criteria and population based utilization standards) and practice standards, the development of training initiatives in those areas, and the cultivation of effective skills and attitudes for relating to reviewers.

REFERENCES

Burns, B.J., & Santos, A.B. (1995). Assertive community treatment: an update of randomized trials. *Psychiatric Services, 46,* 669–675.

Cigna (1991). *Level of care guidelines for mental health and substance abuse.* Hartford, Connecticut: Cigna.

Flynn, L.M. (1994). Managed care and mental illness. In Schreter, R.K., Sharfstein, S.S., & Schreter, C.A. (Eds.), *Allies and advocates: the impact of mental health care on mental health services* (pp. 203–210). Washington, DC: American Psychiatric Press, Inc.

George, R.A., McFarland, B.H., Angell, R.H., & Pollack, D.A. (1995). Guidelines and standards of care for mental health treatments in the Oregon health plan (10th draft). Unpublished manuscript, Portland, OR: Oregon Health Sciences University Department of Psychiatry.

Gerson, S.N. (1994). When should managed care firms terminate private benefits for chronically mentally ill patients? *Behavioral Healthcare Tomorrow, 3*(2), 31–35.

Glazer, W.M. (1992a). Overview of utilization management. *Psychiatric Annals, 22,* 355.

Glazer, W.M. (1992b). Psychiatry and medical necessity. *Psychiatric Annals, 22,* 362–366.

Hausman, W., & Rioch, D.M. (1967). Military Psychiatry: a prototype of social and preventative psychiatry in the United States. *Archives of General Psychiatry, 16,* 727–739.

Hymowitz, C., & Pollock, E.J. (1995, July 13). Psychobattle: cost-cutting firms monitor couch times as therapists fret. Wall Street Journal, p. A1.

Jacobs, C.M., & Lamprey, J. (1991). Emerging trends in utilization review and management. *AAPPO Journal,* 15–22.

Kane, J.M. (1995). Clinical psychopharmacology of schizophrenia. In Gabbard, G.O. (Ed.). *Treatments of Psychiatric Disorders,* second edition, volume 1 (pp. 969–986). Washington, DC: American Psychiatric Press, Inc.

McFarland, B.H., & George, R.A. (1995). Ethics and managed care. *Child and Adolescent Psychiatric Clinics of North America, 4,* 885–901.

McGee, M.D., & Mee Lee, D. (1995). Rethinking patient placement: the human service matrix model for matching services to needs. Unpublished manuscript.

Overall, J.E., & Gorham, D.R. (1962). The brief psychiatric rating scale. *Psychological Reports, 10,* 799–812.

Pomerantz, J.M., Liptzin, B., Carter, A.H., & Perlman, M.S. (1994). The professional affiliation group: a new model for managed mental health care. *Hospital and Community Psychiatry, 45,* 308–310.

Pomerantz, J.M. (1995). A managed care ethical credo: for clinicians only? *Psychiatric Services, 46,* 329–330.

Sabin, J.E. (1994). The impact of managed care on psychiatric practice. *Directions in Psychiatry, 14,* 1–8.

14

Quality Evaluation and Monitoring in Public Settings

JEFFREY BERLANT, DONALD ANDERSON, CHARLES CARBONE, and MICHAEL JEFFREY

It is an axiom that all clinicians aspire to provide quality care. Until recently, however, few have tried to define it, measure it, and, most importantly, subject their own clinical work to scrutiny. One of the mandates of managed care includes the evaluation, monitoring, and improvement of the quality of care to provide a better clinical product than would otherwise occur in unmanaged systems. Systems of care which develop a superior capacity to provide quality care than currently found in unexamined, unorganized practice should, in the managed care scenario, have a competitive advantage and enhanced chance of surviving in the new public sector managed care (PSMC) environment.

KEY DEFINITIONS

Quality. There are several possible components of quality in healthcare. These could include:

- community-standard care (at least average)
- optimal care (superior to average)

169

- scientific care (using technologically sophisticated procedures)
- efficacious care (using practices known to "get patients better' (Berlant, 1992)
- patient or family satisfaction
- avoidance of adverse outcomes
- attainment of positive outcomes

Quality is known only by comparison of actual practices to an ideal standard; to the extent that the ideal standard is approximated, the quality of care is better. To the extent that the standard is related to positive outcomes, outcomes for patients are improved. In the end, quality is multidimensional in nature.

Donabedian's classical definition of quality as involving *structure, process, and outcome* stands as the single most important classification system of quality (Donabedian, 1980). All of these dimensions need to be addressed by a quality monitoring system.

Quality monitoring. Quality monitoring refers to the process of observing, measuring, analyzing, and reporting the quality of practice as it is actually delivered (Fauman, 1992).

Structure, Process, and Outcomes. *Structure* refers to the components or organization of care: What programs are offered? What hours are they open? How many staff are there? *Outcomes* refers to the results or effects of clinical care, including both positive and negative outcomes. *Process* refers to the way in which care is delivered, independent of results. Structure and process analysis consists of comparison of the way in which care is delivered compared to professional standards for the proper methods for care delivery.

Over the years, quality monitoring efforts have emphasized structure, process and outcomes monitoring to differing extents. Because care delivered in strict accordance with the highest standards of professional practice may still result in a negative outcome, and because substandard care may not necessarily result in a poor outcome, in the end, comprehensive quality evaluation must incorporate attention to both.

Standards. Standards are "established principles against which care or health care providers are measured for a specific purpose" (Wilson & Phillips, 1992). Without standards, there is no way to define quality. Although performance can be measured without standards, quality evaluation requires comparison to a standard. For example, in a certain community mental health center, it may take one week to access care by a therapist. If three days is the standard for acceptable access, then one week's delay is poor quality care; if 30 days in the standard, then one week may be very good quality care.

QUALITY EVALUATION OF CLINICAL SERVICES

There are several clinical domains which deserve attention when monitoring quality. Although the following listing is far from exhaustive, a good starting point for a public sector quality monitoring system would be a series of inquiries which address these clinical concerns:

ACCESSIBILITY

- Do patients gain access to needed services?

- What are the barriers to access (e.g. hours and days of availability, eligibility requirements, number of steps in the intake process prior to service provision)?

- Are inpatient services overutilized or inappropriately denied? What about diversion services? Can there be direct admission to day hospital or acute residential services?

- Is there underutilization of outpatient services?

- Do referrals need to go through gatekeepers (e.g. intake workers, PCPs or case managers)?

- Do patients receive referrals to inappropriate or unhelpful treatment assignments or referrals?

- Are there waiting lists or waiting periods for certain services?

- Is there differential access for priority populations (SPMI)? What happens to non-priority publicly funded populations (e.g. AFDC mothers with anxiety or substance abuse)?

- What is the dropout rate between service request and the first encounter with a service provider?

- What is the dropout rate for patients who have seen a service provider?

TIMELINESS OF ACCESS

- What is the interval between request for crisis service and face-to-face evaluation?

- What is the interval between request for non-urgent service and first service needs evaluation?

- What is the interval between first service-needs evaluation and first outpatient service provider visit:

    With a psychiatrist?

    With a non-psychiatric counselor?

- What is the interval between request for inpatient admission and admission to an inpatient service (or to diversion services)?

APPROPRIATENESS

- Is there evidence in inpatient, residential treatment center, partial hospital, or outpatient records of problems in the areas of:
- Diagnosis
- Safety management
- Choice of therapeutic modalities
- Implementation of therapeutic modalities
- Utilization management or level of care determination
- Longitudinal management of care

EFFICACY

- Is there evidence of positive or negative change in areas which need treatment intervention, such as symptom relief, social functioning, treatment compliance, housing stability, substance abuse?

ADVERSE OUTCOMES

- Is there evidence of serious undesired events during the course of treatment, such as mortality, injury to self or others, treatment mishaps, criminal behavior?

THE PURPOSE OF QUALITY MONITORING

Regulatory requirements. Under federal Medicaid waiver regulations for public managed health care demonstrations such as the 1115 waiver, states are required to conduct annual evaluations of the quality of care received by eligible recipients. States may also mandate quality review of their behavioral health managed care programs and mandate that those programs conduct quality audits of contracted providers.

Marketing competition. Behavioral health managed care programs and providers which can demonstrate the capacity to evaluate the quality of care may enjoy an inherent, favorable advantage in the eyes of purchasers of care when compared to programs which have no quality evaluation or outcome data. This is particularly true in the political arena of PSMC, where concerns of consumers, families, and providers for quality services carry greater weight than in the more "bottom line" driven private sector. As quality monitoring/evaluation systems mature and measures for performance benchmarking across programs become more standardized, public mental health programs which have constructed effective quality improvement systems may outperform latecomers.

Provider performance. Detailed monitoring and evaluation of treatment methods and outcomes can, if combined with an adequate risk adjustment system, provide useful information for managing the quality of public programs and networks. Such data can help identify the strengths and weaknesses of individual providers and agencies, thus creating opportunities to channel the flow of patients to providers who would most benefit them. It can also identify problematic providers, who can be either improved (through consultation and training) or removed from the network.

Structured attention to outcomes may also help redirect providers to focus on currently inadequately recognized clinical issues. One recent study found that general health care physicians affiliated with UCLA and Harvard's teaching hospitals underestimated or failed to recognize 66 percent of their patients' functional disabilities (Silberman, 1991). Similarly, MHMA in Massachusetts used quality monitoring data to identify and address a problem with under-recognition of substance disorders in psychiatric inpatients (Callahan et al., 1994).

Quality evaluation at the systems level is essential to monitor and control the performance of public sector managed care organizations (MCOs). Quality measures selected by the public payer, with input from providers and consumers, can significantly influence the actions of the MCO in developing its network. This is especially true if quality measures are linked to financial incentives. A major area of development in PSMC is the refinement of systems-wide quality measures to more accurately reflect important indicators of quality outcomes for public clients (See chapters by Essock and Goldman; Beigel, Minkoff, and Shore).

Benefits for clients or staff. Finally, quality monitoring and evaluation offers the only objective method for protecting patients against systematic underservice in public systems under increasing funding constraints, and particularly in at-risk capitated systems that create incentives for providers to withhold services.

Inadequacies in funding or service-provision practices are difficult to correct if they go undetected. In a similar vein, quality monitoring allows agency staff, who have concern about undertreatment, to become engaged in a process that underscores the agency's commitment to quality service delivery, and not merely the "bottom line".

STYLES OF QUALITY EVALUATION

Policing versus quality improvement models. Proponents of the Deming quality method and other quality improvement models have contrasted the older policing style of quality assurance with the newer style of systematic quality enhancement (Deming, 1982; Laffel & Blumenthal, 1989). The old styles tend to pit practitioners and managers (or providers and MCOs) in an adversarial relationship, resulting in the submersion and covering over of problem areas which need correction. The newer styles argue for a collaboration between managers and practitioners in a mutually supportive effort at rooting out and correcting problems.

Quality improvement models have several variants, but commonly espouse the following principles (Berwick, 1989):

- Recruitment of front-line participants into the detection and correction of quality problems;
- Organizational dispersion of the work of quality improvement;
- Rewards instead of penalties for becoming aware of problems;
- Prevention of problems before they occur;
- Continuous effort at reducing the occurrence of significant problems ("zero tolerance");
- Focus on correction of inefficient/ineffective systems instead of blaming individuals;
- Open display of findings (often using industrial statistical control tools) instead of private criticism of individuals.

METHODS OF QUALITY MONITORING

Current approaches to quality monitoring are in rudimentary stages. In order to help classify systems, as well as to provide an overview of the choices which need to be made in setting up a system, we offer the following dichotomies. In reality, of course, a mixture of each end of the pair may be found in any specific case.

Individual versus aggregate data. Quality monitoring activities can address individual clinical case material or aggregate data regarding program performance (e.g. average length of stay) or systems level data (e.g. inpatient and outpatient utilization) to assess MCO performance.

Inpatient versus delivery system-based reviews. Peer review activities have long been practiced in hospital settings due to JCAHO requirements (JCAHO, 1984). Because of the critical nature of care at the most intensive levels, quality monitoring has appropriately focused on inpatient care. This form of monitoring will no doubt expand to evaluate clinical practice in residential treatment centers and partial hospital programs (Ness, 1994).

The frontier in quality monitoring, however, will be in the area of outpatient and other wrap-around services. In the past, missing standards for documentation, erroneous beliefs that not documenting care provides legal protection for both clinician and patient, more uncertain standards of care for the wider range of care problems seen in outpatient treatment, and the sheer logistics of gathering and analyzing data for the much larger outpatient population have all contributed to minimal growth in this area. Because most care is done at an outpatient level, however, and because good outpatient care may reduce the need for costly inpatient care and other acute services, interest in quality monitoring of outpatient treatment will certainly grow.

Paper-based versus automated data collection. Currently, there are limited computerized applications that permit analysis of information abstracted from paper-based clinical records. In the future, real-time concurrent quality analysis of individual clinical practice may be possible as it is documented; such a system will require development of automated record-keeping methods and sophisticated programming. With regard to program and systems level data, computerized databases, which may be integrated with billing and other financial data, are being developed and used in many systems.

Retrospective versus concurrent review. Most quality monitoring of individual clinical data currently occurs as retrospective reviews of medical records, outpatient office notes, or some other form of standard documentation of clinical work. Concurrent reviews presently conducted in utilization management organizations typically focus on length of stay determinations. Although the quality of care is nominally addressed during these reviews, this focus is poorly conceptualized or developed in most organizations.

Generic versus focused scope of inquiry. Many quality monitoring approaches have attempted to establish a single method for studying the quality of care, no doubt with the intent of arriving at a single set of study variables which can be systematically analyzed in many settings. The result of such efforts, however, can easily be excessively vague or tangential to quality improvement needs (Sanazaro & Mills, 1991).

In the future, mature quality monitoring approaches may be capable of drawing from a wide range of instruments tailored to offer detailed information on a specific problem. Whatever these narrow studies give up in generalizability may be more than compensated for by relevancy.

Process versus outcomes orientation. Older quality monitoring/ evaluation methods often focused on evaluation of compliance of actual clinical practice with theoretical ideals, i.e., with the "process" of care. More recent trends in the field, including JCAHO standards, have shifted the focus towards analysis of the "outcomes" of care, particulary on "adverse incidents". For public behavioral health services, the greatest immediate need is for the development of standards for defining and measuring the "effectiveness" of care. Several organizations are engaged in collaborative efforts to establish a consensus on determining effectiveness. There is, however, no such consensus established in the industry.

Peer review versus best-practices standards. From the perspective of the individual clinician, peer review refers to the process of critical review of one's clinical work by reviewers with similar or superior credentials, training, and experience. Unlike the standardized, uniform, assembly-line production work subjected to analysis by industry quality control, clinical work — especially in the behavioral health field — is a highly specialized form of professional work subject to appreciable amounts of individual variation on the basis of differences in professional theories, patient values and choices, social context, and clinician judgment. Peer review is frequently used to control for these sources of variation.

Peer review might also be applied to community mental health agencies, whose work is also subject to significant amounts of individual variation. Agency peer review might therefore be a useful component of quality monitoring in a PSMC system.

Some managed behavioral health care companies have tried to introduce "best clinical practices" as standards to be used as the basis for comparison in quality monitoring (MCC Behavioral Care, Inc., 1991). Because of unforeseen complexities of care, however, even the best clinical guidelines may be subject to modification in practice. Nonetheless, individual public agencies or networks may find it helpful to develop their own standards of practice, rather than wait for standards to be imposed by others. Public systems may find it useful to adapt state regulatory agency standards and use them as benchmarks for network quality monitoring.

State/Local versus national practice standards. Quality review in PSMC typically occurs locally. In individual programs, regional networks, or statewide systems, state and local standards, as noted above, are readily adapted to this process. Some observers believe that only practitioners in the same community can evaluate the quality of care, and legal standards for clinical practice have traditionally cited a community standard of practice.

Another perspective draws on the growing availability of national standards of practice. National practice standards for behavioral health have been presented by several national clinical organizations, including the American Psychiatric Association, CHAMPUS in association with the American Psychiatric Association and the American Psychological Association, CHAMPUS in association with SysteMetrics for the Tidewater, Virginia, Demonstration Project in Mental Health, the American Academy of Child and Adolescent Psychiatry, the American Society of Addiction Medicine, the National Institutes of Mental Health, the National Institutes of Alcohol Abuse and Alcoholism, and the National Institutes of Drug Abuse. Current textbooks of psychiatry also contain extensive reviews and condensations of the clinical literature to serve as useful sources of national standards. Proponents of national standards point to the persistence of disproved and idiosyncratic local practices as a barrier rather than a stimulus to quality improvement in a community.

Chart audit versus structured instrument approaches to clinical outcome assessment. Because most quality monitoring has relied on retrospective evaluation of paper-based, traditional clinical records, the chart audit stands as the predominant unit for study. The often uneven quality of documentation, including limited comprehensiveness of monitoring and choice of variables for comment, is not conducive to reliable, scientific analysis of practice and outcomes.

Many private sector groups have proposed the use of a wide range of psychometrically validated, structured instruments for evaluating changes in clinical status. These have included some old instruments such as the Global Assessment of Functioning Scale (GAF) and the Brief Symptom Inventory (BSI). Others include newer scales, such as the SF-36 or Basis-32 for the evaluation of general functioning (McHorney, Ware, & Raczek, 1993).

The Health Outcomes Institute, for example, has urged managed care organizations and group practices to use the Health Status Questionnaire 2.0, an instrument closely keyed to the SF-36. Applicable to persons over 13 years of age, the HSQ assesses eight specific health attributes within three major health dimensions: overall evaluation of health, functional status, and well-being. The HSQ measures changes in both health and depression (Radosevich, Wetzler, & Wilson, 1993).

The most ambitious report card effort to date, HEDIS (Health Plan Employer Data and Information Set) 2.0/2.5, developed by the National Committee for Quality Assurance (NCQA), provides standardized measures to assess performance of managed care organizations in several clinical areas, including mental health. The outcome measure it has selected, however, only tracks ambulatory follow-up rates after hospitalization for major affective disorders (Cordgan & Neilsen, 1993; Group Health of America). This measure is extraordinarily limited in terms of the scope of examination (follow-up visits), the diagnostic group which can be examined, the age range (18–64), and follow-up range (within 30 days of discharge). It is also limited insofar as some managed care organizations increasingly use inpatient hospitalization primarily for involuntary treatment, introducing a major confounding factor beyond the control of providers: lack of patient insight and motivation in seeking care due to illness characteristics.

A significant problem with the SF-36, Basis-32, HSQ, and HEDIS is that they may not be sensitive enough to measure clinical outcomes in public sector populations with higher levels of acuity, severity, and chronic disability. The Mental Health Statistics Improvement Program, associated with the Center for Mental Health Services, has attempted to construct a "report card" of standardized outcomes measures. It has recommended ten crucial indicators for tracking mental health services:

- Mental health expenditure per enrollee

- Rates of functional improvement (e.g., missed days at work or school)

- Individual satisfaction/dissatisfaction with received mental health services

- Availability and utilization rate of nontraditional services

- Extent to which services help achievement of client goals

- Rates of negative health/mental health outcomes per enrollee

- Global rating of staff based on knowledge/competence, manner/skill, informed choice in treatment planning, protection of individual rights

- Percent of clients keeping primary staff contact person for one year

- Rate of follow-up after discharge from psychiatric inpatient care

- Rate of population identified with depressive symptoms and referred for treatment, compared with national norms.

The MHSIP effort specifies some outcomes indicators of particular interest to public sector agencies (Center for Mental Health Services, 1994). These include:

PHYSICAL HEALTH

- Suicide rates
- Specific morbidity rates (e.g., neuroleptic malignant syndrome among persons with serious mental disorders)
- Medication side effects

PSYCHOLOGICAL HEALTH

- Distress from symptoms
- Self-esteem
- Psychological development (children)

INDEPENDENCE

- School performance (children)
- Lost work days (adults)
- Impairment from substance use (everyone)
- Percent time working (serious mental disorders)
- Use of restrictive services (serious mental disorders)
- Behavior problems (children)

SOCIAL RELATIONSHIPS

- Family functioning
- Social support (serious mental disorders)

ENVIRONMENT

- Protective home environment (children)
- Homelessness and housing stability (serious mental disorders)
- Linkage to community services (serious mental disorders).

Specific, standard measures of these indicators are not suggested, but are necessary to conduct any cross-organizational comparisons ("bench-marking"). No single instrument has yet achieved universal acceptance as a method for measuring effectiveness of care (Frieden, 1995, March). It is unlikely that any single instrument would ever serve as an adequate measure for all of the multiple dimensions that need attention when evaluating behavioral care outcomes. The behavioral health field has yet to devise a plausible clinical stratification system for controlling for differences in risk

---

Survival Tips

Quality Evaluation and Monitoring In Public Settings

Clinical domains which deserve attention when monitoring quality:
- Accessibility
- Timeliness of access
- Appropriateness
- Efficacy
- Adverse outcomes

PSMC programs and providers which can demonstrate the capacity to evaluate the quality of care may enjoy an inherent, favorable advantage in the eyes of purchasers when compared to programs which have no quality evaluation or outcome data.

Quality monitoring and evaluation offers the only objective method for protecting patients against systematic underservice in public systems under increasing funding constraints.

Quality improvement models have several variants, but commonly espouse the following principles:

- Recruitment of front-line participants into the detection and correction of quality problems;

- Organizational dispersion of the work of quality improvement;

- Rewards instead of penalties for becoming aware of problems;

- Prevention of problems before they occur;

- Continuous effort at reducing the occurrence of significant problems ("zero tolerance");

- Focus on correction of inefficient/ineffective systems instead of blaming individuals;

- Open display of findings (often using industrial statistical control tools) instead of private criticism of individuals.

Because most care is done at an outpatient level, interest in quality monitoring of outpatient treatment will certainly grow.

The greatest immediate need is for the development of standards for defining and measuring the "effectiveness" of care.

Individual public agencies or networks may find it helpful to develop their own standards of practice.

factors which may influence outcomes (Markson, Nash, Louis, & Gonnela, 1991). Furthermore, the practical aspects of using any standardized scale including managing costs, training, data integrity management, coding, reliability testing, and patient/clinician acceptance — have proven formidable, especially in public settings (Nelson, 1981). Nonetheless, it is advisable for public programs to select some methodology for outcome measurement (See chapter by Essock and Goldman).

A CASE EXAMPLE OF QUALITY MONITORING:
THE ARIZONA EXPERIENCE

The following case example illustrates one method for applying quality monitoring principles to programs in a statewide system of care, using retrospective chart audits to examine clinical care within capitated regional public sector agencies.

BACKGROUND

The Division of Behavioral Health Services of the Department of Health Services, State of Arizona (DHS), is responsible for administration of a capitated managed mental health program for recipients of Title XIX Medicaid funds as well as for non-Medicaid recipients with serious mental disorders. It also administers a federal block grant providing for substance abuse treatment for public patients. The waiver for the Title XIX project requires that there be an annual quality monitoring project. As the regulations are interpreted in Arizona, DHS is mandated to conduct an annual independent review using the case file review method in order to evaluate the accuracy of assessment, appropriateness of treatment, and effectiveness of care. The DHS state-wide system consists of six regional agencies (Regional Behavioral Health Authorities, or RBHAs) which are charged with the responsibility of meeting the treatment needs of the defined population. The Department of Health Services turned to the National Behavioral Health Unit of William M. Mercer, Inc. to assist it in carrying out its quality monitoring mandate.

DHS also had strategic reasons for evaluating the quality of care. In order to promote more cost-effective treatment, it wished to reduce the need for care at inpatient and residential treatment center settings by improving the timeliness and effectiveness of outpatient treatment methods. For this reason, and because a prior study had examined inpatient care, it focused on a detailed evaluation of the quality of outpatient care in the RBHAs.

STUDY DESIGN

The study included only Title XIX patients, consisting of 121 SMI adults and 191 children randomly selected from state rolls of those who had undergone intake into one of the RBHAs during the first quarter of 1994. This sample size provided a descriptive analysis of the state operation which would meet a 95% confidence limit ±7% for both adults and children. The RBHAs were found to be proportionately represented in the sample. The study followed the course of all services provided to outpatients during the first 90 days following intake assessment.

Copies of RBHA records, including intake assessment information, case management records, case management team records, and case management status assessment records, were sent along with outpatient treatment records to a national panel of 11 board-certified, senior psychiatrists distributed in multiple geographical locations across the country. These clinicians were experienced chart reviewers, and records were matched by age group with specialty certification. Norquist et al. (1995), have since shown the feasibility and cogency of a very similar methodology, examining the quality of care for the treatment of depressed elderly patients hospitalized. The clinical reviewers used an automated questionnaire which carried them through explicitly defined questions; the data were then compiled and analyzed by a quality editor. To diminish surveillance bias, the reviewers were asked to use a list of 99 common quality of care problems seen in outpatient practice, but were allowed to add additional problems if needed.

STUDY PARAMETERS

The study examined data relevant to four major quality parameters:

- Timeliness of access to services

- Appropriateness of treatment

- Opportunities for improvement in quality of care

- Outcomes of care.

Under **Timeliness of Access to Services**, the study examined the intervals from referral (request for services) to intake assessment, intake to delivery of the first case management services, intake to the first case management team meeting, and intake to the first outpatient clinical service.

Under **Appropriateness of Treatment**, the study examined intake issues (diagnostic adequacy, level of functioning, staff responsiveness to risk level at intake, effect of intake worker credentials on quality of evaluation, and an overall grade for intake performance), case management activities (compliance with designation requirements for case managers, documentation of case manager activity, patient contacts by case managers, contributions to the overall quality of care by case managers, and an overall grade for individual case manager performance), case management team activities (team review of case managed cases, contributions to the overall quality of care by teams, and an overall grade for case management team performance), and outpatient provider activities (overall grade by provider type), and effects of specialty type (mental health only versus dual diagnosis).

Under **Opportunities for Improvement In Quality of Care**, the study examined the frequency and distribution of care problems, and separated out high from low priority issues. The study also conducted a detailed content analysis of the types of problems most commonly seen in the system.

Under **Outcomes of Care**, the study examined efficacy of care, using a Global Clinical Impressions scale, rating the effects of care on an ordinal scale ranging from +1 to +3 for degrees of improvement, –1 to –3 for degrees of deterioration, and 0 for no change. Dimensions analyzed for outcomes included seven major domains:

- Symptom relief
- Dangerousness
- Overall social functioning
- Retention in treatment
- Compliance with treatment
- Facility recidivism
- Need for other community agencies.

The study-also examined adverse events, including detailed indexing of incidents within the following areas:

- Mortality
- Self-injurious behavior
- Assaultive behavior resulting in physical harm
- Physical injury
- Non-lethal medication reactions.

USES OF THE FINDINGS

Because this chapter is mainly concerned with an overview of considerations involved in undertaking quality evaluating and monitoring, the specific findings of the study will not be reported. It is important to note, however, that this study did yield useful data which led to corrective action plans in several areas. The study has resulted in: *policy changes* including changes in the methods by which case management services are distributed in accordance with need stratification, *structural changes* such as the formation of quality monitoring groups jointly staffed by DHS and RBHA personnel, and *procedural changes* such as changing intake evaluation forms to better meet administrative and clinical requirements. Further, the availability of inter-RBHA comparisons has assisted DHS in tailoring technical support services to each RBHA.

QUALITY MONITORING LESSONS LEARNED
FROM THE STUDY

Despite its limitations compared to an ideal scientific research design, the study demonstrated the utility of the peer review model for acquiring comprehensive, relevant, descriptive, and affordable information suitable for planning purposes. A greater appreciation was gained about the complexity of the variants of passage through the system, which should prove useful in future planning for better efficiency of service.

Although the study has provided good baseline data as an initial point for future comparisons, thereby allowing for on-going monitoring of system performance, there is limited comparative data for benchmarking. The greatest weakness of the peer review model seems to be in its limited applicability to cross-system comparisons, since those would be valid only if performed by the same panel of reviewers. However, until the quality monitoring field makes substantial advances in developing consensus on reliable standardized outcomes measurement tools, it is our opinion that no superior alternative is currently available.

APPLICATION TO OTHER PSMC SETTINGS

Because of resource limitations, it may be difficult for individual public sector agencies involved in managed care to conduct quality monitoring studies of this scope and magnitude. Nonetheless, this study's design provides a useful framework that smaller organizations may wish to scale down to adapt to their needs and means. Such monitoring, using fewer quality indicators, an abbreviated survey tool, a smaller sample of clients, and internal panels of peer reviewers, might generate sufficient data to fit their limited budgets. Whether such an abbreviated quality review would be as valid has yet to be demonstrated. In addition to this framework, an adequate PSMC system should have the capacity for collecting and reporting the data, analyzing the data, constructing corrective action plans for quality improvement, and evaluating the results of implementing those action plans.

ADVICE TO PUBLIC SECTOR CLINICIANS AND MANAGERS

Paradigm shifts. Although "quality improvement" initiatives have been in existence for many years, some clinicians and managers may feel uncomfortable with the changes that will be necessitated by increased demands for accountable processes and positive outcomes. Public sector clinicians and agencies, once on the cutting edge of clinical technology, have often been mired in inflexible administrative structures and insulated from the "real world" pressures of the private sector. As a result, there may be particular resistance to objective quality monitoring and proactive quality improvement.

Some clinicians may avoid evidence which suggests that their favored clinical practices are less efficient than others or perhaps even deleterious. Clinicians are trained to be confident in their decision making, even in the face of minimal improvement. Failure to improve may be ascribed to patient chronicity or severity or to a necessary lag period before treatment takes effect. In recent years, these resistances have hindered programatic transitions from the traditional use of day treatment or housing programs for persons with SPMI to more innovative approaches, such as clubhouse, supported housing, and employment programs, which may lead to better outcomes.

In addition, the prior training experiences of clinicians and managers may have engendered methods and attitudes not easily relinquished or modified with a patchwork of new approaches and techniques. Many clinicians therefore treat patients based largely on their initial training, remaining hesitant about changing therapeutic style and doubting the claims of alternative approaches. These attitudes may create resistances, for example, to implementing family and consumer collaboration in treatment planning, in spite of data suggesting that such enhanced involvement would increase consumer satisfaction.

Other clinicians may highly value the importance of autonomy in treatment decisions, having chosen a professional life precisely because of a desire to exercise individual judgment with minimal administrative intrusion or accountability requirements. Others may fear adverse legal, employment, or other consequences as retribution for shortcomings identified in their work. These are legitimate concerns, which every quality improvement system must address with great consideration and care.

Managers may be faced with similar concerns and may find themselves unexpectedly highly invested in defending the organizational structures and processes that they have spent years developing.

Faced with an evolving system of quality improvement, both clinicians and managers must come to terms with any of the above issues that may apply. To do this, practitioners need to make the leap from perceiving quality monitoring as a form of policing (and themselves as potential victims) to a recognition that it is a necessary step towards improving the quality of patient care.

Paradigm shift number 1: Develop routine monitoring and evaluation of performance, learn from poor outcomes and treasure mistakes. In the past, quality assurance focused on individual failures. When there were poor results, offenders were forced to defend their actions. The risks were high: shame if an error were made, and fear and resentment if sanctions were applied. The implicit theory was to find the bad outliers, punish or eliminate them, and then quality would improve.

The new approach requires broader horizons and broader involvement of front-line clinicians in quality improvement efforts. To improve a process, its shortcomings and problems must be systematically identified and characterized, its causes understood, and superior alternative methods devised. Looking the other way, ignoring problems, or minimizing significance all interfere with quality improvement. Although learning about mistakes or poor outcomes may generate regrets, the first step in quality improvement is to find the biggest problems, identify the greatest sources of dissatisfaction, and work together to resolve them. If a mistake occurs, the wisest system response is to invite self-reflection and understanding of the process by which this mistake occurred. From understanding, a plan for changing the system to prevent recurrences can be prepared.

In this new approach, clinicians and managers must recognize that hiding problems will hurt everyone. Over time, the performance of the managed care system will suffer, to the detriment of patients and practitioners alike. Therefore, as a corollary to treasuring mistakes, it is important to identify ways to expose problems in the system. Clinicians must learn and be supported to have the courage to do this. The system must protect clinicians who do. Impulses to blame and punish must be suppressed.

Paradigm shift number 2: Become open to learning better ways from peers. For historical reasons, behavioral health clinicians and managers have often learned to function in a solitary manner, developing a capacity to make decisions independently, privately, and immediately. The resulting sense of self confidence is comfortable — but not necessarily best for the patient. The reality is that every clinician and manager can learn from the experience and knowledge of peers. As the scientific basis for behavioral health treatments increases, as it has dramatically done in recent years, the functional need for specialization and sharing of information grows.

In the new approach, quality improvement requires curiosity and openness to learning new techniques. Instead of hearing a colleague's approach as a threat to one's confidence as a therapist, the clinician must continually ask, "What can I learn to do better?" Feelings of clinical helplessness before difficult problems need to lead to the question, "Does anyone know how to do this better?" Slow clinical progress should raise the question, "Could someone else's approach work better?"

Paradigm shift number 3: Brainstorm collaboratively to design new solutions. Examples of collaborative problem solving are not new. The reorganization of hospital units along the lines of interdisciplinary treatment teams and the formation of integrated, multidisciplinary treatment programs have used group solutions for difficult problems. The extent to which these solutions were created, collaboratively rather than hierarchically, has been notably inconsistent.

In a comprehensive quality management approach, clinicians from many disciplines will routinely have to collaborate and pool creative efforts to generate new solutions. These solutions must be based on a heightened awareness of the complexity of treatment needs and the importance of coordinating the delivery of well designed and well orchestrated treatments by many parties. Organized collective action generates a power that makes possible greater achievements. The willingness to partake in such efforts will be required of all clinicians and managers.

Paradigm shift number 4: Expect change and value experimentation. In the public sector, clinicians and managers have often practiced in systems that protected and facilitated neophobia. The individual clinician or manager could regulate change to a considerable extent in accord with the speed, direction, and method of change which felt comfortable.

In the new approach, clinicians need to expect rapid change in treatment methods. As the quality monitoring and assessment process reveals areas of poor outcome, high expense, or high morbidity, clinicians will have to change old practice patterns, relate to each other differently, and learn new techniques. Those who have not built in an expectation of change, of even revolutionary change, will feel blindsided. On the other hand, those who expect such dramatic change can manage and, to some extent, even welcome it.

Paradigm shift number 5: Replace fear with curiosity and enthusiasm. Organizational change often brings anxiety. The best antidote, in our opinion, is an enthusiasm borne of striving to build a better system of care. Having to consider changing old assumptions and practices may bring self-doubt and resentment — or it may stimulate curiosity. Clinicians and managers need to replace fear with a healthy sense of curiosity and enthusiasm about the end goal: how to help patients and programs improve. The system needs to make it safe for clinicians and managers to be open, self-revealing, willing to learn new approaches. The system needs to provide security for clinicians and managers to admit to mistakes, learn from them, and help improve care.

Paradigm shift number 6: Quality management is participatory. Clinicians need to participate in setting practice standards and to examine and improve documentation practices to facilitate quality monitoring and assessment. Clinicians and managers also need to participate in analyzing data in order to develop corrective plans so that poor outcomes and problems will decrease. Increased partici-

---

Survival Tips

Quality Evaluation and Monitoring In Public Settings

The following paradigm shifts are critical to success:

- **Develop routine monitoring and evaluation of performance, learn from poor outcomes and treasure mistakes.**
- **Become open to learning better ways from peers.**
- **Brainstorm collaboratively to design new solutions.**
- **Expect change and value experimentation.**
- **Replace fear with curiosity and enthusiasm.**
- **Quality management is participatory.**

pation in the quality monitoring process increases staff acceptance of proposed solutions.

CONCLUSION

Quality monitoring and assessment, once a boring, mandated administrative process, may become the source for the most exciting advances in everyday clinical practice. The advances of clinical science mean little if they are not incorporated into effective and efficient ways to practice. In many ways, the path to a better future for PSMC leads from an intensive focus on quality.

REFERENCES

Berlant, J.L. (1992). Quality assurance in managed mental health. In S. Feldman (Ed.) *Managed mental health services* (pp. 201–221). Springfield, IL: Charles C. Thomas.

Berwick, D.N. (1989). Continuous improvement as an ideal in health care. *New England Journal of Medicine, 320,* 53–56.

Center for Mental Health Services. (1994). *Mental health component of a health plan report card: Progress report.* MHSIP Mental Health Report Card Task Force. Washington, DC: Author.

Corrigan, J.M., & Nielsen, D.M. (1993). Toward the development of uniform reporting standards for managed care organizations: The health plan employer data and information set (version 2.0). *The Joint Commission Journal of Quality improvement, 19*(12), 566–575.

Deming, W.E. (1982). *Quality, Productivity, and Competitive Position.* Cambridge, MA: Massachusetts Institute of Technology Center for Advanced Engineering Study.

Donabedian, A. (1980). *Explorations in quality assessment and monitoring: The definition of quality and approaches to its assessment.* Ann Arbor, MI: Health Administration Press.

Fauman, M.A. (1992). Quality assurance monitoring in psychiatry. In M.R. Mattson & G.F. Wilson (Eds.), *Manual of Psychiatric quality assurance: American Psychiatric Association Committee on Quality Assurance* (pp. 57–67). Washington, DC: American Psychiatric Association.

Frieden, J. (1995, March). New survey lets patients assess their own improvement. *Clinical Psychiatry News,* p. 18.

Group Health Association of America, Inc. (n.d.). *Measuring quality: Guide for presenting HEDIS to employers,* Washington, DC: Author.

Joint Commission on Accreditation of Healthcare Organizations (JCAHO): *Accreditation Manual for Hospitals, 1985.* Chicago: JCAHO, August 1984,

Laffel, G., & Blumenthal, D. (1989). The case for using industrial quality management science in health care organizations. *Journal of the American Medical Association, 26*(20), 2869–2873.

Markson, L.E., Nash, D.B., Louis, D.Z., & Gonnella, J.S. (1991). Clinical outcomes management and disease staging. *Evaluation & The Health Professions, 14*(2), 201–227.

MCC preferred practice-guide. (1991). MCC Behavioral Care, Inc.

McHorney, C.A., Ware, J.E., & Raczek, A.E. (1993). The MOS 36-item short-form health survey (SF-36): 11. Psychometric and clinical tests of validity in measuring physical and mental health constructs. *Medical Care, 31*(3), 247–263.

Nelson, R.O. (1981). Realistic dependent measures for clinical use. *Journal of Consulting and Clinical Psychology, 49,* 168–182.

Ness, D.E. (1994). Outcomes assessment in adult psychiatric partial hospitalization. *Continuum: Developments in ambulatory mental health care, 4,* 207–218.

Norquist, G., Wells, K.B., Rogers, W.H., Davis, L.M., Kahn, K., & Brook, R. (1995). Quality of care for depressed elderly patients hospitalized in the specialty psychiatric units or general medical wards. *Archives of General Psychiatry, 52,* 695–701.

Radosevich, D.M., Wetzler, H., & Wilson, S.M.(1993). *Health Status Questionnaire 2.0.* Bloomington, MN: Health Outcomes Institute.

Sanazaro P.J., & Mills, D.H. (1991). A critique of the use of generic screening in quality assessment. *Journal of the American Medical Association, 265*(15), 1977–1981.

Silberman, C.E. (1991). From the patient's bed. *Health Management Quarterly, 13,* 12–16.

Wilson, G.F., & Phillips, K.L. (1992). Concepts and definitions used in quality assurance and utilization review. In M.R. Mattson & G.F. Wilson (Eds.), *Manual of psychiatric quality assurance: American Psychiatric Association Committee on Quality Assurance* (pp. 22–30). Washington, DC: American Psychiatric Association.

Section IV

Clinical Program Issues: Introduction

DAVID POLLACK

This section describes a number of clinical program and service prototypes that make sense in PSMC systems. Many of the service models described have been developed prior to the advent of managed care and its more formal introduction into public sector mental health care. However, it is important to include descriptions of these programs or service ideas for two specific reasons. First, these programs are the most logical to include in PSMC systems, since they emphasize the principles of effective managed care: cost conscious approaches to delivering service to the clients most in need in the least restrictive settings. Second, in some areas of the country, these types of services have only been partially or incompletely implemented; the introduction of managed care offers the opportunity to more fully justify and develop such programs and services.

15

Alternatives to Acute Hospitalization

MICHAEL A. HOGE, LARRY DAVIDSON,
and WILLIAM H. SLEDGE

Over the past two decades there has been slow but steady growth in the development of treatment modalities that are considered potential "alternatives" to hospitalization. The *acute care* function of hospitals increasingly has been shifted to such alternatives as it appears that these satisfy several of the critical elements involved in delivering *managed* public sector mental health services. A managed approach, as we have suggested in a previous work, involves "the organization of an *accessible* and *accountable* service delivery system that is designed to *consolidate* and *flexibly deploy* resources so as to provide *comprehensive, continuous, cost-efficient,* and *effective* mental health services to *targeted* individuals in their *home communities.*" (Hoge, Davidson, Griffith, Sledge, & Howenstine, 1994).

With these goals in mind, it is possible to clarify the value and utility of the non-hospital options for acutely ill individuals. First and foremost, for patients who can safely be diverted from inpatient admission, the "alternatives" appear to be at least as *effective* as hospital care in terms of reducing symptoms and preventing relapse, and may at times produce superior results in terms of improved social functioning (Hoge, Davidson, Hill, Turner, & Ameli, 1992; Kiesler, 1982). Second, these alternatives are *cost-efficient* in that per episode costs can be reduced from approximately 10–50% (Burns, Raftery, Beadsmoore, McGuigan, & Dickson, 1993; Fenton,

Tessier, Contandriopoulos, Nguyen, & Struening, 1982, Hoge et al., 1992), and the diversion of a patient from hospital level care appears to decrease the probability of future hospital admissions (Kiesler, 1982). By virtue of the fact that "alternatives" are typically located in the patient's *home community*, the ongoing involvement of outpatient treaters is more likely, resulting in enhanced *continuity*.

Thus for reasons of effectiveness, cost-efficiency, continuity, and location, the use of alternatives to hospitalization fosters the goals of a managed care approach to public mental health services. Our objective in this chapter is to review three major forms of alternatives to hospitalization that have emerged in the public sector. The first is *day hospitalization* which typically provides 20–30 hours of daytime programming for acutely ill patients diverted or transitioned from inpatient care. The second is *crisis respite care* which involves the provision of shelter and supervision in a time limited fashion. The third alternative involves the provision of *mobile response services* in the form of crisis intervention conducted in patients' homes and in the community. Below we describe these clinical approaches, drawing on the definition of managed care offered above to highlight the functions of each treatment in managed systems of care.

Survival Tips
Alternatives to Acute Hospitalization
For reasons of effectiveness, cost-efficiency, continuity, and location, the use of alternatives to hospitalization fosters the goals of a managed care approach to public mental health services. These alternative services include: **Day Hospitalization**   **Acute Crisis Respite Care**   **Mobile Response Services**

DAY HOSPITALIZATION

Three models of partial hospitalization have emerged over the past 15 years, and since these models differ in terms of functions, staffing patterns, and lengths of stay it is important to distinguish them (Rosie, 1987). *Day care* programs are designed to maintain patients and prevent relapse by providing structured programming that is largely recreational and social in nature. Large numbers of patients are served by few staff, most of whom are not professionally trained, and the average length of stay tends to exceed 1 year. *Day treatment* programs function to reduce symptoms and improve functioning in patients who display marked impairment but are not candidates for hospitalization. Programming tends to be moderately intensive and goal directed, staffing consists of professionals and para-professionals, and lengths of stay average between 3 and 12 months. *Day hospitalization* functions to stabilize acutely ill patients who might otherwise require an inpatient admission (diversion) or would need to remain in the hospital (step-down). The programs are staffed predominantly by professionals and have average lengths of stay that range from 2 to 6 weeks.

As public sector systems have evolved, day care programs increasingly have been replaced by social programs such as clubhouses, and day treatment programs have been supplanted by structured social and vocational rehabilitation programs (Drake, Becker, Biesanz, Torrey, McHugo, & Wyzik, 1994). These changes have occurred because of concerns about the day care and day treatment models, including their cost, long lengths of stay, frequent absence of a goal directed focus, and lack of generalizability for skills learned in office-based settings. In contrast, day hospitalization has emerged as a potentially viable alternative to hospitalization in managed systems of care. Public sector interest in this concept reached its zenith in the mid 1980s when the Massachusetts Mental Health Center published outcome data on their day hospital-inn model, reporting that an average of 72% of all acutely ill patients in the system were managed in this program on any given day (Gudeman, Shore, & Dickey, 1983; Gudeman, Dickey, Evans, & Shore, 1985).

The American Association of Partial Hospitalization (AAPH) offers the most comprehensive set of standards that apply to the design and operation of a day hospital (Block and Lefkovitz, 1994). These standards require that programs be time-limited, offer ambulatory services at a minimum of 20 hours per week over a minimum of 5 days per week, provide a highly structured clinical program that emphasizes "active" or goal directed interventions, all within the context of a "stable therapeutic milieu." The latter implies that there is some consistency to the group of patients and staff who assemble each day in the program. Staffing should be multidisciplinary and intensive with a staff to patient ratio of 1:4 in day hospitals that focus on crisis stabilization.

Psychiatrists must provide "supervision and input" as dictated by the needs of each patient, and must be available to the patients 24 hours a day either directly or through negotiated coverage arrangements.

The AAPH standards prescribe that at least 65% of scheduled program hours involve treatments that specifically address the presenting problems of the patients. Survey data reported by Kiser and Prudden (1994) provide useful norms regarding day hospital programming, and indicate that most partial hospitals for adults rely heavily on groups, including group psychotherapy and skills training. Individual therapy was offered by 67% of the programs represented in the survey, and family therapy by only 40% of the programs. Psychiatric assessment and medication management were key elements of these adult day hospitals while the provision of vocational and pre-vocational services was reported by less than half of the programs in the study sample. These program elements must be offered within a program structure that facilitates rapid admission, immediate treatment and discharge planning, and collaboration with other providers involved in the ongoing care of the patient.

There is a substantial body of research and clinical experience with the day hospital modality which illustrates both the capacities and limitations of this treatment approach. The clinical effectiveness of day hospitals has been demonstrated for those patients who can safely be diverted from inpatient care. There is controversy, however, over the percentage of acutely ill patients that can be diverted, with estimates ranging from 15–72% (Hoge et al., 1992). This variation is probably due in part to the characteristics of the day hospital program, with more intensely staffed and highly structured programs able to manage more acutely ill patients, and to the norms in a given treatment system around taking calculated clinical risks. Conservatism about risk, combined with clinician, patient, and family bias in favor of inpatient hospitalization during crises, has most likely produced the phenomenon of under-utilization which has plagued day hospitals despite their proven effectiveness (Fink, Heckerman, & McNeill, 1979; Fink, Longabaugh, & Stout, 1978). Given the tendency for underutilization to occur, successfully integrating a day hospital within a managed system of care requires implementation of inpatient gatekeeping structures and procedures for early detection of crises so that patients decompensating can be identified and admitted to the program.

Once patients are admitted, research and clinical experience suggests that drop-out and non-attendance rates will be high, ranging from 20–50% (Beigel, & Feder, 1970; Bender & Pilling, 1985; Romney, 1982). Similar percentages of day hospital patients appear to require overnight hospitalization in order to manage acute symptoms (Turner & Hoge, 1991). Attempts to refine selection criteria so as to minimize drop-outs or treatment failures have not been successful, and so program administrators must implement practical clinical strategies such as providing transportation to minimize drop-out and developing "guesting" arrangements whereby patients can be managed in a local hospital overnight.

Despite the clinical and cost effectiveness of day hospitalization there have been growing concerns about this modality in the public sector. Continuity of care is frequently disrupted in systems where patients are rapidly transferred among outpatient, day hospital, and inpatient settings. Since day hospital admission is likely to decrease a patient's contact with outpatient providers, family, and other natural supports, there is concern that the day hospital environment can promote regressive tendencies, disrupt ongoing relationships, and lead to heightened anxiety and symptom exacerbation at the time of day hospital discharge. Lengths of stay for patients diverted from inpatient admission do, in fact, tend to substantially exceed the inpatient length of stay for those not diverted (Creed, Black, & Anthony, 1989), mitigating the potential cost savings. Perhaps of even greater concern is that the majority of day hospital admissions are as a step-down from inpatient rather than diversion (Kiser and Prudden, 1994), raising the possibility that in many instances day hospital services may be complementing rather than substituting for inpatient care, producing higher costs per episode.

Many public sector systems currently use day hospitals as a major element in a managed system of care. To improve care while achieving cost efficiency, day hospitals should function primarily to divert inpatient admissions while maintaining close collaboration with outpatient providers. Connecting day hospitals with residential options such as the respite programs described below will significantly enhance the capacity of the day hospital to serve the diversion function. Expanding operations to 7 days per week also enhances the capacity of the program to manage acutely ill patients as an alternative to inpatient care. To the extent that day hospitals do not achieve this function and this focus, they will be increasingly replaced by some of the intensive outpatient treatments which are emerging as alternatives to partial hospitalization.

ACUTE CRISIS RESPITE CARE

While the term "crisis respite care" is somewhat ambiguous, there is a growing consensus that it refers to the provision of mental health services in a short-term residential setting as an alternative to acute, voluntary psychiatric hospitalization. For the past two decades, the use of short-term residential alternatives to hospitalization has grown steadily in the Western world despite the lack of a coherent definition, purpose, or conceptualization for their use. As employed here, the term acute crisis respite care will *not* include the use of acute hospital stays (or alternatives) to provide respite for family members of severely mentally ill adults (Geiser, Hoche, & King, 1988) or the brief placement of such patients with carefully selected families in the community in order to provide respite to families or residential service providers (Britton & Mattson-Melcher, 1985). Neither will we address "hostel" services (Brook, 1973) which usually function as an alternative to institutionalization for long-stay patients (Gibbons, 1986; Hyde, Bridges, Goldberg, & Lowson, 1987; Simpson, Hyde, & Faragher, 1989).

Acute crisis respite care has been found to be *appropriate* for a wide range of adults with psychiatric difficulties. Most commonly designed for persistently mentally ill adults who experience an acute exacerbation of their illness, acute respite care also has been found to be appropriate for young adults experiencing a first acute episode of major mental illness (Brunton & Hawthorne, 1989), long-stay users of day hospitals (MacCarthy, Lesage, Brewin, Brugha, Mangen, & Wing, 1989), adolescents with psychiatric difficulties (Schwartz, 1989), and individuals in an acute psychiatric emergency resulting from a life crisis (Brunton & Harwthorne, 1989). However, evaluation of crisis respite *effectiveness* has been largely limited to descriptive accounts (Brunton & Hawthorne, 1989; Walsh, 1986), or to comparisons involving non-equivalent patient groups (Brooks, 1973).

Most recently, Sledge and colleagues conducted a controlled comparison in which public sector patients referred for hospitalization were randomized to either standard inpatient care or acute crisis respite plus day hospitalization. Detailed results are reported elsewhere (Sledge, Tebes, & Rakfeldt, in press) but can briefly be summarized as follows; in terms of suitability for the combined crisis respite/day hospital option, 83% of voluntary patients who were deemed to require hospitalization met the eligibility criteria for treatment in the alternative. Clinical effectiveness was comparable, with no significant differences on measures of symptoms, functioning, quality of life, or patient satisfaction. The crisis respite/day hospital option reduced costs by about 20% compared to standard inpatient care.

These data suggest that crisis respite programs, particularly when paired with intensive clinical options such as day hospitalization, can serve as effective and cost efficient alternatives to hospitalization for patients in the public sector. Ensuring the utility of such programs in managed systems of care requires a well functioning gatekeeping process in which patients are screened and triaged appropriately. Without stringent gatekeeping, a crisis respite program may drift toward admitting patients who would not normally be hospitalized, or the program may be used routinely as a "step-down" treatment following brief hospitalization. While these uses of crisis respite may seem to fill important clinical functions, there has been no systematic evaluation of the clinical or cost effectiveness of such approaches.

The creation of a crisis respite program begins with careful specification of the desired function of the program, the target population of patients to be served, and the clinical service system context in which the program is to exist. Once these considerations are resolved, subsequent decisions regarding issues such as location, staffing, and management of crises within the program follow logically.

Using diversion from inpatient admission as the desired program function, the data reported by Sledge and colleagues (Sledge et al., in press) suggest that non-psychotic (i.e., depressed) patients are the easiest and most cost-effective to manage in crisis respite programs, with manic patients being the most difficult to manage given their need for high levels of structure. Psychotic patients can be clinically managed in these programs but cost efficiencies are mitigated by these patients' comparatively high need for supervision and clinical care.

Site selection should emphasize a desire to create a normalized, home-like environment, while locating the program close enough to emergency back-up services such as mobile crisis teams or police assistance. Programs should be set up as a home with separate sleeping quarters and common living, dining, and kitchen areas, paying special attention to securing sharps or other instruments that could be used for assaultive or self-injurious behavior.

With respect to staff selection, the program must be designed so that experienced professionals maintain responsibility for the clinical tasks of assessment, diagnosis, treatment and discharge planning, and crisis management; however, this may be accomplished by affiliating the program with a clinical unit in the treatment system. Many of the daily tasks in a crisis respite program such as supervising or monitoring patients and assisting them with daily living skills are best accomplished with paraprofessionals who are more likely to view these tasks as appropriate to their staff role. Optimal staff to patient ratios are highly dependent on patient acuity, with one staff member for every three patients as a reasonable departure for planning purposes. A minimum of two staff should be on site when patients are present in order to respond to crises or unexpected events.

Crisis respite programs functioning as an alternative to hospitalization must provide intensive clinical treatment either directly or, more often, through formal arrangements with other clinical services. Rapid assessment and strategic interventions such as medication changes, family meetings, and housing location must begin immediately to resolve the crisis which precipitated admission since lengths of stay tend to be very brief, hovering between one and two weeks. There must be clear policies and procedures for managing crises that occur while in the program since patient and staff safety is a primary concern. Ready access to inpatient care must be available for those who continue to decompensate. Substantial efforts must also be made to connect patients with continuing treatments and supports which can be accessed after discharge from the crisis respite program.

MOBILE RESPONSE SERVICES

For the last thirty years, public sector mental health systems have experimented with the use of mobile response services to divert acutely ill patients from hospitalization (e.g., Fenton, Tessier & Struening, 1979; Hoult & Reynolds, 1984; Muijen, Marks, Connolly, Audini, & McNamee, 1992; Pasamanick, Scarpitti & Dinitz, 1967; Weiner, Becker & Friedman, 1967). Regardless of the form such interventions take, these programs have a common goal of bringing assessment and treatment services *to* the patient in his or her setting. This contrasts with both partial hospitalization and crisis respite care, which entail removing patients from their natural environment.

There are three major advantages that have been identified with the use of mobile response services (Mosher & Burti, 1994; Stroul, 1993). The first advantage is that the provision of on-site services allows patients to maintain many of their ties and activities in the community. Interventions performed within patients' own environments are more likely to mobilize natural supports and also more likely to be relevant and effective for that context, minimizing the potential loss of learning that patients experience when trying to generalize skills learned in office-based programs. The second advantage is in the prevention of, and diversion from, hospital-level care. Either through a proactive approach involving early assessment and intervention, or through intensive on-site crisis intervention, mobile response services can prevent deterioration and relapse, stabilize patients, defuse crisis situations, and redirect clients to less restrictive, less regressive and less costly services than inpatient care. The third advantage is the ability of outreach staff to respond to the needs of difficult-to-reach patients who either have not made use of office-based services, such as the mentally ill homeless, or who find it exceedingly difficult to do so, such as the elderly. By engaging these individuals within their own milieu, mobile response services assist and provide treatment to many people who would otherwise remain "unreachable through more conventional approaches" (Stroul, 1993).

Patients in crisis may request help from mobile response programs directly, but often come to the attention of mobile crisis teams through requests for assistance made by family or friends, community providers (e.g., residential counselors), and the police or members of the public when behaviors transgress social norms. Typical situations that involve mobile crisis intervention include threatening or assaulting family members, self-imposed confinement within the home due to paranoia, agoraphobia or other symptomatology, and agitation or disorientation in public places (Gillig, Dumaine & Hillard, 1990).

As an alternative to hospitalization, patients are met at their homes or other community locations and provided intensive services and supports for up to several times a day, several days a week until the crisis is resolved. These services include engagement, assessment, treatment, disposition and follow-up. Engagement, particularly for patients reluctant to accept treatment, is critical, although the crisis nature of mobile responses makes it imperative that a working alliance focused on presenting problems be formed rapidly. Assessment and treatment are conceptualized from an acute care perspective, with a focus primarily on the immediate presenting issues and needs that precipitated the crisis situation. Interventions include the provision of medications and support, as well as a variety of techniques practiced on-site to stabilize the patient's milieu such as conflict mediation, problem-solving, family and community interventions, environmental modification and the mobilization of natural supports such as the patient's friends and co-workers. Stabilization of the acute episode leads to the formulation of a disposition that involves referral and linkage to on-going resources and supports, such as ambulatory psychiatric services, social and vocational rehabilitation programs, self-help and peer support groups, and other medical and social service providers. To ensure crisis resolution and effectiveness in the referrals and linkages made, mobile crisis staff may also conduct follow-up visits to the patient to facilitate the on-going processes of engagement in and use of services and supports.

Mobile crisis teams are interdisciplinary in nature, including psychiatrists and psychologists as well as nurses, social workers and paraprofessionals. Outreach is usually conducted by teams of at least two staff, who may be equipped with communication equipment such as beepers and/or cellular phones to facilitate their immediate response and to arrange for back-up from their own team or for police and ambulance support. Mobile crisis programs vary in terms of hours of operation from 24 hours a day, seven days a week to the more common pattern of maintaining mobile capacity from early morning to late evening each day. These programs are typically operated out of emergency rooms or other acute service components of hospitals and community mental health centers. Most programs set criteria for eligibility for mobile crisis services, targeting specific patient groups within a defined geographic area such as severe and prolonged mentally ill patients currently experiencing acute psychiatric distress, or those patients who will not or cannot access services through other means. Patients typically excluded from mobile services are those whose problems are predominantly related to substance use, violence, or medical problems without co-morbid severe and persistent mental illness. The intensity, frequency, and duration of interventions is driven by the patient's level of symptoms and dysfunction, and can range from a brief interaction to overnight supervision. For situations in which patients do not have supports but will require supervision overnight in order to avoid hospitalization, programs either can provide for mobile crisis staff to remain on the premises overnight or can enter into contracts with other provider agencies to furnish staff for this purpose. Paraprofessional "specials" and visiting nurses can be employed for this purpose, assuming that such an arrangement does not pose substantial risk to patient or staff (Stroul, 1993).

With the continued shift from hospital to community-based treatment and recent changes in Medicaid reimbursement guidelines, states have seen significant increases in the provision of mobile response services over the last few years (Miller & Duffey, 1993). Systems that develop mobile crisis intervention programs may experience a significant decrease in inpatient admissions, with estimates ranging from 23 to 68% (Cohen & Sullivan, 1990; Fenton et al., 1979; Hoult & Reynolds, 1984; Muijen, Marks, Connolly, & Audini, 1992; Smith, Fenton, Benoit, & Barzell, 1976; Stroul, 1993; Tamayo, January, Peet, & Benditsky, 1990). A major concern associated with the development and successful implementation of these programs has been the safety of the staff (Stroul, 1993). Programs differ in terms of criteria for the involvement of police in conducting mobile crisis. Some programs will send staff only to familiar areas in cases in which patients are known not to pose any potential for violence, while other programs will send staff to unknown areas to assess unknown patients, but with police support. Programs also differ in terms of their agreements with police on such issues as who will enter the scene first, be in charge of the intervention, and have final say on the formulation of a disposition. In all cases, however, programs find that developing a working relationship and understanding with the police is essential to the effectiveness and safety of interventions conducted in the community.

DISCUSSION

In this chapter we have focused on a review of perhaps the most common alternatives to acute hospitalization for public sector patients, including day hospitalization, crisis respite programs, and mobile response services. There are a host of other treatments which are less well defined and less studied, such as foster care, home care, "partial" partial hospitalization programs, and intensive outpatient programs (IOPs). While the characteristics of "alternatives" to hospitalization vary (see Table 1), the research findings, although limited, are quite consistent.

These treatment modalities appear to be as clinically effective as hospitalization and cost less, and there is anecdotal evidence that patients may express greater satisfaction with the non-hospital approaches.

There are both philosophical and economic forces which converge to promote the use of treatments that are simultaneously the least restrictive and least costly. Thus, third party payers, external utilization reviewers, and many public sector managers will not only press for patients to be diverted from inpatient care, but will also require that the least intensive and least costly of the appropriate alternatives be selected. As an example, managed care organizations are now beginning to aggressively restrict the utilization of partial hospitalization services in favor of less costly options, such as intensive outpatient treatment. Providers working in managed care environments will need to adopt a cost-conscious approach to utilizing hospital alternatives, while actively advocating for adequate treatment of patient needs, and guarding against under-treatment.

Despite the evidence for clinical and cost effectiveness, there is a nagging question about these alternatives which relates to the ambiguous role of episode-focused, acute care with a patient population that requires continuous treatment. Given the persistent nature of the illnesses treated in public sector systems, the provision of high quality alternatives to hospitalization cannot replace the need for comprehensive and continuous clinical, rehabilitative, and social services (See chapter by Hawthorne and Hough). For many patients the occurrence of an acute episode may reflect the absence or inadequacy of non-acute services, and thus stabilization and return to these inadequate services will provide only an illusory and temporary solution to the crisis. For other patients, their tenure in the community may depend on the availability of highly intensive outpatient services such as assertive community treatment or supported housing. The dearth of such services in many communities means that patients admitted to programs designed as brief alternatives to hospitalization must either be treated in these modalities much longer than planned, blurring program function and eroding potential cost savings, or must be discharged to an insufficient array of continuing treatment services (Bond, 1991). Finally, even when continuing treatment services are adequate, it is a difficult challenge to maintain continuity and consistency of care as patients cross the boundaries between continuing and acute treatment programs.

Alternatives to hospitalization are of demonstrated utility in assisting patients to resolve crises and in engaging patients in a network of continuous services and supports. Without such services and supports these alternatives may replicate the "revolving door" phenomenon usually associated with hospital based treatment systems, in which relatively high cost and intensive services are used repeatedly due to the lack of adequate follow-up care. From this

TABLE 1: Typical Characteristics of "Alternatives" to Acute Hospitalization

	Day Hospital	Crisis Respite	Mobile Crisis
Site	Office-based	Community residence	Patient's home or other community location
Function	Hospital diversion & step down	Hospital diversion	Hospital diversion
Intervention	Structured program focused on clinical stabilization	Supervised shelter combined with crisis intervention	Outreach & crisis intervention
Hours of Operation	Weekdays, 6–8 hours per day	Evenings & nights, 7 days per week	Early morning to late evening, 7 days per week
Lengths of Stay	1–4 Weeks	1–2 Weeks	Single visit to multiple visits per week over several weeks

perspective, alternatives to hospitalization are one, and only one, critical element in any attempt to build a managed mental health system in the public sector.

REFERENCES

Beigel, A., & Feder, S. (1970). Patterns of utilization in partial hospitalization. *American Journal of Psychiatry, 126,* 101–108.

Bender, M.P., & Pilling, S. (1985). A study of variables associated with under attendance at a psychiatric day centre. *Psychological Medicine, 15,* 395–401.

Block, B.M., & Lefkovitz, P.M. (1994). *Standards and Guidelines for Partial Hospitalization.* Alexandria, VA: American Association for Partial Hospitalization.

Bond, G.R. (1991). Variations in an assertive outreach model. In L. Neil (Ed.), Psychiatric Outreach to the Mentally Ill, *New Directions for Mental Health Services, 52,* (pp. 65–80). 52 San Francisco: Jossey-Bass Publishers.

Britton, J.G., & Mattson-Melcher, D.M. (1985). The crisis home: Sheltering patients in emotional crisis. *Journal of Psychosocial Nursing and Mental Health Services, 23,* 18–23.

Brook, B.D. (1973). Crisis hostel: An alternative to psychiatric hospitalization. *Hospital and Community Psychiatry, 24,* 621–624.

Brunton, J., & Harwthorne, H. (1989). The acute non-hospital: a California model. *Psychiatric Hospital, 20,* 95–99.

Burns, T., Raftery, J., Beadsmoore, A., McGuigan, S., & Dickson, M. (1993). A controlled trial of home-based acute psychiatric services. II: treatment patterns and costs. *British Journal of Psychiatry, 163,* 55–61.

Cohen, N.L., & Sullivan, A.M. (1990). Strategies of intervention and service coordination by mobile outreach teams. In N.L. Cohen (Ed.), *Psychiatry Takes to the Streets: Outreach and Crisis Intervention for the Mentally Ill* (pp. 63–79). New York: The Guilford Press.

Creed, F., Black, D., & Anthony, P. (1989). Day-hospital and community treatment for acute psychiatric illness: a critical appraisal. *British Journal of Psychiatry, 154,* 300–310.

Drake, R.E., Becker, D.R., Biesanz, J.C., Torrey, W.C., McHugo, G.J., & Wyzik, P.F. (1994). Rehabilitative day treatment vs. supported employment: I. vocational outcomes. *Community Mental Health Journal, 30,* 519–532.

Fenton, F.R., Tessier, L., Contandriopoulos, A., Nguyen, H., & Struening, E.L. (1982). A comparative trial of home and hospital psychiatric treatment: financial costs. *Canadian Journal of Psychiatry, 27,* 177–187.

Fenton, F.R., Tessier, L., & Struening, E.L. (1979). A comparative trial of home and hospital psychiatric care: one-year follow-up. *Archives of General Psychiatry, 36,* 1073–1079.

Fink, E.B., Heckerman, C.L., & McNeill, D. (1979). An examination of clinician bias in patient referrals to partial hospital settings. *Hospital and Community Psychiatry, 43,* 345–354.

Fink, E.B., Longabaugh, R., & Stout, R. (1978). The paradoxical underutilization of partial hospitalization. *American Journal of Psychiatry, 135,* 713–716.

Geiser, R., Hoche, L., & King, J. (1988). Respite care for mentally ill patients and their families. *Hospital & Community Psychiatry, 39,* 291–295.

Gibbons, J.S. (1986). Care of "new long-stay" patients in a district general hospital psychiatric unit: the first two years of a hospital-hostel. *Acta Psychiatrica Scandinavica, 73,* 582–588.

Gillig, P., Dumaine, M., & Hillard, J.R. (1990). Whom do mobile crisis services serve? *Hospital and Community Psychiatry, 41,* 804–805.

Gudeman, J.E., Dickey, B., Evans, A., & Shore, M.F. (1985). Four-year assessment of a day hospital-inn program as an alternative to inpatient hospitalization. *American Journal of Psychiatry, 142,* 1330–1333.

Gudeman, J.E., Shore, M.F., & Dickey, B. (1983). Day hospitalization and an inn instead of inpatient care for psychiatric patients. *New England Journal of Medicine, 308,* 749–753.

Hoge, M.A., Davidson, L., Griffith, E.E.H., Sledge, W.H., & Howenstine, R.A. (1994). Defining managed care in public-sector psychiatry. *Hospital and Community Psychiatry, 45,* 1085–1089.

Hoge, M.A., Davidson, L., Hill, W.L., Turner, V.E., & Ameli, R. (1992). The promise of partial hospitalization: a reassessment. *Hospital and Community Psychiatry, 43,* 345–354.

Hoult, J., & Reynolds, I. (1984). Schizophrenia: A comparative trial of community orientated and hospital orientated psychiatric care. *Acta Psychiatrica Scandinavica, 69:* 359–372.

Hyde, C., Bridges, K., Goldberg, D., & Lowson, K. (1987). The evaluation of a hostel ward: a controlled study using modified cost-benefit analysis. *British Journal Psychiatry, 151,* 805–812.

Kiesler, C. (1982). Mental hospitals and alternative care: non-institutionalization as potential public policy for mental patients. *American Psychologist, 37,* 349–360.

Kiser, L.J., & Prudden, K. (1994). *Overview of the Partial Hospitalization Industry.* Alexandria, VA: American Association for Partial Hospitalization.

MacCarthy, B., Lesage, E., Brewin, C.R., Brugha, T.S., Mangen, S., & Wing, J.K. (1989). Needs for care among the relatives of long-term users of day care: a report from the Camberwell High Contact Survey. *Psychological Medicine, 19,* 725–736.

Miller, M.P., & Duffey, J. (1993). Planning and program development for psychiatric home care. *Journal of Nursing Administration, 23,* 35–41.

Mosher, L., & Burti, L. (1994). *Community Mental Health: A Practical Guide.* New York: W.W. Norton & Company.

Muijen, M., Marks, I.M., Connolly, J., & Audini, B. (1992). Home based care and standard hospital care for patients with severe mental illness: a randomised controlled trial. *British Medical Journal, 304,* 749–754.

Muijen, M., Marks, I.M., Connolly, J., Audini, B., & McNamee, G. (1992). The daily living programme: preliminary comparison of community versus hospital-based treatment for the seriously mentally ill facing emergency admission. *British Journal of Psychiatry, 160,* 379–384.

Pasamanick, B., Scarpitti, F.R., & Dinitz, S. (1967), *Schizophrenics in the Community: An Experimental Study in the Prevention of Hospitalization.* New York: Appleton-Century-Crofts.

Romney, D. (1982). Patients who drop out of psychiatric day care. *Canada's Mental Health, 30,* 20–21.

Rosie, J.S. (1987). Partial hospitalization: a review of recent literature. *Hospital and Community Psychiatry, 38,* 1291–1299.

Schwartz, I.M. (1989). Hospitalization of adolescents for psychiatric and substance abuse treatment: legal and ethical issues. *Journal of Adolescent Health care, 10,* 473–478.

Simpson, C.J., Hyde, C.E., & Faragher, E.B. (1989). The chronically mentally ill in community facilities: a study of quality of life. *British Journal of Psychology, 154,* 77–82.

Sledge, W.H., Tebes, J.K., & Rakfeldt, J. (in press). Residential alternatives to psychiatric hospitalization. In M. Phelan, G. Strathdee, & G. Thornicroft (Eds.), *Emergency mental health services in the community.* London: Cambridge University Press.

Smith, F.A., Fenton, F.R., Benoit, C., & Barzell, E. (1976). Home-care treatment of acutely ill psychiatric patients: a review of 78 cases. *Canadian Psychiatric Association Journal, 21,* 269–274.

Stroul, B.A. (1993). *Psychiatric Crisis Response Systems: A Descriptive Study,* Rockville, MD: Center for Mental Health Services.

Tamayo, L., January, J., Peet, M., & Benditsky, H. (1990). The systems impact of an urban mobile crisis team. In N.L. Cohen (Ed.), *Psychiatry Takes to the Streets: Outreach and Crisis Intervention for the Mentally Ill* (pp. 121–133). New York: The Guilford Press.

Turner, V.E., & Hoge, M.A. (1991). Overnight hospitalization of acutely ill day hospital patients. *International Journal of Partial Hospitalization, 7,* 23–26.

Walsh, S.F. (1989). Characteristics of failures in an emergency residential alternative to psychiatric hospitalization. *Social Work in Health Care, 11,* 53–64.

Weiner, L., Becker, A., & Friedman, T.B. (1967). *Home Treatment: Spearhead of Community Psychiatry.* Pittsburgh: University of Pittsburgh Press.

16

Integrated Services for Long-term Care

WILLIAM HAWTHORNE and RICHARD HOUGH

INTRODUCTION AND BACKGROUND

One of the challenges of public sector managed care is to address the complex needs of persons with serious and persistent mental illness (SPMI). Although many public sector providers are appropriately concerned that application of private sector managed care treatment restrictions may adversely affect treatment of persons with SPMI, managed care also offers the opportunity for both *programmatic* and *reimbursement* flexibility that in some cases may enhance services to persons with SPMI. The best examples of this have occurred in the development of capitated funding projects for provision of integrated services to this population. This chapter outlines the basic conceptual framework for such a project, a comprehensive, multi-level, integrated services system (ISS) designed to provide long-term treatment and rehabilitation services on a capitation-basis to persons with SPMI.

Because of the capitation method of reimbursement, project managers have the flexibility to design a system that more closely approximates an ideal ISS, without restrictions imposed by fee-for-service reimbursement constraints.

PROGRAMMATIC ISSUES

What are the programmatic requirements of an "ideal ISS"? From a historical perspective, early efforts to provide community-based services to persons with SPMI were facilitated on a national level by the development of the Community Support Program (CSP) in 1978 by the National Institute of Mental Health (Turner & TenHoor, 1978). The CSP described specific functional components necessary for a successful treatment system for persons with SPMI and served as the model for development of many community systems.

Over time, research has increasingly focused on two major elements of such systems as contributing to success: *psychosocial rehabilitation technology* (outpatient and residential) and *intensive case management*.

PSYCHOSOCIAL REHABILITATION TECHNOLOGY

Recent advances in psychiatric and psychosocial rehabilitation technology suggest that persons with SPMI can benefit from specialized treatment systems designed to optimize the potential for improved functional and quality of life outcomes. While the specific mechanisms that produce improved outcomes remain elusive, community-based psychosocial programs have been demonstrated to be more effective than traditional methods of treatment (Brekke, 1988). The ISS described below relies on fundamental psychosocial concepts (Bachrach, 1992), which were operationalized in community-based programs involving residential treatment, supported housing, clubhouses, case management, and the integrated services agency model. Several specific programs which have incorporated these concepts serve as model program components for the ISS.

In their evaluation of a psychosocial residential treatment facility, Hawthorne, Fals-Stewart, and Lohr (1994) found dramatic reductions in hospitalization, significant increases in employment, and significant decreases in homelessness. Clients who graduated from the program were referred to as "alumni" and were closely followed and supported in the community. The study compared outcomes for the year following discharge from the program with the one year mean of the two-year period before admission.

In contrast to the residential treatment model where clients are required to move to more or less supervised housing options, Shern, Surles, and Waizer (1989) describe a supported housing model which emphasizes the importance of permanent housing. In this model, needed support and treatment services for persons with SPMI are designed and provided for the client in the client's home.

Many clubhouse programs have been modeled after the Fountain House program in New York (Beard, 1982; Rosenfield & Neese-Todd, 1993) and emphasize client empowerment and vocational opportunities. Individuals involved in clubhouse programs are considered members, rather than patients or clients.

INTENSIVE CASE MANAGEMENT

A substantial amount of research has demonstrated the utility of intensive case management (ICM) in facilitating continuity, reducing service fragmentation, making appropriate services available, and providing a trusting, consistent relationship for the client with SPMI (Stein & Test, 1980; Intagliata, Willer, & Ergi, 1986). ICM has repeatedly been shown to decrease psychiatric and non-psychiatric hospital use (Bond, Miller, Krumwied, & Ward, 1988; Lipton, Nutt, & Sabitini, 1988; Borland, McRae, & Lycan, 1989). When applied to the "frequent user" sub-population, the method was found to reduce use of emergency psychiatric hospital services and to produce overall cost savings (Quinlivan, Hough, Crowell, Beach, Hofstetter, & Kenworthy, in press). Despite these promising findings, long-term outcome data documenting improved quality-of-life and functioning are scarce. A recent study by Hough et al. (in review) compared intensive case management services with more traditional intensity case management. While clients in both conditions showed less use of hospitals, improved functioning and improved self-perception of quality-of-life over 18 months, no evidence of greater effect in the intensive case management group was found.

Although clearly advantageous, ICM is not always successful in addressing problems associated with fragmentation or lack of coordination of services within the mental health care delivery system. Case management must usually rely on the voluntary cooperation of other providers. Consequently, it may be difficuft to bridge the "gap" created when providers operate with a sense of client "ownership" and the client has multiple providers. Even the best case managers may have difficulty negotiating continuity into a mix of services such as outpatient, socialization or day treatment services, a residential facility or supported housing program, and an occasional hospital episode. Further, fragmentation within the existing system can inadvertently complicate transitions between levels of care.

ICM clinicians also encounter fragmentation that exists between the mental health system and other involved service systems. Hough (in review), for example, found that the largest proportion of case manager time was spent facilitating client access to and use of social service, housing, criminal justice, alcohol and drug, and mental health systems. These and other forms of fragmentation and lack of coordination can unintentionally produce barriers rather than optimize opportunity for clinical, functional, and quality-of-life improvements for clients. Given the advances we have seen in psychosocial rehabilitation technology, it seems reasonable to attempt to achieve far more than reduction in hospitalization and cost savings to the system.

REIMBURSEMENT ISSUES

Problems associated with fragmentation can be compounded by variations in reimbursement mechanisms. Often, the type and frequency of service are influenced by the reimbursing or funding organization. Community-based program services, for example, are generally not reimbursed by third party payers. On the other hand, more traditional providers tend to orient services toward what is reimbursable rather than toward what may optimize outcome potential for persons with SPMI (Reed & Babigian, 1994). While these issues can exert considerable influence on the design and delivery of service, they are based in the mechanics of reimbursement and not the needs of persons with SPMI.

CAPITATION

Given this dilemma, capitated payment has been identified as a possible solution. Despite early misgivings about capitation-based payment systems being used only to control costs (Bloom et al. 1994), there is growing evidence that capitation may also provide a viable method of addressing problems of fragmentation and lack of coordination (Lehman, 1987). While capitation does not automatically address fragmentation, Lehman (1987) specifies that capitation systems may increase flexibility and offer new configurations of services that are better coordinated and less redundant. Capitation, for example, can allow payment to be made for what the clients need when they need it, such as stable housing, which is not usually covered in conventional systems of reimbursement. Also, problems of client "ownership", limiting case management access, multiple providers and treatment plans, can be mitigated by careful engineering at the treatment planning stage. Case managers have considerably more leverage in the mix of providers if they control payment and are required to authorize services. Lehman (1987) suggests that everyone, whether individual providers or agencies, is required to relinquish some autonomy in order to achieve integration of services. The advantages and importance of a single point of responsibility for client care has been emphasized and documented in the literature (Hu and Jerrell, 1991; Shern, Surles, & Waizer 1989).

Capitation-based systems have recently been initiated in a number of states. In their review of the literature on these systems, Bloom, Toerber, Hausman, Cuffel, and Barret (1994) describe various methods used in the design of capitation-based systems established in Pennsylvania, New York, Minnesota, Arizona, California, Colorado, Rhode Island, and Utah.

Another approach to fragmentation is reported by Hargreaves (1992) in his discussion of the Integrated Services Agency (ISA) model in California. In 1988, the California Legislature created capitation-based funding for two ISAs designed and operated specifically for persons with SPMI. These ISA programs have *no restrictions on the use of funds*, but are responsible to provide or pay for *all* mental health services to clients. This arrangement allows for a high level of creativity and flexibility in the provision of services, yet maintains ISA accountability.

Similarly, in Los Angeles County, California, another approach has been implemented, based on the ISA model and incorporating both psychosocial and capitation principles. The Los Angeles County Department of Mental Health has applied this model on a capitation basis to "high utilizers" of the public mental health system. Capitation-based contracts have been executed with community-based provider organizations in several regions of Los Angeles County. These organizations are paid on a capitation basis and are responsible to provide, or pay for, all mental health services required for the client (See chapter by Barbour, Floyd, and Connery).

SYSTEM OVERVIEW

Aspects of each of the program models discussed above are incorporated into the integrated servicer system (ISS) presented, although the integrated services agency (Hargreaves, 1992) and the intensive case management model (Quinlivan et al., 1995) discussed above are more influential. The discussion presents a basic managed-care system comprised of an array of flexible and integrated services. The ISS can be successfully designed into an existing case management system or can be used in conjunction with contracting private services. However, designing an effective system to produce improved outcomes will likely require more than augmented case management or a central authority (Reed & Babigian, 1994; Talbott, 1995). Accordingly, certain system components, which are considered important to the effective functioning of the system, are presented, although, as Bachrach (1992) has pointed out, the underlying psychosocial principles are the most important aspect.

The following discussion is therefore not intended to present the "right" or only way to design and operate a capitation-based system for persons with SPMI, but rather to present some basic guidelines and ideas that we hope will be useful in designing a system customized to the local needs of a community.

The process of planning, designing, and implementing a system for persons with SPMI may best be undertaken in cooperation and collaboration with representatives of local providers, client advocacy groups, and family members. Involving these groups at the planning level will add important and useful perspectives to the design of the system. It will also help to insure a higher level of cooperation and may help overcome resistance from some, such as hospital providers, who may not benefit financially as much as under the traditional reimbursement system. Unlike most forms of payment, capitation can offer the opportunity to share risks and benefits with subcontracted providers. Involving other providers at the planning stage can help to align system goals and facilitate system integration. This planning process will also help ensure that the system is customized to local needs. As Bachrach (1992) has pointed out, a system cannot be "canned" and simply exported to different communities without carefully evaluating and addressing the cultural, social, and economic aspects as well as the unique needs of each community.

SERVICES

Operationally, the ISS relies primarily on a clinical case management model, with application of a psychosocial rehabilitation philosophy. The most important aspect of the ISS is the relationship between the client with SPMI and the staff of a multi-disciplinary team. The team should include the disciplines of psychiatry, psychology, nursing, and social work, as well as specialists in dual diagnosis/substance abuse treatment, and peer counseling. The importance of including state-of-the-art psychiatric involvement on treatment teams has been emphasized as a major factor in seeking improved outcomes (Talbott, 1995). Paraprofessionals and volunteers were found to be particularly helpful in a study comparing the cost-effectiveness of several case management approaches (Hu & Jerrell, 1991). Selected family members as well as clients with SPMI should also be considered for inclusion as team members. The usefulness of family members in a case management system has been documented by Intagliata, Willer, and Egri (1986). Quinlivan and his colleagues (in press), in an intensive,case management program for treatment of "frequent users", demonstrated that selected clients can be effective and helpful as counselors, particularly in working with the more severely disordered clients. The team should also provide or have direct access to other services, such as individual, group, and family counseling and psycho-educational services, vocational services including supported and competitive employment opportunities, educational, and medical services. Linkage with primary care providers, including emergency care should be established as an integral component of the ISS. Similarly, linkage should be established with other systems that may be involved with clients such as drug and alcohol, social services, and criminal justice.

While all members of the case management team should know every client served by the team, one team member will have a more primary and close relationship with each client. We will refer to this team member as the personal service coordinator (PSC). The PSC becomes counselor, friend, collaborator, and advocate of the client as well as the coordinator of care. These relationships are intended to continue indefinitely as determined by the client. Previous clients should always be welcome to return if and when they feel the need. In order to achieve such a relationship, it is important for the case management team members to genuinely like and thrive on working with these clients. It is also of central importance for staff, at all levels of the organization and of all disciplines, to share a philosophy that is consistent with the principles of psychosocial rehabilitation as discussed by Bachrach (1992). Case management teams, particularly PSC staff, should also be culturally competent and able to communicate in the preferred language of the client.

The client and the PSC collaborate on the development of the personal service plan, which is created individually for each client. Each client must be seen as a unique individual, not just as a member of the SPMI population.

Case management teams should be based where they will be most accessible to clients. Each team coordinates the delivery of all services to the clients in its service area. PSC staff should carry a pager or cell phone and be available on a 24-hour basis. Also, an 800 phone number may be a helpful option, allowing toll-free access to the system by clients, their families, other providers, and the community on a 24-hour basis.

Enrollment into the ISS system can be accomplished by marketing the service directly to clients with SPMI. Statutes and regulations relative to enrollment in prepayment plans may vary from state to state and must be carefully reviewed before deciding on a specific enrollment method.

At the time of enrollment, a comprehensive psychosocial and physical assessment should be conducted. At the same time, a crisis intervention and emergency plan should be developed for each client with input from the PSC and family members or other individuals with significant involvement in their lives. By doing this during a time when the client is not in crisis, the client and his/her significant others, as well as the case management team, will be better prepared if a crisis does arise.

PSC staff should maintain regular and structured contact with clients. At the time of enrollment, contact may need to be frequent. With less stable clients, daily contact may be indicated. Occasionally, for short periods, contact may actually be continuous until appropriate arrangements can be made to ensure client safety. On the

---

Survival Tips

Integrated Services for Long-term Care

An array of integrated system components or levels of care should be available in the ISS. These should include at least the following:

psychiatric hospitalization, including involuntary detention; a hospital alternative/diversion program, transitional and/ or long-term residential treatment facility; a clinic, day-treatment, or partial hospitalization program, a clubhouse program, day rehabilitation and socialization services, in-home mental health care, money management, and housing assistance.

The importance of financial and clinical systems integration and the importance of the client's perspective in the design and operation of the system cannot be overemphasized.

other hand, some more stable clients may find frequent contact to be unnecessarily stressful and may request less contact. Tailoring services to individual needs is a key component of the ISS.

SYSTEM COMPONENTS

Integration of Services In a Capitated System

Operational integration of services in the capitated ISS is a centrally important concept. Whether services are provided directly by ISS staff, or by sub-contract, the case management teams will serve to integrate the system components. Integration will be facilitated not only by careful clinical management, a close working relationship between the case management team and the other ISS or sub-contracted providers, and a high level of collaboration between the clients and the case management team, but also by direct control of reimbursement for all service components.

In addition, integration will be further facilitated by the design of subcontractual arrangements with outside providers. Whether subcontracting is by case-rate, fee-for-service, or sub-capitation, the case management team should design and manage the level and intensity of services. This can be accomplished in a number of ways. The role of the case management team could be expanded to include authorization of services, or, they could have a more advisory role wherein authorization and payment decisions would be made further up the administrative ladder. Particularly in larger public systems, contractual relationships are managed at an entirely different level than that of the client and the case management team. Nonetheless, efforts should be made to link these controls more directly to the operational level of the client and case management team.

These contractual arrangements are an important aspect of integrating services and also represent one of the major departures from more traditional case management systems. Most case management systems rely on the voluntary cooperation of other providers in the system, which can vary considerably. Property engineered capitation systems tend to focus and align the goals of system providers. By design, system providers are working toward the goal of helping each client become as functional and as independent as possible. Careful management of resources and an emphasis away from more expensive and intensive services such as hospitals can benefit both the client and the system.

However, this shift in reimbursement systems may also introduce ethical considerations of a different nature than those generated within fee-for-service reimbursement systems. While capitation can offer increased flexibility and creativity which may facilitate improvement in clinical, functional, and quality-of-life outcomes for the client with SPMI, there are no guarantees. As fee-for-service systems tend to be abused by over-utilization of services, so capitation-based systems lend themselves to abuse by failure to provide needed and necessary services and resources. Because most capitation systems are population based rather than service based, the provider receives payment regardless of whether or not a client receives services. This arrangement provides little incentive to seek out difficult clients with SPMI, particularly those who are homeless and may not seek services on their own. The prospect of incurring increased costs for emergency care at some point in the future may not always be an adequate deterrent, especially in the short run.

Case-rate payments, which are service based instead of population based, may provide a viable option in this instance. Specific services, such as hospitalization, are reimbursed on a negotiated rate per episode, regardless of length of stay. The arrangement may also include a form of warrantee, which requires the hospital to provide free or discounted readmissions within a specified time period. Case-rate payments can therefore offer an incentive to seek out and serve clients who may otherwise go without, and an incentive to provide quality services by linking the service to the outcome.

An array of integrated system components or levels of care should be available in the ISS. These should include at least the following: psychiatric hospitalization, including involuntary detention; a hospital alternative/diversion program (See chapter by Hoge, Davidson, and Sledge); transitional and/or longterm residential treatment facility; a clinic, day-treatment, or partial hospitalization program, a clubhouse program, day rehabilitation and socialization services, in-home mental health care, money management, and housing assistance.

Psychiatric hospital services, particularly locked beds, are essential. The case management team psychiatrist should have admitting privileges at the hospital where a client will be admitted if hospitalization is necessary. This will allow for continuity in the client's treatment and continuous involvement of the case management team who will determine the treatment and the length of stay actually necessary in a hospital setting.

Residential treatment services include structured long-term and/or transitional residential treatment facilities for clients who are not stabilized enough to function without on-site staff on a 24-hour a day basis. These residential programs are housed in normal residential neighborhoods, usually in large single family homes, or small remodeled apartments housing from eight to twelve clients. They are designed to provide a supportive treatment setting for clients who are at high risk for hospitalization, and/or who have experienced repeated failures at attempts to live in the community, even with a high level of staff support. The programs are not presented as a place to live indefinitely, but as a place to learn how to live in the community. This level of care may be particularly useful for reintegration of long-term or State Hospital clients back into the community.

Inclusion of a clubhouse type program can serve as the vocational component of the ISS. It can include the operation of supported and competitive employment opportunities as well as house client operated businesses. For example, a clubhouse could actually be the hub or centerpiece of the ISS system with an array of services provided on site. On the other hand, for some communities, the ideal clubhouse may be entirely client operated and simply supported financially by the ISS.

The availability of housing assistance has been demonstrated to be beneficial in the treatment of persons with SPMI (Talbott, 1995) and is considered an essential component of the ISS. Housing can include living independently in an apartment, an independent living facility, or living with one's family. Housing can also be provided in multiple-unit apartment-type buildings. These housing resources may also be comprised of smaller residential units and/or duplex units and should be located in areas where clients have access to services and public transportation. They can be leased by the ISS or can be provided by sub-contract. The most important issue is that these housing resources are made available for clients to rent.

The ISS should be able to eliminate hospitalizations due to problems associated with lack of housing for its clients. Hospitalization can occur simply because a client decompensates when he or she has no money and no place to stay. Often, clients are unable to independently rent an apartment simply because they do not have the required security deposit, first and last month's rent, and the fee for a credit check. This arrangement will allow clients to rent apartment units without these often preclusive cash requirements. Clients can establish a credit history as a tenant by renting from the ISS. Clients who require temporary hospitalization or admission to other more restrictive levels of care would not risk losing their apartments as a consequence.

The PSC should have the flexibility to provide services to the client in his or her home whenever that level of care is most appropriate. Such interventions can sometimes prevent decompensation and reduce the "drop-out" factor from the ISS.

OUTCOME RESEARCH/QUALITY IMPROVEMENT

The use of process and outcome measures to monitor and improve program effectiveness is becoming widespread. Improvement in the outcome of care should be as important as financial considerations in the operation of the ISS system. Failure to link outcomes to the operation of a system can be a costly omission (Reed & Babigian, 1994). It is particularly important in a new system implementation to carefully design an outcome measurement system to provide feedback on provider and system performance. The ability of the ISS to measure and link the outcome of care to system/provider operation is crucial to the successful operation of the system. An effective evaluation system will provide benchmarks from which efforts to improve the quality of services for persons with SPMI can be measured (See chapter by Essock and Goldman).

In concluding our discussion of a system of treatment and rehabilitation for persons with SPMI, there are two centrally important factors that should be emphasized and serve as guiding principles in the process of design. One is the importance of financial and clinical systems integration. A properly designed, capitation-based public sector managed care system can offer integrated, high utility, and cost-effective services within a framework that allows creativity and flexibility.

The importance of the client's perspective in the design and operation of the system is another factor that cannot be overemphasized (Anthony et al., 1988; Marlowe, & Marlowe 1983). In order to maximize opportunities for clients with SPMI to achieve and sustain substantive clinical and functional gains, as well as improvement in their quality of life, the system must be designed to meet the client's needs, and not the needs of the system.

REFERENCE

Anthony, W., Cohen, M., Farkas, M., & Cohen, B. (1988). Clinical care update: the chronically mentally ill case management- more than a response to a dysfunctional system. *Community Mental Health Journal, 24,* 219–228.

Bachrach, L. (1982). Assessment of outcomes in community support systems: results, problems, and limitations. *Schizophrenia Bulletin, 8,* 39–61.

Bachrach, L. (1992). Psychosocial rehabilitation and psychiatry in the care of long-term patients. *American Journal of Psychiatry, 149,* 1455–1463.

Beard, J., Propst, R., & Malamud, T. (1982). The rehabilitation services of Fountain House. *Psychosocial Rehabilitation Journal, 5,* 47–53.

Bloom, J., Toerber, G., Hausman, J., Cuffel, B., & Bartlet, T. (1994). Colorado's capitation plan: an analysis of capitation for mental health services. *Institute for Mental Health Services Research,* (Working Paper #194). Berkeley, CA: Center for Research on the Organization and Financing of Care for the Severely Mentally Ill.

Bond, G., Miller, L., Krumwied, R., & Ward, R. (1988). Assertive case management in three CMHCs: a controlled study. *Hospital and Community Psychiatry, 39,* 411–418.

Borland, A., McRae, J., & Lycan, C. (1989). Outcomes of five years of continuous intensive case management. *Hospital and Community Psychiatry, 40,* 369–376.

Brekke, J. (1988). What do we really know about community support programs? strategies for better monitoring? *Hospital and Community Psychiatry, 39,* 946–952.

Hargreaves, W. (1992). A capitation model for providing mental health services in california. *Hospital and Community Psychiatry, 43,* 275–277.

Hawthorne, W., Fals-Stewart, W., & Lohr, J. (1994). A treatment outcome study of community-based residential care. *Hospital and Community Psychiatry, 45,* 152–155.

Hough, R., Wood, P., Hulburt, M., Quinlivan, R., Tarke, H., & Yamashiro, S. (in review). Using independent housing and supportive services with the homeless mentally ill: an eighteen month outcome study. *American Journal of Public Health.*

Hu, T., & Jerrell, J. (1991). Cost-effectiveness of alternative approaches in treating severely mentally ill in California. *Schizophrenia Bulletin, 17,* 461–468.

Intagliata J., Willer, B., & Egd, G. (1986). Role of the family in case management of the mentally ill. *Schizophrenia Bulletin, 12,* 699–708.

Lehman, A. (1987). Capitation payment and mental health care: a review of the opportunities and risks. *Hospital and Community Psychiatry, 38,* 31–38.

Lipton, F., Nutt, S., & Sabitini, A. (1988). Housing the homeless mentally ill: a longitudinal study of a treatment approach. *Hospital and Community Psychiatry, 39,* 40–45.

Marlowe, H., & Marlowe, J. (1983). The mental health counselor as case manager: implications for working with the chronically mentally ill. *American Mental Health Counselors Association Journal, 5,* 184–191.

Quinlivan, R., Hough, R., Crowell, A., Beach, B., Hofstetter, R., & Kenworthy, K. (1995). Intensive case management: implications for planning, service delivery, and costs. *Hospital and Community Psychiatry, 46,* 365–371.

Reed, S., & Babigian, H. (1994). Postmortem of the Rochester capitation experiment. *Hospital and Community Psychiatry, 45,* 761–764.

Rosenfield, S., & Neese-Todd, S. (1993). Elements of a psychosocial clubhouse program associated with a satisfying quality of life. *Hospital and Community Psychiatry, 44,* 76–76.

Shern, D., Surles, R., & Waizer, J. (1989). Designing community treatment systems for the most seriously mentally ill: a state administrative perspective. *Journal of Social Issues, 45,* 105–117.

Stein, L., & Test, M. (1980). Alternative to mental hospital treatment, I: conceptual model treatment program and clinical evaluation. *Archives of General Psychiatry, 37,* 392–397.

Talbott, J. (1995). Evaluating the Johnson Foundation program on chronic mental illness. *Hospital and Community Psychiatry, 46,* 501–503.

Turner, J., & TenHoor, W. (1978). The NIMH Community Support Program: Pilot approach to a needed reform. *Schizophrenia Bulletin, 4,* 319–344.

17

Psychiatric Interface with Primary Care

DAVID POLLACK AND RUPERT GOETZ

INTRODUCTION

Although health care for mentally ill patients is often inadequate, and although primary care providers (PCPs), sometimes referred to as the "hidden mental health network" (Schurmah, 1985), often provide a substantial amount of mental health (MH) care to public patients, the mental health interface with primary care (MH-PC) has received little attention (Committee on Preventive Psychiatry, GAP, 1980). The advent of public sector managed care has now created incentives and pressure for integration in order to enhance opportunities for PCP gatekeepers and to minimize costly disruptions between mental and primary health care.

Despite clear advantages and compelling need for integration of primary care and mental health care in the treatment of public sector mental health patients (Goldberg, 1995), such coordination of services is commonly lacking. In fact, public sector health and MH services often are more poorly integrated than private sector services due to a series of unique difficulties. The patient with severe and persistent mental illness (SPMI) frequently has no primary care provider (PCP). State mental health and health systems are often distinct agencies. The public system as a whole is facing a budget crisis, yet it is overwhelmed by need. What can sustain or even encourage MH-PC collaboration under such circumstances?

We will first point to some difficulties in existing MH-PC inter-
faces, then cite some examples of "interface management" tools that
have been formulated or implemented to address current problems.
In keeping with the theme of this book, the focus will be on issues of
particular interest to the public sector.

PROBLEMS

To clarify the impact of managed care on the complex public MH-
PC interface, a grid, composed of **access, accountability** (clinical
direction), and **affordability** (cost), and plotted against the perspectives of **patient, provider**, and **system** may be helpful to formulate
relevant questions. This grid provides a preliminary taxonomy of
problems and constitutes a map against which to review the multiple influences of interface management strategies.

Examples of questions at the public MH-PC interface:

	Patient	*Providers*	*System*
Access:	Can I get in?	Where will the patient be seen?	Who will be covered?
Accountability:	Who do I see?	Who is in charge?	What will be covered?
Affordability:	What will it cost me?	Who decides how much to provide?	At what cost, and to whom?

Various models of public sector managed care (PSMC) solve these
interface questions in different ways.

Carve-out. In a MH carve-out, the dollars for MH services are
managed separately from general health dollars. Accountability and
affordability are therefore more directly under control of the MH providers. Access in such systems may still be mediated by primary care
referral, or it may be controlled entirely by the MH system. In some
instances, PCPs may have financial incentives (affordability control)
to minimize specialty referrals and to treat MH problems themselves.
In these models, collaboration, consultation, and coordination between separate MH and PC systems become exceptionally important.

Carve-In. In this model, MH and PC services are under common
management. PCPs are more likely to serve a significant gatekeeping (access) function and to retain more accountability for
"case managing" their patients through various specialty services.
Affordability involves not only attention to controlling direct MH expenditures, but also to controlling all health expenditures. Flexibility and integration may be enhanced, but access and accountability
problems may be more difficult. The value of explicitly setting priorities for what health MH and PC conditions to cover and what
services to provide may be more apparent in this approach.

In the public system, an underlying complicating factor relates to the special populations served by providers. Public patients tend to be more ill and less effective in advocating for themselves. Therefore, some strategies, quite appropriate in the private sector where patients can change plans, may not be appropriate here. Public health and mental health providers, in response to the overwhelming need to provide service to so many patients (and their history of having budgets "managed" or cut back for decades), tend to emphasize advocacy for "sufficient" patient services. This places them at the risk of being accused of fiscal blindness, and thereby becoming less politically effective. The following three sections identify how these issues impact patients, providers, and the health care system as a whole.

PATIENT PERSPECTIVE

From a public patient's viewpoint, the enhanced integration of MH and PC in PSMC can be a mixed blessing. Referring patients to get a PCP in order to access MH benefits and services may increase the probability that public MH patients will receive some primary health care and perhaps will reduce suffering and costs (for conditions that would require more expensive treatment if not properly treated earlier in the course of an illness). However, patients with SPMI may have great difficulty with this requirement. Where can they turn for mental health or primary care? Who will help them select a PCP and obtain a referral? Once patients approach a PCP, will they be welcomed and treated comprehensively or stigmatized and treated superficially?

Once in a provider's office, how can they articulate their needs? Patients with mental disorders tend to express their concern using signs and symptoms based on the type of provider (MHP or PCP) they are seeing and not just on the disorder itself (Schurman, 1985). Can they make and keep their own follow-up appointments, and will they follow medical instructions reliably?

Finally, variations in MH and health benefits may be confusing, with different restrictions or co-pays for different types of services. Who will help patients who are poor or who have SPMI to negotiate and understand these differences?

PROVIDER PERSPECTIVE

Provider issues are no less complex. With regard to access, PSMC arrangements may encourage more involvement of PCPs in coordinating the total care of persons with SPMI, but these same patients are often rejected, discounted, unrecognized, or otherwise under-served by PCPs because of PCP fear, bias, lack of knowledge, or clinical confusion. Consequently, many of these patients receive primary care services, of uncertain quality, from their psychiatrists (Fogel & Goldberg, 1983–84).

Similarly, PSMC arrangements may identify certain community mental health centers (CMHCs) as preferred MH providers to accept referrals from PCPs, yet patients with certain psychiatric disorders who are referred from PCPs may be denied service because resources are limited to persons with SPMI or high acuity (e.g., suicidal) patients (Olfson, 1991). Some have been served in the mental health system, have had negative experiences, and are unwilling to go back. Others have been barred from services because of noncompliance with treatment, dangerous or other unacceptable behavior, or discriminatory practices toward individuals with comorbid conditions (especially substance use disorders). As a result, a significant number of persons with mental health and chemical dependency (MHCD) disorders receive some or all of their MHCD treatment from PCPs, usually with few mechanisms or opportunities for routine linkage and consultation between MH and PC providers.

With regard to accountability, responsibility for patient care decisions, treatment approaches, and outcomes have different meaning for PCPs and MHPs. PCPs maintain intermittent, but open-ended relationships. While PC patients may not be seen very often, a case isn't usually closed unless the patient requests transfer, dies, or otherwise "officially" leaves care. By contrast, MH providers offer a more intense therapeutic relationship. Engagement in this relationship is a prerequisite for treatment. If the patient does not follow through with appointments the case may be closed and re-opening it may require a new "intake" and review of the whole therapeutic plan. How can a passive or frightened patient, or one who is prone to splitting, be jointly managed by the MHP and PCP, and who carries ultimate responsibility for treatment decisions?

Fiscal issues at the provider level relate to who does the gatekeeping and who pays for the care. PCPs may be responsible for authorizing routine MH lab tests (e.g., annual chemistry screens or lithium levels), as well as for trying to minimize use of psychiatric treatment. MH providers may try to shift the cost of neurological or neuropsychiatric evaluations to the PCP. The MHP will be held accountable by the PCP for the cost impact of treatment recommendations and will be challenged to avoid redundant, excessive or unnecessarily expensive orders for medications or lab tests, and to provide clear justification for such orders. This may be particularly emphasized in the public system where multiple levels of providers (MD, NP, RN, LPN) are used.

SYSTEM PERSPECTIVE

MH and PC providers have quite different training backgrounds and clinical cultures. As they pursue integration or collaboration for survival, they must also deal with the changed incentives, which now include the tension between patient advocacy and generally fixed or shrinking budgets. Access issues, which include the questions of a basic benefits package and eligibility criteria, present special problems in the public sector. A simplistic characterization of the situation is the "golden rule": whoever has the gold, rules or "he who pays, plays." In the private sector, whether mental health is integrated (carved-in) or carved out, there is an assumption that a health plan can calculate the anticipated budget necessary to cover the members' health care needs. However, the public mental health system contains many patients who would be considered catastrophic risks in the commercial market, and for whom the public health systems (both mental and physical) provide a safety net. A few patients with SPMI in a large pool of otherwise healthier patients may constitute a reasonably calculable and manageable risk. However, with the advent of PSMC, a large number of patients (or plan members) have needs that are not as easily predicted, and for which there is much less precedent information. Many of these needs also may be labeled social rather than medical. Where do supported housing or certain psychosocial rehabilitation services fit in for the patient with SPMI? Are these "medically necessary" benefits? How do MH and PC providers come to agreement on how to deal with these issues?

Accountability struggles between systems are typified by confidentiality conflicts. Some would argue that the content of psychiatric records may be particularly sensitive for some patients and that it may require special protections not applicable to other medical records. Information about specific psychiatric problems or chemical dependency issues may be misconstrued by others, or even be regulated differentially by statute. Information may also be made available to patients' employers, especially when the employer is providing the health coverage. Medicaid and other public insurance programs may use sensitive information to eliminate entitlements for certain patients (such as substance abusers) whose behavior is considered their own fault and not justification for public support. Do mental health confidentiality rules take precedence over health department rules where such entities are distinct and in conflict?

Survival Tips

Psychiatric Interface With Primary Care
 	
Critical issues:
 	
    Benefit Package Design
    Screening and Prevention Methodologies
    Access and Availability of MHPs
    Confidentiality
    Communications and Collaboration Between PCP and
        MHP
    Gatekeeping and Authorization Conflicts
    Consultation Models
    Quality: How to Monitor and How to Assure
    Financial Incentives: Ethical and Clinical Concerns
    Collaboration: Obstacles and Costs

Finally, there are the issues of cost. Separate funding streams must ultimately be merged (at the patient level, at least) without falling victim to the "combined, therefore cut even more" response of legislators. While still separate, definitions of "medical" and "MH" must be clarified: Is the white blood count being done for medical or psychiatric reasons? Does it come from the PC or the MH capitation rate? Also, if one assumes the value and benefit of improved and effective collaboration between the MHP and PCP to be apparent, how does the system support such collaboration? With such difficulties clearly in mind, we can now turn to some interface management tools that have been proposed as solutions.

SOLUTIONS TO INTERFACE CHALLENGES

Bartlett (1995) has coined the concept of "interface management" as the key to effectively dealing with the many problems associated with the MH-PC interface. The following examples demonstrate how some programs and providers are attempting to manage the access, accountability, and affordability issues encountered within that interface. Access solutions include the development of inclusive benefit packages, the use of effective tools to screen for mental disorders, the introduction of other prevention techniques for primary care providers, and methods to increase the availability of MHPs. Accountability solutions involve the development of appropriate communications and collaboration strategies. It is especially important to attend to confidentiality issues, gate-keeping and authorization conflicts. Likewise, the introduction of consultation and liaison models that address the entire range of patient needs and provider capabilities is critical. Affordability is affected by all of the above, but requires particular attention to the effective management of financial incentives and to system design (carve-out versus integration).

Benefit Package Design. For any comprehensive care system or health plan to be truly effective in addressing the mental health needs of the population, it must first of all recognize that mental health conditions are of sufficient importance in terms of morbidity, mortality, and cost-effectiveness of treatment to include them in the overall benefit package of the plan or care system. In the public sector, where the main focus of treatment is persons with SPMI, it is also essential that primary care needs not be obscured by the mental health needs.

Various attempts at parity, the rallying cry of the mental health community during the health care reform debates, have been proposed or developed around the country. Most have involved increasing the benefit for mental health services (e.g., by increasing the number of outpatient visits or inpatient days allowed) without reference to the type of mental health condition and without attention to their impact on or relationship to other health care conditions or services. Often this approach to parity has involved identifying certain psychiatric conditions as appropriate for the same kind of coverage as other "medical" problems. This has led to a shift of certain "mind" conditions to "body" legitimacy, but has done little to effectively eliminate the false and discriminatory dichotomy of the mind-body split in benefit design.

As noted earlier in this chapter, in any carve-in system in which funding for health and MH services are combined (and therefore in competition), the issue of prioritization of MH spending vis a vis other health conditions is critical. In an attempt to solve this problem, the prioritization approach of the Oregon Health Plan (OHP) was created. The OHP designed a benefit package in which mental health conditions were evaluated and ranked by the same criteria (such as mortality, treatability, and rehabilitation potential) as all other health problems. The result was a prioritized list of conditions to be covered in which mental health was fully integrated and highly valued vis a vis other medical problems. This benefit package identifies a list of conditions which may be covered for payment for Medicaid patients. The Medicaid budget dictates how many conditions on the list are covered.

Among the outcomes of this unique planning effort are the increased awareness by primary care providers of the importance of mental health conditions to the overall health of their patients and the apparent protection of mental health conditions from being selectively eliminated from the range of covered conditions and services (Pollack, McFarland, George, & Angell, 1994). Whether or not the OHP ultimately succeeds, its prioritization approach establishes that parity for MH services within an overall benefit package is possible. Short of the Oregon strategy, systems must identify critical services (e.g., assertive community treatment) and introduce incentives in the benefit design to promote their utilization.

Screening and Prevention Methodologies. With the integration of mental health into organized care delivery systems, the importance of providing comprehensive diagnostic evaluations for all patients becomes more readily apparent. It is especially important to identify any mental health or chemical dependency problems or risk factors in primary care settings and somatic conditions or risk factors in mental health settings. PCPs, always very pressed for time, may have to adjust their evaluation approaches in order to incorporate attention to these issues. This pressure will only become greater in managed care systems. Therefore, when faced with the additional demand to be alert to MHCD problems, PCPs may resist using mandated screening methods, unless they are easy to administer and interpret, are effective in their ability to identify significant MHCD problems, and are combined with ready access to on-site MHCD support or referral to MHPs located in other facilities.

The development of effective methods by which PCPs can screen most, if not all, of their patients for MHCD conditions is one of the more promising areas of activity. Several different research projects (most notable are the Prime-MD [Spitzer et al., 1994] and SDDS-PC [Broadhead et al., 1995]) have been operating to create valid and easily administered screening devices. The best of these involve questionnaires, with fewer than 50 questions, which patients fill out themselves or which can be administered by medical or clerical staff. These forms can be scored by computer and indicate either the MHCD diagnostic area or at risk behaviors that may be of concern.

These screens tend to focus on identifying the conditions that might more likely surface in a primary care setting, such as mood, anxiety, and eating disorders, as well as alcohol and substance use problems. These are crucial mental health concerns, which frequently are not addressed in the public mental health system. More severe psychotic conditions would be more likely to be identified by simple observation of the patient or from reports from the patient's family or others who know the patient. Interpretations of the screening tools may indicate whether a patient should be referred for further psychiatric evaluation and treatment. Preliminary data from trials of these tools indicate a significant number of previously unrecognized psychiatric disorders in primary care patients. Wide distribution and use of these or other similar products may not only make the identification and referral process more manageable, but will raise PCP awareness of the need for addressing MHCD issues. It must be stressed that some studies have shown that merely increasing the ability of PCPs to recognize certain MHCD conditions does not necessarily lead to improved treatment or outcomes for those conditions (Katon & Gonzales, 1994). Effective on-site treatment, consultation, and specialty referral access as described below must also be available.

In the course of defining the mental health components of the Oregon Health Plan, a prevention document was created. This definition of preventive services included age-related tables indicating screening tests, history questions, high risk populations, and specific MHCD problems that might be encountered. As with the development of the prioritized list of covered conditions and services, the prevention document integrated the concept of mental health prevention with other primary care prevention ideas and methods. Each prepaid health plan (PHP) that contracts with the Oregon Health Plan must demonstrate the use of some method of screening for MHCD conditions, either by the use of one of the tools described above or some other method chosen by the PHP.

Access and Availability of MHPs. How can the MHP be available to consult with the PCP when the PCP is providing psychiatric care for certain patients, or when the PCP is seeing a patient who is in the care of the MHP? The expertise of the MHP can be quite helpful to the PCP in understanding the psychiatric aspects of the patient's condition and to prevent under- or mistreatment. Many PCPs complain that, even when they identify MHCD problems in their patients, they are often frustrated in their attempts to refer patients for MHCD services. Community mental health programs (CMHPs) often have long waiting lists or are constrained by narrower eligibility criteria (e.g., restricted to serving only persons with SPMI or acutely ill psychiatric populations). MHCD provider organizations must develop more immediate access for a wider variety of patient referrals. This may require retooling the intake processes to triage referrals into different levels of immediacy (i.e., immediate or urgent, emergent, less severe), but provide enough capacity to serve most, if not all of these referrals.

On-site consultation relationships with larger primary care facilities (and phone consultation availability for smaller clinics and individual PCP's offices) must be developed as an important resource. Devoting time to create and maintain these types of consultation relationships will become a cornerstone of support for the MH-PC interface under managed care.

Confidentiality. It is essential to balance the need to provide and receive pertinent information with the need to protect the patient from unnecessary and potentially damaging intrusions into his/her privacy. For effective clinical management of the patient's care, the exchange of information between PCP and MHP is critical. This may include physical exam findings, lab test results, medication and other treatment plans and effects. It may also relate to the need for the PCP to make decisions regarding the authorization of certain services.

If the PCP and MHP are not working for the same system of care (i.e., an integrated organization, such as an HMO or a PPO), there should be cooperating provider agreements which allow for information exchanges without requiring formal releases of information. If such agreements are not legal or proper, the MHP should have the patient sign a general release at the time of enrollment in services. Such a consent should explain that certain information may need to be exchanged with other entities for the purpose of authorizing care or payment for care. If a release is required and the patient refuses to sign (because of mistrust, confusion, fear, etc.), the MHP should educate the patient about the need for such collaboration. Likewise, PCPs will have to assure that the content of the patient's psychiatric records will be protected and only used for appropriate clinical and treatment authorization activities. If PCPs have access to MHCD records, they must be aware of the potential risks of inappropriate release of sensitive information.

Communications and Collaboration Between PCP and MHP. Beyond the confidentiality concerns, there are major logistical problems that affect the communications between PCP and MHP. If the two providers work for different organizations (even if they work for the same entity, especially if it is very large), the mere process of sending or receiving timely communications may be very difficult and can interfere with the provision of services. If the MHP does not provide sufficient supportive information when referring a patient for primary care services, the PCP may be uncertain of the reasons for the referral and may be likely to give less attention and less than adequate services. The need for both providers to know what medications each is prescribing for the patient is obvious. The need for timely sharing of lab results in both directions is also apparent. If the managed care arrangement is such that the results of tests ordered by the MHP are sent first to the PCP, it is essential to make sure that the results get to the MHP as well.

In some cases, especially when patients are unwilling or unable to receive or obtain care from two different treatment facilities, the services of the one discipline may need to be provided at the site of the other. This requires cross training and consultation-liaison activities in both directions.

The need to collaborate cannot be overemphasized. However, it is also important to avoid having the communications process encumbered by excessive bureaucratic requirements. Requiring that the MHP and PCP contact each other for every treatment decision or authorization can lead to micromanagement situations and will diminish the value and meaning of their communications.

Gatekeeping and Authorization Conflicts. As managed care systems evolve, we are witnessing the advent of capitated funding schemes, risk assumption by providers, constraints on specialist referrals, and the use of gatekeepers. Various conflicts between the PCP and MHP can develop. If the PCP is in a gatekeeping role vis a vis patients referred to or served by the MHP, there is a potential for major power struggles over the proper care of the patient. The MHP must recognize the cost impact of treatment recommendations and avoid redundant, excessive or unnecessarily expensive orders for medications or lab tests. Rather than ordering tests because they are "routinely done," the MHP will have to provide clear justification for such orders. The development of clear and appropriate practice guidelines may help with this problem. How does the MHP deal with the fact that he/she may be dependent on the PCP to decide whether to approve certain treatments (or at least the payment for those services) when the PCP may be presumed to have less knowledge or experience with such psychiatric treatments?

In many managed care arrangements, certain services provided by MHPs may be subject to approval or authorization by a gatekeeping PCP. This is the case in the Oregon Health Plan. The prepaid health plans (PHPS) that serve Medicaid recipients have funds included in their general capitated rates that are intended to cover pharmacy and laboratory services, including those that may be prescribed or ordered by psychiatric prescribing providers.

When this arrangement, which had been designed by the state Medicaid office, was first discovered by the MHPs working in CMHCS, there was a great deal of anger and alarm. The potential for misunderstanding and denial of services for psychiatric patients whose needs for medications and ancillary lab studies would be subject to PCP approval and the cumbersome processes involved in obtaining such approval were considered too great a risk.

Months of negotiations and educational efforts led to compromises on both sides. MHPs are now aware of how to quickly identify the PHP and PCP with whom their patients are enrolled for services. Protocols have been developed in collaboration with the PHP medical directors. After the patient has been identified as a mutual responsibility of the MHP and PCP and a brief treatment plan sent from the MHP to the PCP, certain prescriptions and lab tests can be ordered without need for further authorization. In the event that services outside of the protocols are desired, the MHP sends a brief form requesting authorization to the PCP. The MHP tries to anticipate such requests so that they are not commonly needed on an emergency basis. If there is a significant difference of opinion regarding the approval of such services, the MHP can appeal the decision to the medical director of the PHP.

Although the original reasons for the inclusion of these services in the PHP capitation rate are unclear and subject to debate, the end result has been that MHPs and PCPs have been forced to communicate and collaborate about many more patients than they have ever shared before. It has also afforded the opportunity for PCPs to get a clearer understanding of public MHPs and their patients.

Consultation Models. In order to meet the complex service needs of the wide variety of patients with psychiatric disorders who are enrolled in public sector managed care programs, it will be necessary to develop flexible models of assessment and treatment that take into account the different locations in which these patients may present and the varying ability that they may have to manage working with MHPs or PCPs.

Pincus (1987) has eloquently described the various models of managing the MH-PC interface. These descriptions include a useful vernacular for communicating about the interface. The models vary according to the level of involvement and the types of activities performed by each side of the interface. The more collaborative of these models include the service delivery team, the consultation and service model, and the integrated health care team. Strathdee has identified the attachment-liaison model, which most closely resembles the consultation and service model, as the most effective and popular linkage approach in recent experience in the United Kingdom (Strathdee, 1987; Creed & Marks, 1989). Public sector managed care systems in the U.S. may be most suited to the application of the attachment-liaison model.

For the many patients who surface in primary care settings, it may be useful to provide on-site mental health consultation, assessment, and treatment services. The larger the primary care setting, the more feasible it may be to assign a mental health provider or team to work in collaboration with the PCPs. The preferable model would include an on-site mental health professional (available for a reasonable amount of time each week), who could provide consultation and triage services for patients identified by the PCP as having apparent psychiatric problems. This MHP could support the PCP in providing sufficient assessment to determine if the patient required treatment. The mental health treatment could be provided by the PCP, the on-site MHP, or by referral to an affiliated mental health provider organization. If the on-site consultation is provided by a non-psychiatrist MHP, it should be augmented by a psychiatrist on-site (but probably less frequently) and via phone access, for specific psychiatric medical support, didactic presentations, case discussions, and other biopsychosocial consultative activities. The flexibility and variety of services provided through this type of model, including its increased potential for improving and maintaining the mental health skills of PCPs, as well as the improved knowledge of and access to the mental health system for more seriously affected patients, make this a superior approach.

The issue of cost, which has long prevented this model from being very widely used in the public sector, may be mitigated by the shift in payment schemes from fee-for-service to prepaid (or capitated). The inherent value of providing effective consultation as described here (which has usually been a non-reimbursable service) can be more easily justified, since revenues would not be strictly tied to services for which billings are generated. Further justification for its value would depend on acceptable clinical outcomes and demonstrable cost-offset.

The recent development and publication of DSM-IV PC, the abbreviated and simplified version of the psychiatric diagnostic manual of the APA, oriented to primary care providers, will provide a great deal of support to MHPs and PCPs involved in this interface. Not only will this document assist MHPs who are providing consultation, such that they can more easily communicate with PCPs regarding the patients about whom they collaborate. The DSM-IV PC will also be an excellent teaching resource, as well as being a significant support for the PCPs, themselves, in evaluating and treating persons with mental disorders. Its use by all those involved in the MH-PC interface will become an essential and automatic part of such collaborations.

Simon (1995) has described the essential features of such a consultation-liaison model within a staff model HMO. He describes the range of services as including four distinct, but overlapping components, which require progressively more participation from the MHP and less from the PCP.

The first is the "curbside" consultation which is usually a brief consultation in person or over the phone, usually focusing on a specific question or problem. The patient is probably not seen by the MHP. The consultation may include certain clinical management suggestions for the PCP to consider and may sometimes lead to a later consultation.

The next level of involvement is the one-time consultation, in which the patient will be seen by the MHP, who serves as an expert consultant and who provides support to the PCP in dealing with a specific diagnostic or management concern.

The third type of liaison service is brief treatment or intermittent support and co-management (e.g., alternating visits between MHP and PCP) of selected cases. This should be reserved for cases that are more likely to respond in a few weeks, but may require intermittent follow-up by the MHP. The PCP continues providing the basic health and mental health treatment after the MHP's involvement diminishes.

Finally, there is the option for the case to be transferred to the MHP for specialty care. This should be reserved for the more severe mental disorders. The need for such referral may be readily apparent at the time of assessment, or may be a result of incomplete or failed response to treatment provided by the PCP.

Simon asserts that any practice arrangement that hopes to be clinically effective, convenient, and efficient must have this full range of liaison services available from the same consultant (or team of MH providers) and at the PCP's practice site.

Similar attachment-liaison relationships can and should be developed in the other direction (i.e., PCP into MH settings), not to mention the need for effective collaboration with providers of addictions services (See chapter by Minkoff). Mental health agencies will benefit from on-site and phone based primary care support in the form of direct care, consultation, and training from affiliated PCPs, especially for those psychiatric patients who are unwilling or unable to go to the primary care facility.

Quality: How to Monitor and How to Assure. Quality has become the byword of managed care. Often related to outcomes measures, it should include attention to questions regarding access to general medical services, the impact on the use of general medical services (i.e., if there is any appreciable "medical offset" from the timely and appropriate provision of mental health services), the rate of identification of MHCD conditions in PCP settings, the satisfaction of the various participants (patients, MHPs, PCPs) with the access, service type and quality, and communications. These more meaningful outcomes measures must be developed, refined, and implemented (See chapter by Essock and Goldman).

Financial Incentives: Ethical and Clinical Concerns. The development of incentives for providers to limit services for patients can be very tricky and troublesome. Clearly, these approaches can lead to reduced costs, but care can be compromised. The financial interests of the PCP may interfere with his/her ability or willingness to do the "right thing" for the patient. If the financial arrangement involves a "withhold" for managing specialty referrals or care (one in which the MHP, or the agency for which the MHP works, shares in any funds that remain at the end of the year), there is the additional risk that the MHP may consciously or unwittingly collude in the effort to deny needed care. The concept of double agentry in relation to the provision of care arises here.

On the other hand, some would argue that the present fee-for-service system creates incentives to provide too much care (e.g., via psychosocial rehab or day treatment programs), whether to make a profit, or to subsidize essential but less profitable programs (e.g., outreach or consultation services).

If there is to be, at least for a time, a system in which the MH services are fiscally carved out, how can the incentives be better aligned to support MHP-PCP collaboration? When MHCD services are provided through separate capitation, the PCP incentive is to refer as much as possible to the MHP. Fiscal integration, on the other hand, promotes PCP gatekeeping, with its attendant problems. While increased referrals to MHPs are certainly desirable, some "cross-incentivization" may be helpful. One such model in Oregon has parallel risk pools, one withheld from the PCP and one withheld from the MHP. Surplus funds in the PCP's pool at the end of the year are distributed only to the PCP; but surplus funds in the MHP's pool are shared between the PCP and MHP. This arrangement is intended to reduce the PCP's tendency to "overrefer" and the MHP's reluctancy to refer patients back to the PCP. Judicious use of specialty providers, without overwhelming their capacity, can be influenced by adjusting the distribution formula, thus spreading the risk to both providers more equitably.

Collaboration: Obstacles and Costs. The value and benefit of improved and effective collaboration between the MHP and PCP is apparent. The system should support such collaboration. The cost of extra communication and consultation should be factored into capitation or case rates. The MHP, who is dependent on fee-for-service payments, should obtain reimbursement for consultation or other case supportive activities, even if they are not "billable". Special consultant positions should be created and supported so that the connections with the PCP are not merely seen as a marginal or "catch as catch can" activity. The expense of technological fixes (such as fax communications, computer tracking systems, standardization of forms) required to make these collaborations more accessible and less time-consuming should be supported and included in the overall budget.

CONCLUSION

Clinicians, administrators, and consumers in both settings must be involved in the process to shape the care delivery system. As managed care programs move into the public arena and as behavioral managed care companies compete for local contracts, and as partnerships between PCPs and prepaid health plans develop, clinicians and other mental health advocates must obtain access to the policy makers. PCPs and MHPs must develop the political influence needed so that patients will get good quality care that is characterized by effective coordination amongst the various clinicians involved.

An essential ingredient to the success of MH-PC interface management is the need for previously held beliefs and attitudes to change, for providers of both types to become more respectful of and willing to collaborate with one another. The implications for MH providers include: the need to be sensitive to the training and consultation needs that the PCPs articulate; the need to recognize when confidentiality is essential and when and what communication with the PCP is preferable; and the need to be responsive to the requests of PCPs. We must adjust to a different pace of work. Some assessments and consultation activities may need to be compressed to a few minutes in order to identify the key problems associated with the case or to determine the appropriate level of care needed. We must be willing and able to write much briefer notes, which summarize our findings and recommendations, rather than listing all the details, since PCPs have less time to review such information.

We must become more familiar with comorbid medical problems, the prevalence of pain, and the increased incidence of somatic complaints that are associated with patients seen in the PCP setting. We must be more generalist in our focus, but with the ability to provide specialist consultation when appropriate.

The MH-PC interface illustrates many of the difficulties and opportunities of managed care. Differences between PCPs and MHPs, in regard to their respective cultures and focus on patient care, may contribute to and be absorbed into the broader PCP-specialist control struggle and, likewise, may be affected by the conflicts associated with the blending of the public and private sectors. However, there are numerous shared values and interests that could mitigate against these destructive tendencies. The false dichotomy of mind-body, particularly criticized by PCP and MHP alike, must now be converted into a seamless whole. The opportunities to reintegrate fiscal considerations into medical decisions and to provide preventive and population-based services are especially promising. The concerns of PCPs and MHPs need to be thoughtfully addressed using clear frames of reference. The two specialties, which have matured somewhat separately, will have to learn to collaborate to an unprecedented degree. If this can be accomplished, our patients will be well served.

REFERENCES

Bartlett, J. (1995). *Interface Management*. Presentation at American Psychiatric Association Annual Meeting, Miami.

Broadhead, W.E., Leon, A.C., Weissman, M.M., Barrett, J.E., Blacklow, R.S., Gilbert, T.T., Keller, M.B., & Higgins, E.S. (1995). Development and validation of the SDDS-PC screen for multiple mental disorders in primary care. *Archives of Family Medicine, 4*, 211–219.

Committee on Prevention, Group for the Advancement of Psychiatry. (1980). *Mental Health and Primary Medical Care. Publication No. 105*. New York: Mental Health Materials Center.

Creed, F., & Marks, B. (1989). Liaison psychiatry in general practice: A comparison of the liaison-attachment scheme and shifted outpatient clinic models. *Journal of the Royal College of General Practitioners, 39*, 514–517.

Engel G. (1980). The clinical application of the biopsychosocial model. *American Journal of Psychiatry, 137*, 535–544.

Fink, P. (1985). Psychiatry and the primary care physician. *Hospital and Community Psychiatry, 36*, 870–875.

Fogel, B.S., & Goldberg, R.J. (1983–84). *International Journal of Psychiatry in Medicine, 13*, 185–192.

Goldberg, R.J. (1995). Psychiatry and the practice of medicine: The need to integrate psychiatry into comprehensive medical care. *Southern Medical Journal, 88*, 260–267.

Katon, W., & Gonzales, J. (1994). A review of randomized trials of psychiatric consultation-liaison studies in primary care. *Psychosomatics, 35*, 268–278.

Olfson, M. (1991). Primary care patients who refuse specialized mental health services. *Archives of Internal Medicine, 151*, 129–132.

Pincus, H. (1987). A framework for Assessing the Interface between Mental Health and Primary Care. *General Hospital Psychiatry, 9.*

Schurman, R.A. (1985). The hidden mental health network: Treatment of mental illness by nonpsychiatric physicians. *Archives of General Psychiatry, 42,* 89–94.

Simon, G (1995) *Mental health and primary care liaison in a staff model hmo.* Presentation at the American Psychiatric Association Annual Meeting, Miami.

Spitzer, R.L., Williams, J.B., Kroenke, K., Linzer, M., deGruy, F.V. 3rd, Hahn, S.R., Brody, D., & Johnson, J.G. (1994). Utility of a new procedure for diagnosing mental disorders in primary care: The PRIME-MD 1000 study. *Journal of the American Medical Association, 272,* 1749–1756.

Strathdee, G. (1987). Primary care-psychiatry interaction: A British perspective. *General Hospital Psychiatry, 9,* 102–110.

18

Integration of Addiction and Psychiatric Services

KENNETH MINKOFF

INTRODUCTION

"In the era of managed care, providing cost conscious dual diagnosis treatment requires a 'retooling' of the addiction and mental health system". (Mee Lee, 1994). Addiction and psychiatric treatment have traditionally been provided in separate, non-integrated service systems, in both public and private sector settings. The estrangement of the addiction system from mainstream mental health has its origins in the development of the 12-Step recovery movement-over 50 years ago-as an alternative to usual medical treatment of addiction, which was essentially non-existent. As a consequence, distinct agencies-and funding streams-have emerged at each level of government. In 1990, more than half of all states had separate state departments responsible for addiction and mental health services; the remainder had separate divisions within a single department. (Ridgely, Goldman & Willenbring, 1990)

This separation of addiction and psychiatric services is so commonplace that practitioners have come to accept it as "normal". Clinicians are often trained in addiction *or* mental health, but not both, and rarely experience themselves as competent in treating both types of disorders. Moreover, the two systems of care have distinct-and apparently irreconcilable treatment philosophies or techniques (Ridgely,

Goldman & Talbott, 1987), and practitioners rarely feel comfortable operating in both systems.

The mental health system, for example, tends to be organized more according to a medical model, with a heavy reliance on "scientific" treatment methods-particularly medication-to provide "relief" for specific symptoms. The addiction system, by contrast, tends to rely heavily on recovering peer counselors, "spiritually-oriented" self-help recovery programs. Medication usage is minimized or avoided, and the focus of treatment may be to allow patients to be confronted by painful feelings or situations rather than to "enable" them by providing relief. Each system tends to focus on its own illness as primary, and to relegate the other illness to secondary status. As a consequence, each system tends to devalue and invalidate the treatment offered by the other. (Minkoff, 1994)

This rift between addiction and mental health services has had considerable impact on the evolution of the public sector mental health system. Although substance abuse services were included in the original federal community mental health center mandates, many CMHCs did not invest heavily in developing addiction services. Even where such services were developed with federal seed money, state funding often was dedicated only to mental health services; state addiction funds were only rarely targeted for CMHCs. In the 1970's and 1980's, as the community mental health mission focused more heavily on the seriously mentally ill, interest in addiction services in public mental health continued to decline. In the last decade, increased recognition of the prevalence of substance abuse among the seriously mentally ill has begun to reverse that trend, but more with regard to development of targeted dual diagnosis services rather than addiction services.

As a result, public sector community mental health programs rarely offer primary addiction treatment, and when such treatment is offered, it is usually not integrated with other CMHC services. Thus, one agency may provide both addiction and psychiatric programs, but the programs may be as unable to collaborate as if they belonged to separate agencies. Lack of integration is particularly reinforced in *public* agencies by the rigidity of separate public funding streams for addiction and mental health services, so that public programs often experience less flexibility than private programs in creating innovative integrated program structures.

With the advent of public sector managed care, however, there has been increasing pressure on public mental health delivery systems to become more integrated. Public sector managed care-like private sector managed care-incorporates responsibility for *both* mental health and substance abuse services. Consequently, the managed care organization (MCO) (however constituted) has a strong interest in managing both primary addiction treatment and primary mental health treatment, as cost effectively as possible, and is much less likely to be tolerant of the clinical and cost-inefficiencies inherent in the fragmented public delivery system.

The advantages and disadvantages of integrated programming, from a care management perspective, are as follows.

ADVANTAGES OF INTEGRATION

Assessment and Triage

Non-integrated intake systems require that the patient's "primary" diagnosis be identified *prior to* assessment. Increasingly, however, patients present for treatment, in both outpatient and emergency settings, with a confusing clinical picture involving both substance-related and psychiatric difficulties. Such patients are better serviced by assessment clinicians who are trained in evaluation of *both* types of disorders, and can make appropriate dispositions accordingly-after the assessment.

In addition, appropriate care management includes an important gatekeeping function, in which patients at risk for hospitalization receive crisis evaluations to determine appropriate levels of care, and to initiate diversionary interventions where appropriate. Public mental health programs frequently have significant expertise in performing such evaluations for psychiatric patients, but have little expertise in assessing addicted patients. In Massachusetts, when MHMA (the Medicaid management company) contracted with Department of Mental Health funded crisis teams to provide 24-hour triage for MHMA patients, the contract required the crisis teams to triage addiction patients as well, a task for which they were largely unprepared. Competence in addiction triage requires familiarity with the ASAM (American Society of Addiction Medicine) Patient Placement Criteria (Level I-outpatient; Level II-intensive outpatient; Level III-medically monitored inpatient detox; Level IV-medically managed intensive inpatient) (Hoffman, Halikes, Mee Lee, & Weedman, 1991, p. 11), for example, and other methodologies for determining level of care for substance abusing patients. Lack of such competence makes it more difficult to refer addicted patients to non-hospital levels of care, such as outpatient detox, partial hospital, and residential detox and rehabilitation, and may result in over-reliance on more expensive hospital-based programs.

Programs, Treatment of Dual Diagnosis

Increasing data on the high prevalence of comorbidity in psychiatric populations (Regier et al., 1990), and particularly public-sector psychiatric populations, indicates that within the cohort of patients served by public sector managed care, dual diagnosis is an expectation rather than an exception (Minkoff, 1991). There is growing evidence that such patients are more effectively treated in integrated settings in which both the psychiatric and substance disorders can be treated simultaneously. (Drake, Bartels, Teague, Noordsy, & Clark, 1993). Lack of integration often results in "ping-pong therapy" (Ridgely et al., 1990) in which the patient becomes a "system misfit" (Bachrach, 1987), bouncing back and forth between both service systems. From a care management perspective, this is the antithesis of cost-effectiveness: it is *more expensive* and *less effective.*

While many public mental health systems have begun to develop substance abuse services for people in programs for treatment of chronic mental illness, there are particular gaps in service delivery for individuals with substance dependence who also have associated psychopathology that does not represent a chronic psychiatric disability but prevents successful involvement in generic addiction treatment. When integrated programs to address such "complicated chemical dependency" are not available, patients are likely to experience a succession of unsuccessful and costly hospitalizations in both addiction and psychiatric settings.

Network Development: One Stop Shopping

Managed care organizations have shown an increasing preference to contract with -and manage- networks with fewer and more comprehensive providers, rather than to manage larger networks of smaller, more specialized providers. According to Mee Lee (1994, p. 266), managed care programs "will increasingly take on the characteristics of a single system of addiction and mental health care combined under one behavioral health administration and treatment team". In this type of environment, integrated providers have a competitive advantage, and public sector providers that fail to provide comprehensive services risk losing significant contracts to more aggressive and flexible private sector organizations. One-stop shopping may also be advantageous to clients and families, particularly public-sector clients, who tend to be less mobile and flexible in seeking services and may be better served if family members with diverse problems can be treated under the auspices of a single provider.

DISADVANTAGES OF INTEGRATION

Reduction of Choice and Flexibility

Narrowing the provider network to include primarily integrated providers is likely to reduce clients' ability to choose providers. This will have particular impact on those clients who wish to be served in generic addiction or mental health settings, but not in integrated settings. This suggests that most networks will retain the flexibility of using non-integrated providers.

Risk of Attenuation of Treatment Quality

Provision of integrated addiction and mental health services by cross-trained staff creates the risk that the quality and focus of the separate addiction and mental health interventions may suffer. Addiction treatment, which tends to require a great deal of consistency and intensity, is particulary at risk of being weakened by the flexibility" of psychiatric settings. Managed care organizations working with integrated programs may still wish to separately assess the standards and quality of psychiatric services and addiction services within those programs.

On balance, it appears that the advantages of integration-from a *clinical* as well as a *managed care* perspective-outweigh the disadvantages. This has probably been true for some time, certainly with regard to the *clinical* needs of dual diagnosis clients, but managed care is now creating a stronger *financial* impetus to promote integration. Given the significant systemic and philosophical barriers described earlier, how can service integration be implemented?

IMPLEMENTATION

Creating a program structure that offers an integrated continuum of addiction and psychiatric services is a step-by-step process that requires a broad commitment on the part of program management, and involvement of the entire organization in the analysis of the problem and development of solutions. In this regard, it can be beneficial to approach integration from the perspective of total quality management (TQM), inviting participation in organization wide

---

Survival Tips

Integration of Psychiatric and Addictions Services

Development of an Integrated Philosophy

Organizational Assessment

Implementing Integration:

Create an organization structure that promotes integration
    Consider a merger or partnership.
    Assess interagency gaps and enhance services to address them.
    Maintain a long-range plan for integration, and avoid marginalization of services.

Develop customer-oriented program models to initiate integration
    Integrated assessment and triage
    Engagement group program
    Active substance abuse treatment groups
    Acute dual diagnosis day treatment
    Integrated psychiatric & addiction inpatient/residential programs
    Integrated case management

Provide ongoing psychiatric and addiction training to all staff.

problem-solving from all levels and categories of staff, with a clearly defined mandate from management, and parameters to assess both process and outcome for the "integration project team" at each stage. Regardless of the process utilized, however, the stages proceeding toward integration can be clearly defined.

STAGE I: DEVELOPMENT OF AN INTEGRATED PHILOSOPHY

Develop an integrated philosophy that provides a unified framework for conceptualizing addiction and psychiatric treatment, and develop a coherent mission statement for the organization based on that philosophy.

Minkoff (1989; 1991) has described a model for integrating the treatment of serious mental illness and addiction based on the following principles: When mental illness and substance disorders co-exist, each disorder should be considered *primary*, requiring its own specific treatment appropriate to the level of severity of the disorder.

1 Serious psychiatric disorders and addictive disorders are both forms of primary chronic biologic mental illness, for which assessment and treatment can be conceptualized using a disease and recovery model.

2 Each disease has its own specific stabilizing treatment (e.g., medication for mental illness, 12-STEP programs for addiction); both types of diseases are characterized by denial, shame, guilt, despair, and stigma, which create barriers to treatment initiation and continuation; for both types of illness, treatment focuses on recovery of the *person* who has the disease, not recovery from the disease, proceeding through phases of acute stabilization, engagement in ongoing treatment, participation in active treatment to achieve prolonged stabilization (maintenance), and rehabilitation and recovery.

3 Comprehensive programming for psychiatric and addictive disorders involves developing a *system* of care, in which each programmatic element addresses the needs of a specific population, defined by the acuity, severity, disability, level of motivation, and phase of recovery associated with each disease (Minkoff, 1991).

Based on this conceptual framework, each public sector program can develop a customer-focused mission statement regarding integration that is (a) specific to its own programmatic mandate and (b) designed to address the needs of both consumers and managed-care payers regarding access, one stop shopping, and comprehensive continuum of programming for each disorder-and for dual diagnosis.

A sample mission statement for an outpatient program might read as follows:

> The mission of our program is to provide a comprehensive continuum of outpatient services for individuals with primary substance disorders and primary psychiatric disorders, separately or in combi-

nation. Access to services should be seamless with regard to type of disorder, and initial evaluation should integrate both psychiatric and addiction assessment capability. The quality of addiction or psychiatric programming should be comparable to that provided in generic addiction or psychiatric settings. Each program element should define its capacity to treat dual disorders, and integrated treatment capacity for all types of dual disordered patients should be available within our continuum, with minimum interprogram barriers to continuity of care.

Once the mission statement and philosophy are developed, it is important to create a process for disseminating the mission throughout the staff and creating opportunities to identify resistances and work them through. Common resistances include:
   We are already burdened enough; why take on more?

1 Addicts (or psych patients) are undesirable and will contaminate our program.

2 We (e.g., the psych team) are willing to do this but they (e.g., the addiction team) are impossible to work with.

3 We don't have the knowledge or skills to do this, and we believe that we never will.

At this stage, in order to resolve these resistances, organizational leadership must: (a) Consistently identify the clinical and competitive advantages of program integration; (b) Model equal validation of addiction and psychiatric clinicians and treatments; (c) Promote the perception that all staff *can be trained*, while encouraging open discussion of anxieties and needs, and identifying ongoing opportunities for training; (d) Emphasize that integration ultimately *reduces* clinician burden due to enhanced skill and reduction in duplication of treatment effort.

STAGE II: ORGANIZATIONAL ASSESSMENT

Assessment of both the *structure* and *function* of the organization in relation to the integration mission is essential in order to plan the implementation process.
   Questions to address in the assessment process include:
   Does the organization structure reinforce or inhibit integration? Is the organization of addiction services comparable in stature and intensity to the organization of psychiatric services, or is one disorder given "secondary" status within the organization hierarchy?

1 For substance and psychiatric disorders separately, how comprehensive is the continuum of care offered by the program, and to what extent are gaps in the continuum available in other programs? For example, for substance disorders, does the program offer detoxification (outpatient, residential, hospital); engagement or pre-motivational programs active addiction treatment (outpatient, individual, group, or family; intensive outpatient

treatment; day or evening treatment; residential or hospital services); relapse prevention programs; programs for special populations (pregnant/parenting woman; HIV positive individuals; methadone maintenance); pharmacological interventions (Antabuse, naltrexone, etc.)? Similar assessment can occur for the psychiatric continuum.

2 To what extent does each program model accommodate the needs of individuals with dual diagnosis? What level of psychiatric complexity or acuity can be accommodated in each phase of addiction treatment? To what extent can outpatient mental health providers address the needs of psychiatrically symptomatic abusers who are not yet ready for substance abuse treatment? To what extent are specific substance abuse interventions available for individuals with serious psychiatric disorders and chronic psychiatric disabilities-integrated case management, premotivational programs, active treatment programs for substance abuse, and addiction treatment? What types of program barriers exist to accommodating dual diagnosed patients (e.g., addiction program won't accept patients on medication, psych program discharges active substance users)?

How seamless is the *clinical intake* and *triage* process? How readily can psychiatric, addicted, dual diagnosis, and diagnostically unclear patients be accommodated at a single point of entry that can assess both disorders simultaneously?

To what extent are staff cross-trained? To what extent do psychiatric clinicians perceive themselves to have-and actually do have-addiction expertise, and vice versa?

Based on the results of the assessment, the program can begin to develop an action plan, and proceed to implementation.

STAGE III: IMPLEMENTING INTEGRATION

STEP 1   Create an Organization Structure that Promotes Integration

As noted earlier, public sector mental health agencies fall into two broad categories: those that offer minimal (or no) substance abuse services, and those that have distinct addiction treatment components within the larger agency. There are more formidable challenges facing each type.

For the mental health agency that currently offers no substance services, the prospect of developing a full continuum of addiction services is daunting. Usually, there is a neighboring substance abuse program to which clients are referred, and there is appropriate resistance to duplicating services. Effective strategies are as follows:

Consider a merger or partnership. Developing a strong agency affiliation between a mental health and addiction program creates an immediate competitive advantage in the world of public sector managed care. Increasingly, agencies that were once at odds are forming formerly unthinkable partnerships to enhance the comprehensiveness of service mix.

Assess interagency gaps and enhance services to address them. With or without a merger, there will exist many patients in either system who require services in the "other" system, but who are unable or unwilling to engage with two systems simultaneously. In mental health programs with minimal substance services, a reasonable first step is to develop a range of low-intensity services that clients can access readily, and which may facilitate ultimate access to addiction treatment. Examples of such services are: a) pre-motivational/educational groups, b) family education programs, and c) active treatment groups. Each of these programs should have separate services for seriously mentally ill clients and for anxious/depressed/personality disordered clients. See below for more detailed program descriptions.

Maintain a long-range plan for integration, and avoid marginalization of services. A common error in psychiatric programs seeking integration is to hire some addiction clinicians and charge them with responsibility for addiction programming, without further structural or clinical integration. Although such a plan permits offering some addiction services, the services remain marginalized within the psychiatric milieu and therefore lose considerable effectiveness. The addiction clinicians (often counselors) are not empowered in the system, and no one (especially physicians) has to listen to them. Clients quickly recognize that the program does not take addiction seriously, because most of the staff have no addiction expertise, and rely heavily on the counselors to provide all addiction services. This impedes rather than enhances integration.

The recommended alternative is to develop a clear mandate that *all* staff will become trained in addiction programming, and identify a concrete list of competencies that will be mastered. Addiction program coordinators must be provided with *comparable* status in the organization's formal versus informal structure to psychiatric program coordinators, and given authority to oversee the clinical performance of all staff treating patients with substance disorders. The primary role of the addiction coordinator(s) is to involve *all* the staff in addiction treatment; staff must be required to participate in training, take patients as assigned, and demonstrate competencies (as in running groups). The program must resist the temptation of assigning all addiction clients to the addiction counselor in order to develop a stronger addiction milieu in the long run.

For agencies that already offer both types of services, similar principles apply.

Both divisions must be accorded equal status, and report equally to a manager strongly identified with the integration project. It could be unwise, for example, to have addiction services headed by a counselor, and mental health services headed by a psychologist; or to have the agency clinical director *also* be the mental health services director, and have addiction services report to him or her.

Clearly mandate the role of each program component in serving dual diagnosis clients. Typical addiction programs, for example, can work with patients with psychiatric complications other than serious

mental illness or disability with the provision of appropriate training, policies concerning use of psychotropic medication, and psychiatric consultation and support. Similarly, psychiatric programs
can provide a range of substance abuse interventions to the seriously mentally ill with appropriate training and support.

*Develop successful structures for interprogram collaboration, resource
sharing, and cross training.* "Successful" means that the initial interventions should be designed to guarantee success-small rather than
grandiose, with attainable objectives. Development of *one* jointly
staffed dual diagnosis group-or *one* cross consultation staff ex-
change-is a good place to begin.

STEP 2 Develop Customer-Oriented Program Models to Initiate Program Integration

Based on the systemwide assessment described earlier, specific
areas can be identified where small scale programmatic innovation
can have a large impact on the agency's ability to respond to refer-
ents and clients in a more integrated fashion. Examples of such programmatic interventions are listed below.

Integrated Assessment and Triage

In order to respond appropriately to managed care referrals, initial
phone triage or assessment should readily accommodate clients
with any combination of psychiatric and/or substance disorder
presentation. Intake and assessment clinicians should be trained to
be receptive to patients with primary substance disorders, and to
encourage them to enter treatment at the time of request. Assessment instruments can be structured to provide equal space and
weight to substance and psychiatric history and symptoms.

Engagement Group Program

Providing initial substance education to clients who present with
psychopathology and substance abuse, but who are not either ready
for or in need of formal addiction treatment, can be accommodated
in educational engagement groups. Those groups use peer influence
to help individuals openly discuss their substance use, acquire
information, and hopefully make better choices. Sciacca (1991),
Noordsy and Fox (1991), Kofoed, Kania, Walsh, and Atkinson (1986)
have described the application of those groups in a variety of psychiatric settings. In most clinic settings, engagement groups can be
designed for specific subpopulations: e.g., seriously mentally ill;
nonpsychotic; adolescents; and so on.

One advantage of those groups is that they can be best led by
psychiatric clinicians with relatively little substance abuse experience. The leader needs to join the group in facilitating the learning

process rather than actively trying to harangue members into becoming abstinent.

Active Substance Abuse Treatment Groups

A portion of the clients who enter engagement programs will advance to seeking active treatment to reduce or discontinue substance abuse. These individuals are often *not* substance dependent, but rather are in need of concrete skills and techniques to change harmful patterns of substance use. Leaders require some specific training in how to teach those techniques. As with engagement groups, active treatment groups can be geared to specific subpopulations.

Acute Dual Diagnosis Day Treatment

In a managed care environment, intensive addiction treatment is increasingly provided in short-term day and evening treatment settings. Generic addiction day treatment can be enhanced to accommodate a broader range of psychopathology concomitantly with addiction, including anxiety, depression, PTSD, and personality disorders, by providing staff training and psychiatric consultation, as well as collaboration with individual psychotherapists who can discuss emotionally charged issues within a context that reinforces the need for sobriety to be a priority for any psychotherapy to have value.

Integrated Psychiatric and Addiction
Inpatient/Residential Programs

Minkoff (1989) has described an integrated psychiatric and addiction unit in a general hospital, where a full addiction group program coexists with a full psychiatric program and all staff are cross-trained. Such units represent the ultimate in one-stop shopping for managed care payers. As public sector recognition of the prevalence of dual diagnosis has increased, so has acceptance of the need for addiction treatment in mental health settings. In Massachusetts, a DMH acute psychiatric unit has recently implemented a full addiction group program, to accommodate the many patients admitted with primary substance dependence. Similar capacity can be developed in crisis residential programs, through staff training and through linkage with appropriately intensive outpatient addiction treatment programs.

Integrated Case Management

Public sector managed care often encourages the development of creative case management for recidivist clients. Drake, Antosca, Noordsy, Bartels, and Osher (1991) have described a continuous treatment team (C.T.T.) model for providing integrated case management outreach to dual diagnosis patients. The availability of ongoing case management that can simultaneously address substance and psychiatric disorders enhances outcome by providing continuity for the patient through multiple diverse treatment episodes, maintaining a consistent stance that combines empathic detachment, and ongoing support. Such case management models can be initiated in any setting by organizing existing case management clinicians into teams that encompass a range of psychiatric and substance expertise, and developing a framework by which they can share their expertise in working with their combined caseload.

STEP 3   Provide Ongoing Psychiatric and Addiction Training to all Staff

Continual training, both through formal lectures, individual supervision, and case conferences, is essential to upgrading the level of skill- and integration-throughout the agency. The agency must commit to training as many staff as possible to develop skills in both areas, and to use better trained staff to train others. Note that although *some* training precedes implementation of new programs, the most effective learning can only occur *after* staff have begun to try new and unfamiliar tasks. Staff often report that they learn more with each successive repetition of training material as they continue to gain clinical experience in new areas. This process of skill development in integrating psychiatric and addiction expertise must continue over many years, before staff are likely to report a significant increase in self-identification as "dual disorder' experts.

CONCLUSION

In summary, public sector mental health programs must increasingly recognize the importance of integrating psychiatric and addiction services in order to respond competitively to the demands of managed care. This chapter has outlined a step by step approach to accomplishing this task, by addressing, in sequence, organizational philosophy and mission, agency structure, clinical programs, and staff development.

REFERENCES

Bachrach, L.L. (1987). The context of care for the chronic mental patient with substance abuse. *Psychiatric Quarterly, 58*, 3–14.

Drake, R.E., Antosca, L.M., Noordsy, D.L., Bartels, S.J., & Osher, F.C. (1991). New Hamsphire's specialized services for the dually diagnosed. In K. Minkoff & R.E. Drake (Eds.) *Dual Diagnosis Of Major Mental Illness And Substance Disorder* (pp. 57–67). San Francisco: Jossey-Bass.

Drake, R.E., Bartels, S.J., Teague, GI.B., Noordsy, D.L., & Clark, R.E. (1993). Treatment of substance abuse in severely mentally ill patients. *Journal Of Nervous And Mental Disease, 181*, 606–611.

Hoffman, N.G., Halikes, J.A., Mee Lee, D., & Weedman, R.D. (1991). *Patient Placement Criteria For The Treatment Of Psychoactive Substance Use Disorders*. Washington, DC: American Society of Addiction Medicine.

Kofoed, L., Kania, J., Walsh, T., & Atkinson, R.M. (1986). Outpatient treatment of patients with substance abuse and coexisting psychiatric disorders. *American Journal Of Psychiatry, 143,* 867–872.

Mee Lee, D. (1994). Managed care and dual diagnosis. In N.S. Miller (Ed.) *Treating Coexisting Psychiatric and Addictive Disorders* (pp. 257–269). Center City, MN: Hazelden.

Minkoff, K. (1989). An integrated treatment model for dual diagnosis of psychosis and addiction. *Hospital And Community Psychiatry, 40,* 1031–1036.

Minkoff, K. (1991). Program components of a comprehensive integrated care system for serious mentally ill patients with substance disorders. In K.

Minkoff, K. & R.E. Drake (Eds.) *Dual Diagnosis Of Major Mental Illness And Substance Disorder* (pp. 13–28). San Francisco: Jossey-Bass.

Minkoff, K. (1994). Treating the dually diagnosed in psychiatric settings. In N.S. Miller (Ed.) *Treating Coexisting Psychiatric And Addictive Disorders* (pp. 53–68). Center City, MN: Hazelden.

Noordsy, D.L., & Fox, L. (1991). Group intervention techniques for people with dual disorders. *Psychosocial Rehabilitation Journal, 15,* 67–78.

Regier, D.A., Farmer, M.E., Rae, D.S., Locke, B.Z., Keith, S.J., Judd, L.L., & Goodwin, F.K. (1990). Comorbidity of mental disorders with alcohol and other drug abuse. *Journal Of The American Medical Association, 264,* 2511–2518.

Ridgely, M.S., Goldman, H.H., & Talbott, J.A. (1987). *Chronic Mentally Ill Young Adults With Substance Abuse Problems: Treatment And Training Issues*. Baltimore: Mental Health Policy Studies, University of Maryland School of Medicine.

Ridgely, M.S., Goldman, H.H., & Willenbring, M. (1990). Barriers to the care of persons with dual diagnosis: organizational and financing issues. *Schizophrenia Bulletin, 16,* 123–132.

Sciacca, K. (1991). An integrated treatment approach for severely mentally ill individuals with substance disorders. In K. Minkoff & R.E. Drake (Eds.) *Duan Diagnosis Of Major Mental Illness and Substance Disorder* (pp. 69–84). San Francisco: Jossey-Bass.

19

Services for Children and Families

ROBERT F. COLE

As with the rest of the American health care system, the specter of change is hovering over mental health. The national reform legislation that failed to pass in 1994, has left behind it a much more vigorous market-oriented reform movement that is rapidly changing the face of health care. This shift is symbolized by a wastebasket of techniques referred to as "managed care". It includes a wide range of practices that have been used by health care purchasers, most aggressively and skillfully by large national employers, to control costs of health care by distributing financial risk to the delivery systems and to improve quality by holding health care delivery systems accountable for the outcomes of treatment. The techniques and approaches represented by managed care are probably neither good nor bad, but the shift to managed care can certainly be considered a crisis because there is danger that things could go terribly wrong if these techniques are not skillfully applied by purchasers. There is an opportunity to make improvements that are long overdue.

This chapter focuses on the opportunity side of this crisis because the improvements that are needed are so massive that they outweigh the perils that "change" presents. This is true because of the basic policy disconnect for child and family mental health which has had a disastrous effect on the lives of children and their families (England & Cole, 1995). I will discuss this policy disconnect and the opportunities to correct it that come with the shift of managed care.

I will cover new (and old) techniques and the revision of theory and practice for child and family mental health that might emerge if we manage this shift well.

In the spirit of this volume I will try to point out how survivors, the dedicated child and family mental health advocates and clinicians, can weather the storm best by moving wholeheartedly with the paradigm shift.

No one can claim certainty about these matters. All that is offered here is a combination of crystal ball predictions and some familiarity and informed guesses about how things are changing — it all needs to be tested and reassessed as the process of change proceeds. The frame of reference from which these comments are made is the experience of a movement of reform which has developed in the decade of the eighties with the Ventura County California child mental health system (Cole & Hanson, 1988), the North Carolina Willie M. consent decree, Child and Adolescent Service System Program (CASSP) fostered by NIMH (Stroul & Friedman, 1986), the Robert Wood Johnson Foundation's Mental Health Services Program for Youth (Cole & Poe, 1993), and the child and family mental health services grants by the federal Center for Mental Health Services (CMHS). These efforts have created new models of service delivery which have in some cases become pilot programs for child and family mental health under managed care, modeling integrated funding and care management under capitated funding.

THE POLICY DISCONNECT

Somehow we have backed into a policy for child and family mental health care that is, in every respect, perverse. No one has made a formal policy but the operative policy is that we have artificially limited the traditional mental health benefit so that it runs out close to the time when it is most needed. This can leave a critical hiatus in care just as a child's condition goes from bad to worse and as a family's tolerance and strength are most vulnerable. Public funding is withheld until there is a full-blown crisis and the home situation has fallen apart. Then the resources are divided unevenly among five or six public agencies, none of which, by itself, is equipped to provide intensive care and all of which have a great incentive to shift responsibility to other agencies. This fragmentation of responsibility, effort and resources for children with serious or severe emotional disturbance (SED) and their families is characteristic of the process of forming American social welfare policy one advocacy group and one entitlement at a time. Other populations with special health care needs face similar problems of negotiating fragmented social welfare programs, but for child and family mental health the inevitable instability of this arrangement is crucial.

An additional aspect of this policy disconnect is a traditional mental health benefit structure that leads to a treatment disconnect for children with SED and their families. This results in overuse of highly expensive inpatient resources and diminished ability to create complex systemic interagency family-based treatment plans that facilitate family and community integration for the child. The traditional "unmanaged" public sector mental health benefit has reflected the private sector benefit structure by limiting reimbursement to inpatient hospitalization and general outpatient services. This service specific benefit may inadvertently create barriers to effective treatment.

As an example, consider the case of a 15 year old boy with attention deficit disorder, learning disabilities with poor school performance, substance abuse, depression, and impulsivity. He comes from a family burdened with the painful problems of an abusive alcoholic stepfather. The boy goes into crisis after a family argument, with an eruption of violent rage followed by expressions of intense suicidal ideation. In the traditional "unmanaged" system, he is likely to be referred for psychiatric hospitalization, which may last 4–6 weeks. He receives a comprehensive inpatient evaluation and milieu-based interventions, but seems to decompensate when discharge planning is brought up, leading to a prolongation of the hospitalization. Coordination with the family and with involved educational and social service agencies is complicated by their geographic distance from the hospital and by the perception that the boy should now be "owned" by the mental health system. Finally, after a lengthy and expensive hospitalization, the boy is returned home (usually at the point that benefits have run out) to an unstable family situation which is a likely breeding ground for rapid readmission. Services defined by benefits and diagnostic codes have been provided, but no one has the responsibility for "care". The care needed for the episode has not been managed nor is it likely that the persistent disability will be effectively managed throughout the child's developmental years.

MANAGED CARE: AN OPPORTUNITY TO RE-CONNECT POLICY AND TREATMENT

The sweeping changes that are coming with the shift to managed care provide an opportunity to correct this flawed system in two ways: first, by integrating the efforts of categorical agencies that share the responsibility for child and family mental health; and, second, by eliminating the split between private and public health care sectors for mental health services, by incorporating the flexibility of privatized managed care systems into care management. The former depends on how the states reconfigure health and related social services expenditures as they move the publicly funded health care into managed care arrangements. The latter depends on how they go about purchasing health care. Will central bureaucracies like Medicaid agencies purchase "managed care" using current public purchasing practices? Or will public health authorities work through local and regional purchasing sponsors capable of allying with other health care purchasers such as large employers or small employer purchasing coalitions, to adopt joint policies regarding risk adjustment and flexible case management for high-need plan members?

How managed care affects child and family mental health services will be played out in fifty different stories as the each state proceeds in its own way. There will be different degrees of success in the pursuit of a coherent policy and in the attempt to create one health care system for all. For surviving advocates and professionals, the items to watch are 1) the coherent development of the delivery system as an integral part of the organized system of care; 2) the shift in practice to encourage home and community based services; and, 3) the shift of roles for professionals trained in traditional mental health disciplines to adopt more flexible, family-oriented interventions.

POLICY PREREQUISITE: COHERENT SYSTEMS OF CARE INTEGRATED INTO THE LARGER SYSTEM

Coherence in a system of care for children with SED and their families means that the resources "hold together" and are provided as directly and straightforwardly as possible from the family's viewpoint. In most communities the artificial limits on traditional health benefits and the fragmentation of responsibility place child and family mental health at less than ground zero.

Managed Care Products. So far managed care's contribution has been focused on behavioral health "products" that have been offered by the purchasers as a "carve-out" of the overall health benefit or "carved-in", i.e. separated by the plans and subcontracted to the behavioral health companies. Private sector behavioral health companies have extended their reach dramatically in the last few years through a set of product features that might be called "vanilla" managed mental health. Its scope does not go beyond what was covered under the traditional artificially limited indemnity benefit, although, because of the assumption of risk, providers can often exercise flexibility in the provision of services.

The basic approach involves controlling cost and focusing effort through application of basic utilization review techniques: preadmission screening and concurrent review; the development and management of a network of individual providers, groups, or agencies who work for the companies under contractually defined arrangements for compensation and compliance with practice protocols specified by the company. These products are organized through a central phone bank of clinicians who oversee the screening and review processes. It is recognized that a degree of tension between the network clinician and the reviewer is very important in providing good judgments and quality care (Feldman, 1992).

The experience of basic managed mental health for children and families is, on the one hand, earlier and more focused intervention for employed members, and, on the other, a more efficient depletion of benefits and subsequent referral to public sector agencies, especially in cases of severe disability. Managed care has not dealt with the need for effective early intervention and prevention, nor with the need for "intensive care" for children with SED, who require continuous care. More effective approaches for children with SED in the public sector will require family and child centered services that promote interagency coordination and continuity at the client level. Likewise, an effective approach to early intervention and prevention will require health plans to develop special support systems for high risk families by partnering with the early childhood community. These partnerships could utilize the resources of child and family mental health delivery systems in a targeted, less expensive, and less stigmatizing fashion.

Managed behavioral health plans have just begun to develop "intensive care" products that provide this type of integrated care management, i.e. tightly organized services to provide continuous care for populations with identified disabilities. This requires a shift from reliance on traditional institutional care in residential treatment centers or hospitals to developing intensive, individualized care based in the home and family through a variety of wrap-around services.

As publicly funded health care and special needs populations are moved into managed care, it seems likely that plans will need to develop special purpose systems of care, much as they develop relationships with centers of excellence for complex procedures and specialized tertiary care facilities which have the capacity to care for them. This will require adequate risk-adjustment methodologies so that purchasers can provide adjustments to premiums for members who choose specific plans.

This kind of risk-adjustment is being modeled in King County (Seattle), Washington, where the public mental health authority has hired US Behavioral Health to administer their "case rates": a system of six rate tiers priced to meet the needs of designated mental health clients. This is a regulation of a resource allocation process that could be more effectively negotiated among professionals in an organization that is at risk for the whole population. But it is a constructive interim measure which will establish the experiential base for setting rates and calculating risk.

For child and family mental health, the introduction of risk adjustment mechanisms will open the way to adequately fund different levels of care, especially for those children who require continuous care. The source of these risk adjustment dollars will likely come from the budgets that currently finance residential and specialized care for these children: i.e., the agencies that share responsibility for children's mental health. Because of access problems ingrained in the Medicaid program, resources for these special health costs were placed in these agencies. When the dollars and services of this assortment of child focused agencies is integrated, and when overreliance on expensive impatient care is reduced, there should be sufficient savings to achieve "parity" for mental health conditions and benefits with other diseases and disabilities.

What surviving child mental health providers may conclude from these developments is that a new organizational format for child and family mental health services is emerging. Traditional mental health agencies will be modified in relation to it, but will be substantially different from the child guidance clinics, mental health centers, hospitals, residential programs, day programs, and group practices of the past.

In the past, clinicians were paid by the services provided in an encounter and billed through the fee-for-service system. This artificial concept of "service" became more real than good sense could justify: it obscured the immediacy and flexibility of the caring process. The new organization, the "care management entity", can be a svelte, but effective operation. It will have a minimal administrative structure that will balance financial and clinical issues in all decision-making. Its core staff will be a team of care coordinators who orchestrate the formation of multi-disciplinary care teams around each child and family. The team produces a plan of care, and the plan of care mobilizes the provider network through authorization of individually tailored services. These organizations can operate substantially at risk, as well as accepting traditional fee-for-service patients, and will have the flexibility to provide genuinely "intensive" services in home and community settings.

As plans and behavioral health organizations begin to create intensive and continuous care products for this and other special needs populations, they are likely to rely on these kinds of organizational models.

HOMEWORK: THE SHIFT TO HOME AND COMMUNITY CARE SETTINGS

Reference has been made to the importance under managed care of individualized services and the translation of intensive care to home and community settings. The fact is that the move to managed care, if directed skillfully by purchasers, can support the movement to reform child and family mental health. The reform recognizes the fact that "kids do better in families", even kids with SED, when the families have adequate supports. This is not a trivial matter, because the professional community in the last several decades has questioned the value of the family's contribution. Families were blamed, discounted as "dysfunctional", and children have been separated from them through placement and institutionalization on a dramatic scale. MCOs will recognize the value of family care because, on the one hand, it comes without staffing three shifts, and a family can receive a lot of supportive services before the costs come anywhere close to that of residential care. On the other hand, there is real evidence that kids do better in families and positive outcomes increasingly are the operational goal for successful MCOS.

Intensive care in home and community settings requires a whole new approach to service delivery. Services have to "work for families" and may look much different than they have in the past. Outreach and access issues will govern the way they are offered. A course of psychotherapy will not necessarily take place in a clinic; it may begin over coffee at a restaurant across from the single parent's apartment. Respite care, or flexible in-home care, or mentoring may be critical factors in keeping the child at home. Schools may emerge as providers of individualized educational programs for the seven hours of programming for which they are responsible. The school's contribution will be seen as integral to the whole community-based clinical strategy.

An excellent example of this type of clinical and programmatic innovation is the Home-based Family Stabilization Services (CASSP 1987). In these programs, teams of family-oriented clinicians engage with the family and with all involved agencies at the time of crisis. They provide a combination of family-oriented crisis intervention, often in the home, plus ongoing multi-agency systems coordination to develop a treatment plan that mobilizes resources to minimize utilization of hospital or residential care. MCO benefit plans pay for this service either directly, on a per-case or per-hour basis, or through riskbased payment mechanisms that encourage the providers to control cost and improve outcome through the creation of these models of care management.

In the case example cited earlier, the availability of this type of intervention would result in a very different outcome. Instead of hospitalization, the 15 year old boy would probably be held for 1–2 days in a crisis stabilization bed, while the family stabilization team organized a systems intervention to engage the client, family, school, and, other potential resources for social and treatment support. Emphasis would be on returning the boy to his home quickly, providing the family with intensive family crisis intervention in the home, with 24 hour availability to additional crisis services, to maintain safety while a long-term support plan is being developed. Such an intervention is not only less expensive and more normalizing than traditional hospitalization, but there is a much better potential for successful outcome.

In spite of the changes in the format of services, seasoned clinicians and the clinical methods with which they were trained will remain essential assets of service delivery under managed care. The individualized plans of care must meet medical quality assurance standards and be imbued with the methodical articulation of the goals of the interventions and regular periodic assessment of their results. As the issues strengths and needs of the child and family change, the plan of care will change as well. In particular, as intensive care efforts are constructed, the clinical strategy will take on the character of organizing a "treatment milieu" in the home and community setting. The language of wrap-around has made this traditional clinical methodology most accessible, building on the image of a string of services that can be "wrapped around", so a child can function well in normal settings.

Surviving advocates and professionals will recognize the positive possibilities in these changes. Traditional child care agencies with large investments in real estate and institutional programming will face substantial staff development challenges to adapt to these new programming modalities. As payment methods change, it will be easier for these agencies to adapt because their practice has been largely shaped by the way they have been paid, i.e. so much for a "slot" in a standard day program, or a "bed", or a fifty-minute therapy session. There have been and will be dramatic decreases in the use of some of these traditional services. This change will be painful for some, but creative adjustments to the kind of service delivery that works for families, with practical immediacy and real flexibility, will open possibilities for which many dedicated professionals and advocates have been fighting for a long time.

ROLE CHANGES FOR CLINICIANS

To a large extent, the roles clinicians have played in the various mental health disciplines have been shaped by institutional and organizational modalities which managed care is in the process of rapidly abandoning. Survivors will find new roles in the new delivery systems. The traditional training venues for the mental health disciplines (eg., inpatient, outpatient, partial hospitals) worked because they could become the economic base of the training program. Psychiatric residents and other trainees in psychology, social work, and nursing could be minimally supported and they provided an inexpensive workforce for these programs. This worked because it was paid for by a fee-for-service reimbursement system within which there was almost no accounting for cost or quality of outcomes.

The professional expectations of the trainees in these disciplines have been shaped by this experience. Private practice in psychotherapy is the ideal; positions in respected institutions are quite acceptable. Few aspire to work in dwindling state hospitals; few have entered into new forms of programming in CMHCs for persons with SPMI or in systems of care for children with SED and their families. The move to managed care will require medical effectiveness: interventions that work at reasonable cost. The traditional services, outpatient, inpatient, and partial hospital, are certainly necessary components of an effective delivery system, but few would argue that they are sufficient for child and family mental health without an array of home and community supportive services to complement them.

This change of role will be profoundly challenging to many of the best child and family mental health clinicians. Survivors will recognize the place of dearly held values in the new visions guiding the emerging delivery systems. They will move easily from traditional contexts into new home and community settings and be able to respond directly to the considered needs of children and families.

The contribution of seasoned clinicians is critically needed and includes the refined art of clinical judgment in understanding mental health problems and the clinical method that conceptualizes treatment strategies and monitors progress toward defined treatment goals. The dysfunctional policy for child and family mental health has left the field in disarray with the burden of the work in the hands of line workers with very uneven preparation and background. The "non-system" has not arranged human capital and expertise effectively. Once we transcend our resentment and suspicion, highly trained clinicians will have an essential role in creating the new special needs systems of care. The themes operative in this transition of roles are four: homework, teamwork, coaching, and management.

Homework. If children do better in families, it is necessary to recognize that families are the front line of direct care and treatment. We may need to temporarily work with surrogate families, but families must be the field of focus, for better or worse. Surviving clinicians and advocates may be entering new territory. The change will require them to be sensitive to and respectful of the domain of the family and careful in entering it. The strengths of the family members must be recognized and they must be seen as respected colleagues in the treatment of the child.

Teamwork. Home and community care requires clinicians who have always held decisive authority in institutional settings to re-orient themselves to membership on a team. Effective teamwork assumes a mutual dependency and shared vision of the goal. The clinician in private practice, however skillful, has a limited reach. The same clinician, as a team member, works in concert with the rest of the team and can affect a wider array of critical factors.

Coaching. On a one to one basis, the treatment team needs seasoned clinicians to function as "clinical coaches", helping team members to conceptualize clinical strategies and guiding concerted efforts to implement them. This is not the role of the autocratic "boss", but more the expert trainer whose authority is established by working hard for the team and by bringing an in-depth perspective to the issues.

Management. The new special needs systems of care will need seasoned clinicians to provide clinical management which guides the process of treatment undertaken by the multi-disciplinary team. This management function insures that the interaction of the child, family, "helpers", and other care givers is open and constructive. The clinician manager oversees the allocation and organization of resources for the whole delivery system.

Profile of the Survivor. Child and family mental health under PSMC will have an even greater need for highly skilled clinicians than in the past, because these skills are precisely what can make managed care arrangements work. What will be difficult for many child and family mental health clinicians is that much of the current system, such as payment methods, agency and institutional bases, treatment conventions, and interagency relationships, will be profoundly changed or even swept away as PSMC practices are implemented. These traditional structures represent professional security, so their loss can be very threatening.

The profile of the surviving child and family mental health provider is that of one who can willingly move with the paradigm shift to family-focused care. This requires integration of the services and resources of all responsible agencies in an individualized treatment strategy that wraps services and support around every aspect of the child and family. This necessitates a multidisciplinary perspective and a fluency in the languages and traditions of child welfare, juvenile justice, substance abuse, special education, as well as health and mental health. Surviving providers will either join with the new service delivery organizations that orchestrate effective individualized care; or they will be proactive in helping their agencies or organizations participate in care offered by MCOs. They will consciously adapt new roles in relationship to family caregivers and in relationship to other members of the care team. With confidence in their refined diagnostic judgment, their conceptualization of treatment strategies, and the organization of treatment processes that their training has given them, they will carefully and indirectly support and guide their partners in the caring process. The rest of the decade will require their best efforts and could be the most productive years of their professional lives. But when they think about it, the surviving providers will realize that they have succeeded by carrying old wine in new wineskins.

REFERENCES

Cole, R.F., & Hanson, G., (1988). *Referencebook on the service system for mentally disordered children and adolescents in Ventura County,* California. Roseland, NJ: National Program Office, Mental Health Services Program for Youth,.

Cole, R.F., & Poe, S., (1993). *Partnerships for care: systems of care for children with serious emotional disturbances and their families.* Interim Report of the Mental Health Services Program for Youth. Washington, DC: Washington Business Group on Health.

Child and Adolescent Service System Program (CASSP), (1987). Series on community-based services for children and adolescents who are severely and emotionally disturbed. Washington, DC: CASSP Technical Assistance Center, Georgetown University,

England, M.J., & Cole, R.F., (1995). Children and mental health: how can the system be improved?, *Health Affairs, 14,* 3.

Feldman, S. (Ed.), 1992. *Managed Mental Health Services.* Springfield, IL: Charles C Thomas.

Stroul, B.A., & Friedman, R.M., (1986). *A system of care for severely emotionally disturbed children and youth.* Washington, DC: Georgetown University Child Development Center.

Stroul, B.A., (1988). *Home based services.* Series on community-based services for children and adolescents who are severely emotionally disturbed. Washington, DC: Georgetown University Child Development Center.

20

Time-Sensitive Treatment in Community Mental Health Settings

KAREN JOAN LUDWIG and DAVID A. MOLTZ

INTRODUCTION

As health care financing and delivery in the United States change rapidly and radically, mental health agencies in the public sector, like all other providers, are being challenged to fundamentally reconsider how most effectively to meet the psychotherapy needs of the populations they serve. In this process it is crucial that new initiatives are considered and implemented in a thoughtful and coherent way, so that changes derive from and express the values and beliefs of the agency.

In this chapter we will consider one such agency, and its transition from long-term to time-sensitive therapy as the primary treatment modality. We will describe the approach that we developed, and its strengths as we have utilized it. The approach does not stand alone; it is equally important to understand the context and the process of change. Therefore, we will also describe how the transition was planned and implemented, how it incorporated and expressed the agency's long-term goals and objectives, and how a clinical culture that supported these changes was shaped.

THE CONTEXT

Shoreline Community Mental Health Services is a community mental health center located in midcoast Maine. In 1989, after years of management difficulties, the agency was in danger of closing. Program development had virtually ceased. A small day program provided services for 8 to 10 individuals. There were no case management or housing services, and crisis services were minimal. Outpatient clinicians worked in isolation, doing long-term individual therapy and providing the best services possible to their own clients, but not addressing the six-month waiting list for services.

At this point the volunteer Board of Directors, with support from the State Department of Mental Health, began to rebuild the agency's management structure. A new management team, in collaboration with the Board, assessed the present state of the agency, the needs of the community, and anticipated trends in mental health financing. From this assessment several long-term goals emerged:

1) *To serve the needs of the community.* Shoreline's catchment area of 85,000 individuals is geographically large and extremely varied. Although the area is relatively homogeneous racially and ethnically, there is wide variation economically and by class. We agreed that as a community mental health center Shoreline should serve the needs of all residents of the catchment area, including those who were not currently receiving services, and that this would require a wide variety of programs and of approaches.

2) *To provide comprehensive and integrated services for people with mental illness.* The management staff was in agreement that the agency's resources should be directed toward those most in need of services, and that serving people with mental illness was the highest priority. We knew that community-based services for this population must be comprehensive, and that they must be integrated, both with each other and with services to the rest of the community.

3) *To prepare for managed care.* Although managed care had barely begun in Maine at that time, it was clear from national trends that in a very few years it would be the predominant form of health insurance. If we were to be ready with an efficient and accountable system of care, we would have to begin to shape our service delivery system immediately.

4) *To ensure the survival of the agency.* In order for the agency to continue to serve the community, it would have to develop strongly as a business and financial entity. This meant becoming more cost-effective, expanding the size and diversity of operations, and assessing and addressing the actual needs of the community, with a focus on customer satisfaction.

These four goals, while discrete and diverse, were seen as complementary rather than contradictory. And it was clear that each would be supported by a shift to time-sensitive, focused treatment as a primary modality.

Five years later, Shoreline has developed a full range of services, and has a staff that is competent in providing time-sensitive therapy. Accomplishing that transition involved questioning our assumptions about the nature of problems and of change; developing a clinical approach; enlisting the staff in the process of change; and creating an environment that would support and maintain the changes.

Survival Tips
Principles of Time-Sensitive Psychotherapy
Mental illness is a biopsychosocial phenomenon.
Individuals and families have strengths and resources which can usefully be acknowledged and mobilized.
The individual is more than his or her illness or problems.
Individuals live in families and communities, and can best be understood and assisted in their social context.
Therapy is most effective when it is focused, and is oriented toward achieving clearly defined goals.

THE CLINICAL APPROACH

When it became clear that the agency needed to move from long-term to more time-sensitive treatment, we considered a variety of models. We found the ideas of de Shazer and the Milwaukee Brief Family Therapy Center (de Shazer, 1985; 1988) and of Michael White (Epston & White, 1992; While, 1986; White & Epston, 1990) to be especially useful, and we did utilize several models in training our staff; but in the end we decided that it would be better to define an *approach* rather than to adopt a particular clinical model. That is, we articulated a set of guiding principles and beliefs about therapeutic change, rather than a particular vehicle or model for change.

We made this decision for several reasons. First, we were working with an experienced staff of talented clinicians, and we believed that it was important to support them in utilizing their particular skills and experiences in the process of change. We also believed that change, whether for clients or for clinicians, is best accomplished by engaging the individual's strengths and resources, rather than by imposing external mandates. Secondly, we wanted to develop an approach that would be useful across the range of clinical services, such as community support or crisis services, rather than a model that would be useful only for outpatient therapy. Finally, we strongly believed that the clinical model must be flexible enough to be adapted to the particular client, rather than the client being asked to adapt to the model. We were concerned that espousing a particular model would lead to a "one-size-fits-all" practice that would not be sensitive to the needs of the client.

For all these reasons, we set out to develop a clinical approach that would guide clinicians in their work, and at the same time would allow them to draw from a variety of clinical models which they found helpful and appropriate. Our approach is defined by the following principles:

1. Mental illness is a biopsychosocial phenomenon, the product of complex and ongoing interactions between the individual's biology, psychology and interpersonal environment (Engel, 1977, 1980; Moltz, 1991, 1993).

2. Individuals and families have strengths and resources which can usefully be acknowledged and mobilized.

3. The individual is more than his or her illness or problems.

4. Individuals live in families and communities, and can best be understood and assisted in their social context.

5. Therapy is most effective when it is focused, and is oriented toward achieving clearly defined goals.

Mental illness is biopsychosocial. Because mental illness is the resultant of the interaction of biological, psychological and interpersonal factors, it can be affected by interventions on any of these levels. "Either/or" arguments about etiology are irrelevant and distracting, and are usefully replaced by questions of interaction and mutual effect. Each of these factors is important, and can support or constrain changes in each of the others.

For people with serious mental illness, psychotherapy is one component of a comprehensive, integrated approach. When appropriate, it is offered in conjunction with other services, not alone.

> A 41 year old man with a long history of schizophrenia and social isolation refused any services other than infrequent medication visits. He could not tolerate other activities because of paranoid thinking and delusions which prevented social interaction. After several years of trying different medicines, he benefited from clozapine to the extent that he could begin to participate in social activities at the Community Support Program. He then requested and was able to utilize psychotherapy, with the goal of learning to differentiate real memories and experiences from fantasized ones.

Strengths and resources. The focus on strengths and resources underlies all of our beliefs and practices. Therapy, rather than focusing on problems and deficits, becomes a process of identifying and mobilizing resources in the individual and the family which can be utilized in developing solutions to their presenting problems.

This change has profound implications for the course of psychotherapy, especially for individuals with mental illness. It allows a focus on the individual's successes in withstanding the effects of the illness, and the fostering of a self-perception as strong and competent rather than as helpless and failing. Family members can be acknowledged for their struggles against the encroachment of the illness on their lives. Success and achievements, rather than failures and incompetence, become the objects of therapeutic exploration.

> A 45 year old man with schizophrenia was interviewed with his mother following admission to a psychiatric inpatient unit. He had been living at home, without treatment, for the five years since his last hospitalization. Both he and his mother had been committed to keeping him at home in spite of increasing delusions and hallucinations, and both were feeling helpless and demoralized because of their inability to accomplish this. When the interviewer expressed interest in how they had managed to succeed for as long as they did in spite of the intensity of the symptoms, both mother and son came alive, and began speaking with enthusiasm about how they had worked together so effectively for so long.

This strength-based approach lends itself naturally to time-sensitive therapy. Rather than working to repair early trauma or to resolve intrapsychic or interpersonal conflicts, the therapist helps the individual and the family to recognize and to apply resources that they already possess. This process may start in the therapy office, but the most important changes occur in the course of the client's life, and therapy becomes a process of tracking and validating the changes as they unfold.

> A twelve year old boy with a long history of school phobia was seen with his father for treatment. They were invited by their therapist to reflect together on incidents in which the boy had been able to "tame the Worries" which generally restricted his life. They also talked together about other times when he had been able to differentiate between these "Lesser Worries" and "Genuine Problems" for which he needed his father's assistance. Father and son began to keep a log of times when the boy was able to recognize and resist "sneaky attempts by the Lesser Worries" to keep him from a desired activity, as well as times when he could call upon his father to help him to overcome a particulary big "Genuine Problem." The boy soon returned to school, and father and son agreed to stay on the alert to identify and resist attempts by the "Lesser Worries" to take over the boy's life again. (See also White, 1989b.)

The individual is more than the problem or illness. While mental illness is irreducibly biological in part, the individual is also more than the illness. We have found Michael White's practice of "externalizing the problem" (1989a) to be extremely useful. "It is not the person who is ... the problem. Rather, it is the problem that is the problem." (White, 1989a, p. 6). When the illness is externalized, resources can be mobilized to limit and control its impact. Rather than identify the individual or the family as part of the problem, the therapist can join with them in a "therapeutic triangle", an alliance against the illness and its effects (Fig. 1)

> A 45 year old man was hospitalized because of delusional jealousy concerning his wife. During the hospitalization he was treated with low doses of antipsychotics. Couple sessions focused on the strengths

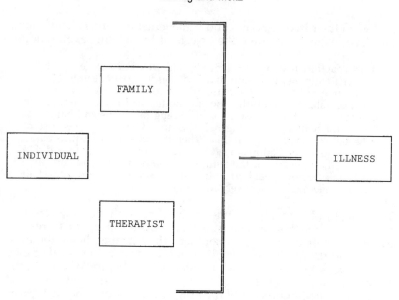

Figure 1 The Therapeutic Triangle

and caring that had kept the couple together for 18 years, and on how he had been able to keep his jealousy from dominating their relationship. However, discharge was impeded because he would not acknowledge that the jealousy was irrational, and his wife was afraid to have him come home unless he did. In a pre-discharge couple session a consultant told the man that he had "a touch of paranoia" which explained his jealousy. When the man said that he was sure of the evidence of his wife's infidelity, the consultant replied that paranoia can make a person certain about things which in fact were not true. He also said that the couple clearly had a very strong relationship, but that the paranoia was "sitting there between you" in spite of their efforts to keep it from dominating them. The man appeared quite relieved, and said to his wife, "I guess this lets you off the hook, and it lets *me* off the hook. I guess the problem is the paranoia." He was discharged soon after this meeting, and on follow-up the couple was doing well.

While externalizing the problem can be useful for all clients, it is especially helpful for individuals with serious mental illness, who have often come to identify themselves with their condition. Externalizing the illness and separating it from the person can be the first step in controlling it and its effects, and offers the individual the possibility of experiencing mastery rather than deficiency and incompetence.

Individuals live in families and communities. If illness is truly biopsychosocial, it can best be understood and approached through the individual's social context. Family members are deeply affected by the illness, and can also be important allies in the struggle against it. Often the most effective way to assist individual clients in managing and overcoming their difficulties is to include the important people in their lives as consultants and participants in the work. These individuals are usually family members, but can also include friends, employers, clergy, health providers, and others identified by the client. They are seen not as part of the problem but as resources, individuals who may become part of the solution.

> A 17 year old girl returned to school after a two year absence because of a serious illness which required an organ transplant. Her deepest concern was that she was now "different", and that her former friends had "deserted" her. Her counselor requested that she invite her friends to a session. Five friends who agreed to attend spoke of their concern for the girl, and asked her why she had resisted their attempts to include her in school activities. The girl, who had not recognized these invitations, began to accept them, and she soon returned to a full schedule at school.

Since family members are often intimately involved with the individual, they can be a source of important information and insight. They can also benefit from information about the illness and about treatment as they help the individual to master the illness. Therefore family members are included whenever possible in treatment planning and review, and are invited to participate in psychiatric evaluations and medication reviews as well. They are encouraged to become involved with the local affiliate of the National Alliance for the Mentally Ill, and to take a course offered by members of the Alliance on "Living With Mental Illness." They may also be invited to join a multiple family group offered by the mental health center. These groups, made up of individuals with mental illness and their family members, can be very helpful in developing a social context based on mutual support and problem-solving. The more the individual and the family know about the illness, the more they can bring their resources to bear on it.

When clients are viewed in the context of their social systems, the nature and goals of therapy shift. Progress is measured in relation to the individual's natural systems, rather than evaluated in terms of the relationship to the therapist or what happens in the therapy room. The goal of therapy becomes assisting the client to define or modify a relationship to his or her natural systems which will facilitate improved and stable functioning.

Therapy should be focused. When there is clear agreement on specific, well-defined goals, and when the treatment process remains focused on achieving those goals, therapy becomes both more effective and more accountable. This is not a new idea (see de Shazer, 1985, 1988; and many others), but it is often the most difficult change to make for a clinician who has been trained in long-term therapy. It implies and requires a different set of assumptions about the nature of problems and the nature of change. From the first encounter the therapist works with the client to define the specific problems to be addressed, and to develop specific, well-defined goals which will direct the course of treatment. The therapy that results is a different approach, and not simply a condensed (and therefore second-best) long-term treatment.

A focused, structured approach to treatment is useful across the range of clinical problems, but it is especially helpful for persons with mental illness. Individuals who have problems organizing their thinking, maintaining attention and concentration, or tolerating the anxiety that may be produced by an unstructured, ill-defined situation often do very well with an approach that is focused, structured and well-defined. Family members also find it useful to have clear goals toward which to work.

When goals are clearly defined in this way, therapy becomes time-sensitive without the necessity of specifying a particular number of sessions or length of treatment. As the work progresses, sessions may be scheduled at increasing intervals, in order to maintain contact and continuity; or therapist and client may agree to "suspend" treatment, leaving open the possibility for other treatment episodes as needed in the future. In focused, well-defined treatment, the work continues until the goals have been met, and then it ends.

CASE EXAMPLE

Evelyn W. was a 27 year old woman with a long history of treatment and a variety of diagnoses. Her previous contacts with therapists had been difficult and antagonistic, with Evelyn feeling unheard and unhelped, and her therapists feeling stymied by her unwillingness to consider her own role in her difficulties, and her proclivity for loud and public protests when she felt that her needs were not being met.

One year prior to her most recent request for services, Evelyn's boyfriend was convicted of sexually molesting her six-year old son. She was distraught about the trauma to her son, and about her inability to protect him. She became increasingly agitated and disorganized, and began experiencing psychotic symptoms. Evelyn voluntarily requested psychiatric hospitalization in the community, but instead she was committed involuntarily to the State psychiatric institution, where she stayed for two weeks. Following discharge she lost two jobs in succession, including one at which she was harassed by fellow employees after a local newspaper published a front-page article in which she recounted her experiences of hospitalization.

Evelyn's current presenting problems were anger and upset concerning the hospitalization and its consequences. She reported that the anger had affected all of her relationships, and that she was unable to control or modulate it. She said that her life was being consumed by ruminations about her involuntary treatment, and about being labeled mentally ill. She felt that she needed intensive therapy, and requested meeting for two hours twice a week to address these problems.

The therapist noted that Evelyn's recounting of her hospitalization had a hypnotic, mesmerizing quality. She listened empathically to Evelyn's account, initially asking questions only to clarify the effects of the hospitalization on her life. However in the first session she began to work with Evelyn to separate her experiences and symptoms from herself. They agreed that the goal of their work together would be to reduce the effect of those past experiences and memories on her present life. They also agreed that one step in decreasing the impact of the memories would be to limit sessions to a maximum of one hour weekly, with a reduction in frequency as Evelyn made progress in reclaiming her life from her symptoms. At the end of the session, the therapist suggested a behavioral "experiment" to help limit the ruminations.

At the next session, one week later, Evelyn seemed calmer. She said that the experiment had worked poorly, but she had found other ways to harness her disturbing thoughts, and she felt that she was more in charge of them than she had been previously. She agreed to continue to work on this, and to meet again in two weeks.

In the next meeting her therapist became curious about how Evelyn had managed to resist the label of "mentally ill person" that had been applied to her. Evelyn spoke of her earlier work with people with mental retardation, and of her commitment to their full participation in the life of the community. As she focused on her experiences of advocating for others, she began to see her potential for struggling more effectively against her own experiences of victimization.

Following this meeting, Evelyn decided to accept a job in the town where she had been hospitalized. She had previously worried that she would become engulfed by her memories if she did this, and had avoided even visiting the town. However she now felt that successfully accomplishing this would help her to resist the definition of herself which had been imposed by the hospitalization.

Over the next two years, Evelyn met with her therapist an average of once every three months. The therapy continued to focus on Evelyn's ability to reclaim her life from the consequences of her hospitalization, and there were many examples of this to notice. She filed a suit with the State Human Rights Commission challenging the dismissal from her job following the article about her hospitalization. She wrote letters to former co-workers and supervisors who had called her "crazy," challenging them to better understand mental illness. She started a support group for parents whose children had been sexually abused. She was able to overcome the effects of her previous experiences to such an extent that she was promoted to a leadership position in her new job. Evelyn often wrote letters to her therapist in the time between appointments; the therapist promptly responded, using the opportunities to encourage Evelyn's evolving definition of herself as a competent, successful person (White & Epston, 1990).

During this period Evelyn called to schedule an appointment whenever she felt that she needed help with a particularly difficult experience of intrusion of her past hospitalization in her current life. When such an incident occurred, Evelyn and her therapist explored strategies and resources that she could use to manage her symptoms until she could "gain the upper hand" again. In addition to internal resources, Evelyn was encouraged to consider using medication, crisis services, support groups, and readings to help her in her struggles.

At the end of two years Evelyn lost the discrimination case against her former employer. However, she discovered that she no longer needed a formal ruling to free herself from the definition of being mentally ill. She believed that she was a successful, competent person, and at the same time that she had an episode of mental illness, from which she had now recovered. After two years Evelyn terminated treatment, with the understanding that she could return at any time if she found herself again in need of consultation.

Although this example involves outpatient therapy, we have found that the principles outlined above can be as usefully applied in our programs for Crisis Intervention, Community Support, Substance Abuse and Psychiatric Services. The approach provides a common clinical philosophy which facilitates integration and interchange between these programs.

It should also be apparent that these principles are very compatible with group work. Multiple family groups focused on a particular illness (McFarlane, 1990) are one example utilizing this approach. Groups for people with mental illness using a "narrative" approach (O'Neill & Stockell, 1991) are another. Application of these principles in a group format can provide highly effective and efficient treatment for a wide range of problems.

IMPLEMENTING THE APPROACH

Throughout the process of defining and implementing this approach, we have chosen whenever possible to encourage and facilitate, rather than to mandate, its use by the clinical staff. We began by defining the values and beliefs described above, and by clearly stating our goals and objectives for the agency. Because of the overlap and complementarity of our long-term goals, we were able to frame this discussion in terms of clinical issues, such as increasing access to services and providing services to more individuals and families, rather than as a response to the mandates of managed care.

Earlier in this paper we discussed our decision to define an approach to therapy rather than adopting a particular model. For similar reasons, we decided whenever possible not to impose a specific limit on the number of sessions offered to clients. Reflecting our belief that individuals do best when they are encouraged to apply their own resources and strengths to solving problems creatively, we insisted only that clinicians make themselves responsible for helping their clients in the most efficient way possible, and that they be accountable for approaching well-defined problems in a focused way. We assumed that firm but gentle pressure in the direction of developing necessary skills and trying these approaches with a variety of clients would allow each clinician to develop a level of comfort and facility which would grow over time, and that utilization of the basic philosophy of treatment could include many different approaches and models. When in a given case a specific limit on the number of sessions was imposed by the payer, this was seen as an additional impetus to use focused, goal-driven treatment, but not as the primary motivation.

In spite of this relatively low-key approach, some of the clinical staff had serious reservations about the changes. This was expressed primarily by the more senior clinicians, who were very experienced in long-term individual psychodynamic therapy and were reluctant to give up a mode of practice in which they believed and in which they felt competent. Much of their resistance was expressed as ethical concerns about providing less adequate, "superficial" therapy to their clients. We responded by questioning the ethics of providing long-term treatment when short-term might be as effective, and of offering intensive services to a very few people and none at all to many others.

Some clinicians felt challenged and excited by the changes, and took to the new approach easily. Others struggled successfully to make it their own. Still others decided that they were not willing to adapt to the new expectations, and chose to leave the agency. This allowed us to recruit new staff who were more comfortable with time-sensitive approaches.

It was vitally important in accomplishing this transition that adequate training be provided. It is not enough to tell clinicians to work more briefly; they need to learn and understand the assumptions underlying the work, as well as specific skills, and they need training and supervision which is organized and coherent over time.

We developed an ongoing staff development program around two training goals: to teach outpatient therapists to work with people with mental illness, and to teach all our clinical staff the philosophy and techniques necessary to provide strength-oriented, time-sensitive treatment.

This training took place in a variety of formats. We sponsored several day-long workshops presented by outside experts, on topics such as working collaboratively with people with serious mental illness and their families; brief family therapy; stigma and discrimination as they affect people with mental illness; and narrative therapy. All clinical staff attended these events. We organized study groups in which we read relevant literature, role-played clinical situations, and presented cases to each other which illustrated problems and, increasingly, successes which clinicians were experiencing. Biweekly staff development presentations on a variety of clinical topics were chosen for their contribution to understanding and applying the approach.

Clinical supervision and consultation consistently supported the time-sensitive approach, as well. Supervision focused on applying the general principles of the approach to the particular case. The process of supervision also reflected these principles: supervisors encouraged the strengths and successes of their supervisees, rather than focusing on mistakes and deficits in their work.

Many of the staff development presentations were geared to business and support staff as well as clinicians. We believed that the shift to a strength-oriented approach was so fundamental that all staff had to understand and support it. How a client is greeted by the receptionist can have as powerful an impact as anything that happens in the therapy session, so it is important that the receptionist be operating from the same assumptions and beliefs as is the therapist.

The full and ongoing participation by the staff in all these training activities was crucial to the success of our project. For a "clinical culture" to develop which will support and facilitate change, there must be a common "language" which is shared by everyone involved. These ongoing, agency-wide trainings provided that language.

WHERE WE ARE AND WHERE WE ARE GOING

By most measures, we have been successful in making the transition to a more time-sensitive and accountable system of care. Shoreline now provides a wide range of services, including a 24 hour/7 day mobile crisis intervention team; adult and adolescent crisis stabilization units; housing supports and case management; dual diagnosis services; and child, adult and family therapy services including group, individual and family therapy. Services for people with serious mental illness, including psychiatric services, are fully integrated in all these programs.

The initial wait for services is sometimes as long as a month, but individuals in crisis or with urgent need can be seen the same day. Between 1989 and 1993 the number of individuals served annually in Shoreline's Child, Adult and Family therapy program (not including crisis or community support services) increased by 93%, while the number of visits per year increased by only 18%. The average number of visits per client in that program went from 17.3 to 10.6 in that time. Clinicians have frequently been surprised by how ready clients have been to define and work toward clear and achievable goals; at times it has seemed that clients have had an easier time with this than have clinicians.

At the same time, we continue to be challenged to develop new ways to meet the needs of the populations we serve. As private managed care plans increase enrollment and Medicaid becomes managed as well, we will have to become increasingly skilled in providing time-sensitive treatment to a larger proportion of our clients. As provider networks and capitated contracts become established we will have to assume risk and learn to manage the care we provide ourselves. And as the State increasingly focuses its resources on individuals with mental illness, we will have to find ways to meet the needs of the large number of individuals and families in our catchment area who neither meet the State's criteria for services nor are covered by private insurance or Medicaid, but who experience very significant psychosocial and psychological distress.

As we meet these challenges it will be necessary for us to continue to examine our values and beliefs, and to work to develop the skills and resources necessary to meet the needs of the people we serve. The work that we have done in developing our clinical approach will form a foundation as we proceed.

REFERENCES

de Shazer, S. (1985). *Keys to solution in brief therapy.* New York: W.W. Norton.

de Shazer, S. (1988). Clues: Investigating solutions in brief therapy. New York: W.W. Norton.

Engel, G.L. (1977). The need for a new medical model: A challenge for biomedicine. *Science, 196,* 129–136.

Engel, G.L. (1980). The clinical application of the biopsychosocial model. *American Journal of Psychiatry, 137,* 535–544.

Epston, D., & White, M. (1992). *Experience, contradiction, narrative & imagination: Selected papers of David Epston & Michael White, 1989–1991.* Adelaide, S. Australia: Dulwich Centre Publications.

McFarlane, W.R. (1990). Multiple family groups and the treatment of schizophrenia. In H.A. Nasrallah (Ed.), *Handbook of schizophrenia* (pp. 167–190). Amsterdam: Elsevier Science Publishers.

Moltz, D.A. (1991). Families with affective disorders. In F. Herz (Ed.), *Reweaving the family tapestry: A multigenerational approach to families* (pp. 286–308). New York: W.W. Norton.

Moltz, D.A. (1993). Bipolar disorder and the family: An integrative model. *Family Process, 32,* 409–423.

O'Neill, M., & Stockell, G. (1991). Worthy of discussion: Collaborative group therapy. *Australian & New Zealand Journal of Family Therapy, 12,* 201–206.

White, M. (1986). Negative explanation, restraint, and double description: A template for family therapy. *Family Process, 25,* 169–184.

White, M. (1989a). The externalizing of the problem and the re-authoring of lives and relationships. In M. White, *Selected papers* (pp. 5–28). Adelaide, S. Australia: Dulwich Centre Publications.

White, M. (1989b). Fear busting & monster taming: An approach to the fears of young children. In M. White, *Selected papers* (pp. 107–113). Adelaide, S. Australia: Dulwich Centre Publications.

White, M., & Epston, D. (1990). *Narrative means to therapeutic ends.* New York: W.W. Norton.

Section V

Advocacy, Evaluation, and Training

DAVID POLLACK

In order to ensure that PSMC systems meet the expectations of the various stakeholders involved, it is essential that consumers and families have adequate input into the planning and implementation of care delivery systems. The growing consumer and family movements have also articulated a number of roles for their constituents in the actual delivery and evaluation of services. Will managed care organizations honor the gains that consumers and families have made and include them in meaningful ways?

Outcomes assessments are critical to determining the success of these new and relatively untested programs. How can the goals of PSMC systems be measured? Will there be enough money within the budgets for service systems to provide for meaningful evaluation? Will research into the adequacy and efficacy of managed mental health care services be well designed, funded, and implemented? The need to maintain the numbers and skills of the mental health workforce seems to come into direct conflict with the demands of managed care systems to provide services efficiently. How will training of mental health professionals be maintained or altered with the changes implied by managed care?

This section attempts to address these extremely important questions and to point out the ways that advocacy, evaluation, research, and training needs can be successfully promoted.

21

Family Advocacy Issues

LAURA LEE HALL and LAURIE M. FLYNN

INTRODUCTION

Radical changes in the public mental health system, resulting from public sector managed care (PSMC) and privatization initiatives, have created significant challenges for family and consumer advocates. As we struggle to adapt to the new language and technology, as well as the new private sector orientation, of key decision makers, we must continue to advocate for access and quality services for persons with severe and persistent mental illness.

Effective advocacy and system monitoring in a changing system requires education, clearly stated principles, and tools appropriate for shaping decentralized, competitive, private sector, and outcome-driven systems. This chapter describes the efforts of The National Alliance for the Mentally Ill (NAMI), representing over 140,000 family members and consumers nationwide, to develop advocacy tools befitting the managed care era. Our goal is to inform not only family members and consumers of our efforts, but to inform providers and planners as well, in order to foster more effective provider/family/consumer collaboration in advocacy and system monitoring activities. The chapter begins with an overview of NAMI's managed care advocacy portfolio and then details our *National Report Card* on PSMC.

NAMI'S MANAGED CARE ADVOCACY PORTFOLIO

NAMI's managed care portfolio addresses the reality of today's public sector:

- It tells our members what managed care is, so as to empower their advocacy.

- It describes clear and unequivocal values and principles that must be upheld in changing systems.

- It recognizes the need for advocacy tailored to the specific approaches of states and local areas.

- It is developing a research base to inform our members, other advocates, and policy-makers as to what is working and what is not.

With all of these activities, NAMI is working to shape the evolving "managed care" face of the public mental health system, for the betterment of people with severe mental illnesses.

Effective advocacy requires a foundation of knowledge. Consequently, one of NAMI's first managed care projects was the publication of *Mental Illness and Managed Care: A Primer for Families and Consumers* (Malloy, 1995). Even as policy-makers, providers, and others involved in the public mental health system scramble to learn the alphabet soup of managed care acronyms — HMO, PPOs, POS, IPAs — consumers and family members must familiarize themselves with the methods of managed care. NAMI's Primer provides "basic information about managed care and the implications of managed care in public-sector mental health services."

NAMI's *Primer* is just a starting point. However, ongoing education of families and consumers is essential. Managed behavioral health care is a complex subject, and it is continually evolving. Further information is needed on the evolving organizational models of managed care, the ways in which different systems perform, the identity and track record of managed care organizations, contracting terms, oversight mechanisms, and others. In addition to the *Primer,* NAMI has established an in-house staff position to provide technical assistance to state and local NAMI chapters (affiliates) on managed care and relevant policy issues. This state outreach function will regularly provide written materials to NAMI's state and local affiliates; will answer telephone inquiries; will review policy documents developed in the states and counties (e.g., draft RFPs and contracts), and will help coordinate knowledge-sharing among our affiliates.

While advocacy strategies may change, the basic principles of quality service systems are a constant. In essence, a system serving people with severe mental illnesses should be a system that partners with and is accountable to consumers and their families, and provides comprehensive, appropriate, and effective treatment and supports. NAMI has produced a set of core "managed care" principles, which translate our values into specific statements relevant to the ongoing PSMC reform efforts. These principles emphasize system accountability, comprehensive services, meaningful participation of consumers and family members, and a focus on individuals with the most severe disabilities.

Health care reform, in general, and reform of the public mental health system, in particular, have become increasingly decentralized in the 1990s. States, counties, and regions in the U.S. are setting policy, contracting for services, and collecting data. The devolution or localization of health policy development from national to regional or local arenas means that advocacy must be increasingly devolved as well.

NAMI has an advantage in this decentralized world. As a grassroots organization, with 1,100 affiliates in all 50 states, NAMI is positioned to shape the managed care revolutions in state public mental health systems. NAMI's national office is working to support and enhance our membership's advocacy capability. In addition to the education and outreach activities described above, NAMI has just awarded its first grant program to state affiliates — *State Initiative Grants for Managed Care Advocacy.* This competitive award, open to all state affiliates, provides up to $30,000 per year for advocacy projects focused on managed care. Five state affiliates, in Iowa, North Carolina, Maine, Texas, and West Virginia, received funding this year. Each state has developed unique advocacy plans, suited to the status of local managed care policy and other unique aspects of the state and its NAMI affiliate. For example, the Texas AMI's grant money will be used to support member education, as managed care in Texas' public mental health system is still very early in its evolution. Maine's AMI is setting up a regional network of AMIs, to share information on managed care and advocacy tactics. Given the close geographic proximity of other New England states, a regional network is especially suitable for a regional managed care advocacy strategy. The AMI in Iowa is developing a statewide family and consumer monitoring system, an advocacy tool befitting a state in which Medicaid managed care is being actively implemented.

The effective shaping of managed care in the public mental health system will require more than education and grassroots advocacy. New information, stemming from research, is a critically important component of NAMI's managed care agenda. NAMI is organizing three different projects, the results of which will inform our advocacy and the evolution of managed care in the public mental health system.

NAMI has spearheaded and continues to lead a project focused on outcomes in behavioral health care. This multi-year project — the *Outcomes Roundtable* — sponsored in partnership with Johns Hopkins University, American Psychiatric Association, Center for Mental Health Services, Eli Lilly and Company, National Depressive and Manic-Depressive Association, National Institute on Alcohol and Alcohol Abuse, National Institute on Drug Abuse, National Institute on Mental Health, and the Washington Business Group on Health — is a multidisciplinary and multi-stakeholder group united to develop outcomes measures that will improve the quality of care and life for the estimated 52 million people who suffer from psychiatric and addictive disorders.

In addition to sponsoring meetings, the *Outcomes Roundtable* includes three task forces, whose aims are: (1) to develop principles for consumer outcomes assessment; (2) to pilot test outcome measurement tools and to review outcome measurement instruments for how well they abide by stated principles; and (3) to disseminate information on the *Roundtable's* work, so as to inform evolving mental health care delivery systems, including those in the public sector. The first task of the *Outcomes Roundtable,* the development of principles for outcome assessment, has already been completed. The twelve enumerated principles uphold the importance of a sound scientific basis to outcome measurement, the inclusion of input from consumers, their care-giving family members, and providers, and linking outcomes to clinical processes.

The work of the *Outcomes Roundtable* is directly relevant to managed care. Outcome measurement and performance, which is consumer-focused, clinically relevant, and scientifically sound, will provide the basis for judging the quality of managed care, balancing the cost-containment incentives that currently prevail in such systems. Families and consumers will have the tools to assure that managed care organizations provide quality care: care that produces the best outcomes for individuals with severe mental illnesses.

NAMI has recently joined forces with the Milbank Memorial Fund to develop a model Request for Proposals (RFP) and contract for managed care organizations in the public mental health system and serving people with severe mental illnesses. As states and counties increasingly contract out the management and provision of public mental services, an important lever of influence is the RFP and contract by which such arrangements are shaped. The most rapidly growing activity of the managed behavioral health care industry is that of "risk-based contracting," in which companies provide and manage services for a set population, at some level of risk. "Risk contracts have a measurable impact on costs of, access to, and effectiveness of services" (Frank, McGuire, & Newhouse, 1995). Contracting for services and their management, especially risk-contracting, clearly can control for costs. This practice also presents the risk of inadequate services. Thus, the specifications in the RFP, and the ultimate terms of the managed care contract, are critically important in delineating definitions of medical necessity, specific services covered, target populations, outcome measurements, provider networks, grievance procedures, and other mechanisms involved in the management of the mental health delivery system. Working with the Milbank Memorial Fund, NAMI will seek to provide model RFP and contract language, to shape the next generation of managed care contracts, so that they are maximally responsive to and responsible for people with severe mental illnesses and their family members.

The third research project that NAMI is undertaking is *A National Report Card: Managed Care and People with Severe Mental Illness.* This study, funded in part by the Ittleson Foundation, will provide a national snapshot of PSMC policies and practices in the U.S. public mental health system, and PSMC's impact on people with severe mental illnesses and their family members.

For consumers, family members, and the general public to understand managed care's impact on people with severe mental illness, three broad domains bear scrutiny: (1) the public policy platform upon which managed care is built; (2) the experiences of patients and their family members in these systems; and, (3) the policies and practices of both public and private MCOs themselves. Building on a series of national assessments of public mental health system performance, including evaluations of state programs and the criminal justice system (Torrey et al., 1990, 1992), NAMI's *National Report Card* will consider all three of these domains and will submit policy recommendations.

The first section of the *National Report Card* will provide a summary of state policies regarding PSMC. For each state, NAMI will provide information on the design and oversight of PSMC systems, the identity of MCOs in the public sector, and key responsibilities of the MCOs. Information will also be provided on the number of individuals served by PSMC systems and the financial resources involved.

For several states, including Massachusetts, Tennessee, Arizona, and Iowa, the *National Report Card* will provide a more in-depth look at PSMC. In each of these states, we will describe the evolution of managed care policies, key decision makers and processes, the models of managed care in place, and evaluation studies relevant to the managed care systems. Based on these case studies, we will analyze the lessons teamed to date.

Part two of the *National Report Card* will directly probe consumer and family member perceptions and experiences of managed care, via a survey of NAMI and the National Depressive and Manic-Depressive Association (NDMDA), the two largest consumer organizations concerned about serious mental illnesses. The survey data, which will be the first of its kind, will be supplemented by extensive interview of family members and consumers around the nation.

The third part of the *National Report Card* focuses on the policies and practices of managed care organizations themselves. This section most closely resembles what are popularly known as health care report cards — "published information about the quality of care provided by health plans" (US GAO, 1994). Our report card survey, which focuses on the largest managed behavioral health care organizations, asks for information on product lines and practices, treatment guidelines, family and consumer involvement, the comprehensiveness of services, and approaches to outcome management. By providing a baseline of information, we anticipate that this report card survey will be revised in the future and adapted to managed care organizations in specific regions and states around the country.

REPORT CARD QUESTIONS FOR MANAGED BEHAVIORAL HEALTH CARE ORGANIZATIONS

While monitoring of the quality of care provided by health care organizations and providers has been underway since at least the end of World War II, the publishing of such data, in the form of "report cards" is a relatively new phenomenon (U.S. GAO, 1994). It was launched by the publication of data concerning hospital coronary artery bypass surgery mortality rates, as analyzed by the Health Care Financing Administration (HCFA) in the late 1980s. Since that time, corporate purchasers of health care have been the driving force behind measures of quality and report cards for competing plans. Without measures of health care quality, the only measurable factor by which corporate purchasers could decide on a health care plan was its costs, a measure not indicative of overall value. Following the leadership of corporate purchasers, legislation in several states mandates the publication of information on health care plan performance. Government bodies and large health plans have developed their own measures and report cards.

Report card measures typically include information on the resources and organizational arrangements in place to deliver care, the processes of care, service utilization measures, outcomes of treatment, and patient satisfaction data. Such data raise a variety of issues, including concerns about the accuracy of reported information, the actual link between report card measures and treatment quality, and the standardization of measures used across plans and providers (U.S. GAO, 1994). In response to this last concern, the National Committee for Quality Assurance (NCQA) has been coordinating efforts to create a standardized set of indicators, which led to the Health Plan Employer Data and Information Set — HEDIS. Over 60 indicators are included in HEDIS for five areas: quality, access and patient satisfaction, membership and utilization, finance, and health plan management activities (NCQA, 1995). Results from the first assessment using the HEDIS indicators were published in early 1995 for 21 large health plans. Since then, NCQA is in the process of adapting the HEDIS instrument for managed care organizations with Medicaid contracts (NCQA, 1995).

Existing report cards raise at least three other concerns especially relevant to people with severe mental illnesses and their family members. First, while information from report cards should benefit not only health plan purchasers and administrators but also consumers themselves, "the needs of individual consumers have not been well communicated to report card developers" (U.S. GAO, 1994). As a consequence, existing report cards may not provide the kinds of information relevant to consumers in their enrollment decisions and advocacy efforts.

Secondly, outcome measures especially relevant to consumers and their family members are generally not included in existing report cards. For example, HEDIS does not include measures that directly reflect the outcomes of care. While several factors argue against the inclusion of many outcome measures in current report cards — including the infancy of this science, the uncertain link between various outcome measures and clinical interventions, and the lack of standard measures used across health plans — the development of this field is imperative for meaningful and true performance-based assessment. Indeed, research and pilot studies in several state public mental health systems are underway, which point to the ultimate ability to assess health plans on the basis of their outcomes (Lehman, 1995).

The third concern raised by existing report cards is their limited consideration of mental health. For example, the first draft of the *Medicaid HEDIS* included relatively few questions pertaining to mental and addictive disorders (NCQA, 1995). Questions especially relevant to severe mental illnesses are all but absent from existing report cards. In the last year, the Center for Mental Health Services (CMHS) and the American Managed Behavioral Healthcare Association (AMBHA) have been developing report cards of their own focused on mental and addictive disorders (CMHs, 1995; AMBHA, 1995). AMBHA's report card, aimed at developing standardized measures for members of this industry association, focuses heavily on performance indicators that are measurable; the results of their pilot study will only be reported for all responding managed care organizations; they will not be reported for individual companies (AMBHA). In contrast, CMHS' effort has resulted in a series of performance indicators that, while reflecting the values of consumers and mental health experts, are not easily measurable with industry databases. CMHS plans to test its report card in the near future.

Questions developed by NAMI for its report card seek to correct the deficiencies of current report card projects. Our report card puts forward questions that are answerable by industry databases, building on measures developed by NCQA and AMBHA. It also asks for background information on the organizations, so as to educate consumers and family members about the industry players. It expands on other report cards, by asking a series of questions pertaining to consumer and family involvement in managed care organizations. It focuses on the most severe of mental illnesses. While standardized outcome measures are not requested, information on the kinds of outcomes used, how they are measured, and how such data are used are requested. Responses from the MCOs will set the stage for future outcome reporting. Early drafts of the report card questions were sent out for review to nearly 30 consumers, family members, researchers, clinicians, and managed care industry representatives.

While the piloted version of NAMI's report card survey will be pared down, the ideal model that we prepared covers 8 domains, including: information on contract portfolio; organizational information; the definitions and numbers of individuals with severe mental illnesses; treatment protocols and the management of clinical decision-making; consumer and family member involvement; availability and use of comprehensive care; and, outcome measurement. This comprehensive version of the report card forms not only a template for our and other report card efforts but also may be an outline for RFPs and contracts for public entities who are contracting with managed care organizations. Furthermore, we will publicize the report card instrument, in hopes of making clear NAMI's values and expectations for PSMC.

Given the early stage of PSMC, and of the report card process, NAMI will not use report card responses to rate managed behavioral healthcare organizations in a best to worst fashion. Such ratings can be worrisome, given the immature science of report cards and performance indicators. Rather, with this first version of NAMI's report card, we intend to simply profile respondent MCOs, and to describe for our members the practices and policies of MCOs serving people with severe mental illnesses.

CONCLUSION

As managed care expands through the public mental health system, consumers and family members, in collaboration with clinicians and provider organizations, must play a pivotal role, so that existing systems are reshaped for the benefit of people with severe mental illnesses. While managed care brings with it positive opportunities for change in the public mental health system, including improved technology, efficient and appropriate resource management, and the elimination of a two-tiered discriminatory system of care — it also brings with it risks of insufficient care for the most severely ill and a lack of accountability to the public. NAMI is working, through education of its members, enhanced state advocacy, and research, to assure that these changes lead to a better service system.

REFERENCES

American Managed Behavioral Healthcare Association, (1995). *Performance measures for managed behavioral healthcare programs.* Washington, DC: Author.

Center for Mental Health Services (1995). *Mental health component of a health plan report card: phase ii progress report.* Rockville, MD: Author.

Frank, R.G., McGuire, T.G., & Newhouse, J.P. (1995). Risk contracts in managed mental health care. *Health Affairs, Fall,* 50–64.

Geller, J.L. (1995). When less is more; when less is less. *Psychiatric Services: 46,* 1105.

Lehman, A.F. (1995). Measuring quality of life in a reformed health system. *Health Affairs, Fall,* 65–72.

Malloy, M. (1995). *Mental illness and managed care: a primer for families and consumers.* Arlington, VA: National Alliance for the Mentally Ill.

Mechanic, D., Schlesinger, M., & McAlpine, D.D. (1995). Management of mental health and substance abuse services. *The Milbank Quarterly,* 73(1),19–56.

National Committee for Quality Assurance. (1995). *Medicaid HEDIS: An adaptation of the health plan employer data and information set 2.0/2.5* (Draft). Washington, DC: Author.

Smith, R.G., & Mandersheid, R.W. (1995). Principles of consumer outcomes assessment. *Dialogue on Outcomes on Mental and Addictive Disorders, Fall:* 1–2.

Torrey, E.F., Erdman, K., Wolfe, S.M., & Flynn, L.M. (1990). *Care of the seriously mentally ill: A rating of state programs. Third Edition.* Washington, DC: Public Citizen Health Research Group and National Alliance for the Mentally Ill.

Torrey, E.F., Steiber, J., Exekial, J., Wolfe, S.M., Sharfstein, J., Noble, J.H., & Flynn, L.M. (1992). *Criminalizing the seriously mentally ill: The abuse of jails as mental hospitals.* Washington, DC: National Alliance for the Mentally Ill and Public Citizen Health Research Group.

U.S. General Accounting Office. (1994). *Health care reform: "report cards" are useful but significant issues need to be addressed,* Washington, DC: Author.

22

Self-Managed Care: Meaningful Participation of Consumer/Survivors in Managed Care

INTRODUCTION

To date there has been minimal participation of consumers/ survivors* in decisions involving the management of managed care organizations. Unlike departments of mental health, which are public entities, and often have significant consumer/survivor involvement, most managed care is directed by private companies which are obligated only to serve their customers. The recent trend toward contracting out Medicaid mental health and substance abuse services to managed care companies has blurred that public/private line. Consumer and family advocacy groups, which had previously focused on state mental health authorities to influence policy, are now aware that in many cases, the arena of decision making has moved to the

---

*I will use the term consumer/survivor or person first language for persons who have been labeled mentally ill. Most consumers prefer people first language such as "a person who is in recovery" or "people who have been labeled mentally ill."

283

state Medicaid authorities. In those states, of which Massachusetts is the earliest and most prominent example, advocacy groups now need to find ways to participate directly in the policies formulated by these Medicaid authorities and managed care organizations (MCOs).

Despite this shift of decision making, the advent of public sector managed care (PSMC) can afford new opportunities for the involvement of consumer/survivors in the mental health system for two reasons:

1. Under the waiver process the previously rigid HCFA rules for Medicaid reimbursable services can be relaxed by the states, thereby allowing funding of nontraditional alternative services (e.g., peer counseling, acupuncture).

2. There is increased interest in money saving self-help approaches in a capitated, managed care environment.

This chapter will describe areas of potential collaboration between consumer/survivor groups and MCOs and their provider networks and the ways consumers can and should participate in the various aspects of PSMC (see Table 1). One of the first steps is the initiation

TABLE 1

How Consumer/Survivors Can Participate in Managed Care

Consumer Values
1. Use of People First Language
2. Self-Determination as a Shared Value
3. Cultural Competence

Consumer Roles
4. MCO Consumer Councils
5. Involvement in Preparation of MCO Proposals
6. Peer Support and Peer Counseling
7. Supporting Consumer-Run Services
8. Participation in Quality Improvement, Outcomes Measures, and Consumer Satisfaction Surveys
9. Consumers as Trainers and Educators

Consumer-Oriented Policies
10. Medical Necessity Criteria and Alternative Clinical Services
11. Increased Credentialling Flexibility
12. Voluntary Alternatives to Hospitalization

Consumer Rights
13. Adequate Confidentiality Safeguards
14. Informed Choice
15. Human Rights Protection and Grievance Procedures
16. Participation in System Reform and Planning

of dialogue between these groups. This process has started in a variety of public and private settings and its progress will depend on the willingness of the MCOs to accept the principles of the consumer/survivor movement, and for both groups to develop mutual respect and trust, as well as a common purpose which goes beyond financial concerns.

PRINCIPLES OF THE SELF-MANAGED CARE MODEL OF RECOVERY

Currently, the consumer/survivor movement is defining its own concept of managed care, the self-managed care model of recovery. Presently, many consumer/survivors are emotionally and spiritually isolated; successful recovery requires connectedness with others and respect as human beings are essential. Until we are respected and addressed in people first language, our efforts to recover meaningful roles of work, family, and play in society will always be blocked by restrictive and destructive societal attitudes.

In order to successfully manage one's care, consumer/survivors need hope, understanding, and meaning in their lives. Consumers must be allowed to speak for themselves, to be listened to, and to be allowed to have a legitimate and respected voice in articulating their goals and desires. They must not be denied the opportunity to experience love, hope, courage, self-esteem, pride, and meaning, many of which are feelings and experiences that so-called "normal" persons take for granted and which they often presume are not within the capability of consumer/survivors.

The ultimate principle consumer/survivors want is meaningful participation in their own mental health care. This principle is clearly stated in Article 4 of the Alma-Ata Declaration of the World Health Organization (1978): "People have the right and the duty to participate individually and collectively in the planning and the implementation of their health care."

WHAT IS MEANINGFUL CONSUMER PARTICIPATION?

People in recovery are acutely aware of differing levels of participation because to be labeled mentally ill means one is not considered a credible participant in community life. In fact, to be called "crazy" in popular usage is to be discredited and discounted. Consumers are subjected to overt discrimination in insurance, housing, jobs, health care, and education. These abuses are inconsistently and infrequently protected by the Americans with Disabilities Act (ADA) because such protection requires disclosure of the disability by the individual, an act which many consumers are afraid to do, because of the very risks of discrimination associated with being known as a person with mental illness. The ADA can not protect consumers against the most devastating discrimination which occurs in the subtle social exclusions experienced daily. Consumers are sensitive to societal and professional "mentalism": how others change the topic of discussion, shift attention away from them, ignore or refuse to inform them, exhibit coldness of response, distance themselves socially, fail to respond to questions or suggestions, and deny them the ability to impact decisions.

Consumers are also acutely aware of how meaningful their input may be. The criterion for meaningful consumer/survivor participation is their formal inclusion in planning and evaluative bodies, in positions of interpersonal significance such that their opinions are reflected in the group's decisions, i.e., to make a measurable difference. Consumer/survivors should be more than window dressing to make a committee look good. They should be people who have had first hand experience with mental illness, who have a sufficient sense of self and the experience with the mental health system to feel able to contribute, and who are in communication with consumer groups. Individual consumers should not be isolated as the sole representative on such committees or boards. There should be at least two consumer/survivors on any board or policy setting body, to provide peer support and to reduce the risk of tokenism and co-optation.

HOW CONSUMER/SURVIVORS CAN PARTICIPATE IN MANAGED CARE

Consumer Values

Public sector MCOs and their provider networks need to understand the most important values which consumers in recovery want to see in an organization.

1. Use of People First Language

There may be nothing which upsets consumer/survivors of psychiatric disabilities more than the objectification of being called "the mentally ill," because the unconscious message that underlies it says "you're not a person; you are part of the mentally ill." The use of diagnosis to avoid or deny the consumer's identity as a person robs him or her of a sense of spirit and a sense of soul. This is why nearly every discussion between consumer/survivors and professionals begins on the theme of language and labels. Clinicians and administrators, and anyone else working with people labeled mentally ill, should ask themselves, "how would you like to be addressed?"

2. Self-Determination as a Shared Value

Public sector MCOs can engage people in recovery by acknowledging that self-determination is a shared value. Self-determination has not classically been a goal of the mental health system. MCOs can actually play a big role in system reform. From my own experience and that of others, an essential ingredient to recovery from psychiatric disability is having a voice, being able to play a major role in treatment and care decisions for oneself. This starts with treatment planning and is an excellent opportunity to change the way practice occurs. Best practices should incorporate self-determination as an element.

3. Cultural Competence

Cultural competence in the broadest sense is associated with understanding, recognizing, and valuing the cultural diversity of people from all different backgrounds. Cultural competence also applies to understanding people's belief systems. People with psychiatric disabilities often have a variety of beliefs that are not shared by the "majority" culture. These should not immediately be labeled as delusions unless there is clear evidence for such a judgment. To distinguish a belief from a delusion, it is extraordinarily important to be culturally competent. For example, a Native American or native Puerto Rican who sees the image of a dead relative may be experiencing culturally appropriate mourning, not a hallucination.

CONSUMER ROLES

Significant roles are associated with meaningful participation as described above. The following list identifies ways, especially in the public sector, that people in recovery can play active and important roles not only in their own recovery, but in that of other people, and in that way to facilitate system reform that honors peer support and self-help. These roles must involve significant participation, which means that consumers' views are listened to, that they are seen as credible, and that they have an impact on the decisions that are reached.

4 MCO Consumer Councils

It is essential for managed care organizations, their partners, and providers to establish consumer councils with real impact. The National Empowerment Center aided the establishment of a consumer council to the Massachusetts Division of Medical Assistance and the Mental Health Management of America (MHMA), the MCO that has been administering the Massachusetts Medicaid contract. In certain respects this has been a good beginning. The council focused on informed consent policies and drafted documents to present some of these findings to providers. A genuine consumer council needs to have broad authority to look at all of the functions of the MCO and its providers.

5. Involvement in Preparation of MCO Proposals

There is no substitute for having people who are in recovery be directly involved in the preparation of bids for contracts. Otherwise the language, the concepts, and the understanding will lack a dimension of consumer sensitivity, because of the continuing lack of widespread education, training, and consciousness raising of administrators, clinicians, and society as a whole.

6. Peer Support and Peer Counseling

Peer support has been shown to be very effective in helping people to recover from psychiatric disabilities. However, until the Medicaid waiver process occurred, states were obliged to use only professional staff. The waivers and contracts that are being set up with MCOs allow a new flexibility to find ways to reimburse people for their work as peer counselors. Peer counselor training programs have been established in California, Oregon, Colorado, New York, and Massachusetts. The mental health system should begin to adopt more of the approaches that have been used in the substance abuse field, where it has been long recognized that people who have been through recovery from substance abuse are often very effective counselors.

7. Supporting Consumer-Run Services

Consumer-run services are different than peer counseling, although peer counseling may be a key component of such programs. In the past ten years, many programs run by people in recovery from psychiatric disabilities have emerged. Many of these services have been funded by the federal government, through the Community Support Program of the Center for Mental Health Services (CMHS) and by state mental health departments. These services are cost effective and user friendly. Many consumers feel more comfortable in a setting where the administrators and staff have been through similar experiences. Such programs can immediately decrease stigma and discrimination felt by consumers. Under the previous Medicaid structure, it was (and still is in some areas) difficult to fund this type of service. Hopefully, future Medicaid contracts will encourage the development and use of these services.

8. Participation in Quality Improvement, Outcomes Measures, and Consumer Satisfaction Surveys

In the mental health center where I work, I have incorporated the participation of people in recovery as valued members of all of our quality improvement teams. They play an important role in recommending useful services and policies that might not otherwise be mentioned and can provide immediate and direct feedback to program directors about what happened in the preceding day in a crisis service or residential program.

Consumer satisfaction surveys need to be reviewed, edited and, wherever possible, administered by people in recovery. Better information is obtained when people are interviewed by peers, because there isn't the same fear of possible retaliation or disappointment by the service provider.

With regard to outcome evaluation, traditional measures such as length of stay in hospitals or symptom reduction do not adequately measure the recovery experience. People in recovery have cited that better indicators of positive outcome include: having a sense of meaning in one's life, feeling that one is respected, forming and maintaining relationships that are important and meaningful, and having the sense that life is worth living. With CMHS support, consumer/survivors have helped to construct a report card for managed mental health services which reflects these consumer based indicators.

9. Consumers as Trainers and Educators

Many people who are in recovery from psychiatric disabilities have participated in or organized workshops and have given talks improving the awareness and consciousness of the recovery experience to a wide range of clinicians, administrators, family members, and other consumers. Consumers have a lot to offer. The experiences that consumers have had in dealing with medication, hospitals, residential programs, and therapy can be most valuable information for health care providers to hear and incorporate into their appreciation of the impact of their activities. But, for this to happen, i.e., for consumers to have a significant training role, clinicians and MCOs must recognize that we do have a lot to teach and that clinicians have a lot to learn. The National Empowerment Center conducted a conference in 1994, called "Learning From Us", during which 88 health care professionals, administrators, and family members participated in workshops that were planned, organized, and carried out by people in recovery from psychiatric disabilities. The evaluations were extremely positive and we look forward to providing more workshops in the future.

CONSUMER-ORIENTED POLICIES

10. Medical Necessity Criteria and Alternative Clinical Services

It is important to broaden the concept of medical necessity and practice guidelines, and to incorporate a variety of alternative or non-traditional healing and treatment modalities. "Medical necessity" is a crucial term under any third party reimbursement scheme because it defines what services will be covered. The term has been narrowly defined under HCFA rules as "habilitative" not rehabilitative, meaning that only medically oriented services would be reimbursed. Under the new state waivers it is now possible for states to more broadly define medical necessity. In recognition that recovery involves much more than symptom reduction, medical necessity criteria need to include the concept of social and human necessity. Oregon and Iowa have included rehabilitation in their criteria of medical necessity, which may allow providers to address rehabilitation and recovery needs, such as work, education, housing, and financial support, as well as symptom reduction. MCOs and providers need to consider and allow the inclusion of alternative and non-traditional clinical services, such as acupuncture (which is frequently being used for detox and recovery from substance abuse), biofeedback, meditation, massage, and other stress reduction approaches. There need to be more opportunities for clinicians to provide these services, regardless of the setting. This would allow clinics, day treatment centers, and residential programs to increase consumers' choice options and enhance recovery and rehabilitation more effectively.

11. Increased Credentialling Flexibility

In the past, only highly credentialled individuals with professional degrees in social work, nursing, psychology, or psychiatry were allowed to be reimbursed for providing Medicaid services. People in recovery from psychiatric disabilities often have not had either the opportunity, the time, or the resources to obtain advanced degrees. There need to be more inclusive credentialling criteria for consumer peer counselors and consumer case managers to be regarded as legitimate providers, whose services would be reimbursable. These criteria could be similar to those used within substance abuse treatment systems to provide credentials for recovering users in recognition that recovery experiences may contribute to clinical effectiveness.

12. Voluntary Alternatives to Hospitalization

The first emphasis here is on voluntary and the second on alternatives. There is a powerful intersection between the cost concerns of MCOs and the expressed preferences of people in recovery from psychiatric disabilities. People in recovery generally want care in the community, as close as possible to where they live. They do not want services in institutional settings. Psychiatric hospitals are extremely expensive, restrictive, and dehumanizing. The move towards community support, community care, consumer-run alternatives, has occurred primarily in the public sector. Numerous successful hospital alternatives, such as "specialling" a person in crisis in the home, providing respite in a specialized apartment, or "home sharing" with the family of a peer, have been developed and described (see chapter by Hoge, Davidson and Sledge).

CONSUMER RIGHTS

13. Adequate Confidentiality Safeguards

Consumer rights are essential to the recovery process because without a protection of rights there can be no sense of equality. Without a sense of equality and respect there cannot be meaningful recovery. The public mental health system has paid a lot of attention to consumer rights and human rights, though it has a long way to go. Private sector providers have less experience in this area and may be more prone to abuses of consumer rights. One of the most important consumer rights is confidentiality. With the advent of large computerized data banks and impersonal clinical record systems, concern about who has access to intimate psychiatric records is one of the greatest fears of people seeking mental health care. Consumer/survivors want to be assured that mental health providers employ active measures to safeguard confidentiality, such as the use of unique identifiers that avoid the accidental release of the person's name or social security number. In addition, releases of information should specify who is to receive the information, the type of information desired, for what purpose, and for how long. Blanket or open-ended releases are not acceptable. Releases should be signed by the consumer every time that information is requested.

14. Informed Choice

Informed consent or, preferably, informed choice is a broad area applying to all of medical care, which recognizes the right of patients to make adequately informed decisions regarding their own care. If we are genuinely going to move towards a system in which the person is capable of making informed choices, then we need to think very carefully about how information is presented. We need to realize that any procedure, any medication, and any kind of therapy is not done *for or to* someone, but is done *with* the person and with the assumption that the person needs to *collaborate* in the treatment decision.

Consumer/survivors have worked diligently in Massachusetts, through the Consumer Advisory Council to DMA and through M POWER, a state consumer/survivor group to address informed choice issues. These bodies have jointly been developing guidelines which hopefully will become regulations, requiring clinicians to document efforts to promote informed choice in a variety of clinical situations.

15. Human Rights Protection and Grievance Procedures

It is critical to have overall human rights protections and consumer grievance procedures, which are accessible and clearly delineated. Whenever a person is a patient in any mental health program or facility, he or she should receive written and oral information regarding client rights, how to access an ombudsperson regarding rights issues, and how to file a grievance. If any rights violation occurs, consumer/survivors need to be able to start the grievance or complaint procedure promptly, without confusing or tedious obstacles to the initiation of the complaint, and with a swift and courteous response from the program. There must also be clear grievance procedures which apply to any denial or restriction of services.

16. Participation in System Reform and Planning

Another important means to protect consumer rights is for consumer/survivors to participate directly in mental health policy development at the local, regional, state, and national levels. Consumers need to be included and allowed to influence Medicaid authority and MCO decisions directly. This point will be illustrated next by looking more closely at Massachusetts.

In 1991 Massachusetts obtained a 1915b Freedom of Choice waiver from HCFA which allowed the state to restrict the choice of providers and to set many of the other rules for its Medicaid program. Without significant consumer or DMH participation, the state decided to have its Medicaid office develop its mental health policy. The Medicaid office introduced an RFP seeking a private MCO to administer the Medicaid mental health and substance abuse program. In 1992 MHMA won the bid. In 1993 the state quietly created a new entity, the Division of Medical Assistance, to specifically oversee its Medicaid programs and become the State Medicaid Authority. In recent years, there had been significant consumer involvement in policy formation by DMH, with no involvement of consumers in Medicaid policy. In 1994 consumer/survivors, under the auspices of the National Empowerment Center, started a Consumer Advisory Council for DMA's mental health program. The council's work led to consumers having input into the RFP for the next phase of the project. The new RFP reflects an ever greater shift of authority from DMH to DMA, with funding and authority for crisis and acute inpatient services being transferred to DMA. Five national MCOs submitted bids. After significant petitioning, consumers were allowed to form an advisory review board. Consumers reviewed a portion of each bid, giving recommendations to the primary reviewers.

Massachusetts is a useful example because the state's early move towards PSMC and experience thus far is being viewed as a model for other states to consider. Though MHMA saved the state millions of dollars, mainly by limiting inpatient detox and psychiatric admissions, there has not been significant consumer participation in the evaluation of the program's impact on long-term recovery, quality of life, and consumer satisfaction.

The following suggestions are primary tasks for consumer/survivors to consider as they take on the rather daunting responsibility of trying to influence public policy.

1. Identify what stage the state or county has reached in health care reform.

2. Find out where the decision-making authority is: with Medicaid authority, with the mental health authority, with the legislature, or some combination of these.

3. Identify the key people involved in the decision process and lobby for consumer/survivor participation in those decisions.

4. Form a committee of consumer/survivors interested in influencing health care reform and connect that committee to a state-wide consumer/survivor group.

5. Strengthen the state or regional consumer/survivor group. The larger the group the greater its influence.

6. Emphasize the cost-effectiveness of self-help, peer support, and voluntary consumer-run community based alternatives to institutional care.

CONCLUSION

Health care reform and PSMC initiatives pose opportunities and risks for consumer/survivors in their quest to improve the care they receive and to have a greater voice in the system of care. There are opportunities to shift the focus away from a system that encourages surplus dependency to one that facilitates the growth and recovery of people with psychiatric disabilities, so that we can take more responsibility for our lives and lead more productive and independent lives in this society. Organizations such as the National Empowerment Center and state-wide consumer/survivor groups are important resources of people and information to promote this dramatic shift.

23

Outcomes and Evaluation: System, Program, and Clinician Level Measures

SUSAN ESSOCK and HOWARD GOLDMAN

INTRODUCTION

Is it cost effective? This is the question being asked by payers, providers, and consumers about mental health care. The "it" can be an isolated treatment within a larger system (e.g., the use of an expensive antipsychotic medication) or an entire system of care (e.g., a carve-out of Medicaid services to a managed care vendor). Because managed care attempts to control costs while delivering appropriate care, questions of cost effectiveness are central to all stakeholders. This chapter emphasizes the evaluation of the effectiveness component of the cost-effectiveness equation.

One of the particular challenges of evaluating effectiveness in a public sector managed care (PSMC) environment is that there are multiple stakeholders (taxpayers, legislators, consumers, providers, public mental health authorities), each with its own perspective. Any measure of effectiveness therefore demands a consensus from all stakeholders in order to be fully validated. Thus, although each stakeholder maintains a unique perspective on cost (to that stakeholder), they all must somehow agree on what outcomes are most important and on how to measure them.

Consequently, this chapter focuses on the measurement of outcomes particularly relevant to PSMC systems, the incentives for different stakeholders to promote and monitor different measures of effectiveness, and contractual aids for evaluating (and influencing) the performance of managed care providers. Public sector concerns about outcome evaluation differ in two important respects from the concerns of the private sector: (1) The public sector has the critical responsibility of protecting the public trust. State and local mental health authorities use outcome assessment to assure that the varied interests of the whole society are addressed and balanced in the policies and practices relating to service delivery. Equity, fairness, due process, liberty, and societal protection are all special concerns of the public sector. Although these *may* be the concerns of a private managed mental health care provider or payer, these *must* be the concerns of a public mental health authority. (2) As a corollary to its broad societal concern, the public sector has responsibility for the entire population, especially individuals who are indigent and those who are most vulnerable and most impaired. The special problem of outcome evaluation in the public sector is to be able to address the broadest of societal concerns for the entire population with the same specificity and rigor as practiced in the private sector.

A FRAMEWORK FOR EVALUATING MENTAL HEALTH SERVICES

A traditional approach to assessing the quality of care divides the concept of quality into assessments of the structures, processes, and outcomes of care (See chapter by Berlant, Anderson, Carbone, & Jeffrey). These concepts can be applied both to evaluation of individual programs and to evaluation of entire systems of care. At the program level, structures of care are the elements which comprise a program: the staff, the building, the equipment, the fiscal and other resources. Examples of questions to ascertain structural quality include: Are enough appropriately trained staff present? Is the physical plant adequate?

Similarly, at the systems level, structures of care delivered by a PSMC system include components such as: access phone lines, emergency service teams, provider networks, contracted service types, available hospital beds, MIS systems, billing systems, and appeals procedures. Questions that address the effectiveness of such MCOs include: Are there adequate numbers of geographically accessible providers? Are there service models available for all covered diagnoses? Are there sufficient numbers of contracted hospital beds? The meeting of structural standards is not sufficient to prove that care is adequate, but failure to meet minimum structural standards implies that care is inadequate.

Processes of care at the program level are the services, therapies, or other interventions provided by a program's staff to clients. Processes are the outputs, as opposed to the outcomes, of care. Assessing the adequacy of processes of care involves creating standards for who should receive what type of service and then comparing the actual services delivered to those standards. Standards may be based on research findings or consensus. By either route, performance expectations can be specified which define the expected processes of care. For example, one expectation of a crisis intervention program might be that it be available at all times and the program's performance can be monitored to evaluate whether it meets these expectations.

Similarly, at the systems level, processes of care in a PSMC system refer to the types and quantity of interventions provided system-wide. Evaluation of such processes of care might include questions such as: How is the timeliness of hospital admission influenced by the pre-certification process? Is reduction in inpatient utilization accompanied by corresponding increases in outpatient utilization? How are utilization patterns related to demographics and diagnosis, and how has this changed from the previous system? Are there reports of barriers to access or premature discontinuation of benefits? Are all emergency services truly available at all times?

Processes of care relate directly to what a program or system of care is designed to *do*, hence process measures have great appeal as a means of evaluating whether a PSMC program is providing the expected services. However, assessing whether services result in the desired outcomes for the client is beyond the scope of process measures. Process measures are an important means of describing the functioning of programs, but they do not address the functioning of clients.

Outcomes of care are those changes in client functioning which clinical and programmatic interventions are designed to produce. Assessing changes in functioning requires measurements both before and after the introduction of the intervention. Clients can be assessed both individually, or as cohorts, defined at the individual program level or at the systems level. Questions at the individual client level include: Is symptomatology reduced? Is level of functioning improved? Is community tenure lengthened? At the program level, questions might include: Is the rate of rehospitalization for program members reduced? Is the rate of employment increased?

Similar questions can be asked at the systems level, as well as broader questions, such as: Is the rate of homelessness for managed care recipients reduced? Are there increased reports of incarceration in jails or prisons? Is the rate of referral to long-term. institutional psychiatric care affected? Are other non-psychiatric medical costs reduced? Because many factors might influence clients' outcomes in any of the outcome dimensions just listed, evaluations of PSMC programs and systems must be designed carefully to ensure that the outcomes being measured are influenced by the program features being studied rather than the impact of another program or system in which the client is also receiving services.

LIMITATIONS OF THE STRUCTURE-PROCESS-OUTCOME APPROACH

All outcomes other than improvement in the lives of members of the target population in question are proxies for the extent to which the provider/vendor is fulfilling its mission.

Proxies can fool you. Measures of structures (e.g., counting program types), processes (e.g., number of clients seen), or "indirect" outcomes (e.g. those not central to a program, such as increased time between hospitalizations) may lead to false assumptions about the services' impact on clients' lives. A program count may make services look rich when the programs are actually functioning so poorly that they have little impact on clients' lives. The programs may see many clients, but they may not be people with serious mental illnesses. Clients may average long times in the community between hospitalizations, but the hospitals' front doors may be so tightly shut that people who would benefit from admission cannot get in. Proxies may be useful for program management, but one must always keep in mind that they are simply proxies for client outcomes and not the real thing. The further a measure is from the primary source, i.e., the client, the more one must contend with alternative explanations for the results. As much as possible, outcome measures should focus on outcomes directly relevant to the client's areas of disability and the functional impairments the disability produces.

In addition, performance measures, whether for internal monitoring or external review, can stifle innovation. The more structures and processes of care are set in stone, the less flexibility an organization has in offering novel, flexible, client-centered approaches to meeting clients' needs. A balance must be struck between measuring performance by agreed-upon standards and constraining flexible approaches to care via rigidly prescribed approaches (e.g., addiction treatment services can only be provided by traditional addiction treatment providers, not in integrated psychiatric-addiction treatment settings).

WHY OUTCOME MEASURES ARE NECESSARY

Performance and outcome measures help offset the economic incentives to undertreat that are inherent in PSMC capitated systems. When payment is fixed, the only way to meet revenue targets is through cost efficiencies. Although these cost-control incentives can promote good care by encouraging cost-effective treatment in mobile crisis services, less restrictive residential or day hospital settings, and to reduce the use of expensive settings such as emergency rooms and hospitals, just saying "no" can also be a cost efficiency, and MCOs must be monitored to make certain that appropriate services are not being withheld.

Because resources are limited, PSMC systems must demonstrate that they produce acceptable clinical outcomes for acceptable costs. MCOs must evaluate their contracted programs for clinical results. This requires documentation not only of who receives what and from whom, but with what effect, and for what cost. Measures of the structure and processes of care help evaluate what it takes to get what outcome. Too often, however, information is collected only on the structures and processes of care but not on outcomes, thereby encouraging inferences about outcomes on the basis of assumptions about processes.

For this reason, it is vitally important that outcome measures truly measure outcome, and not merely structure and process. There are many reasons why process and outcome measures may get confused. First, we are accustomed to asking whether employees, including providers of mental health services, are "doing their job," or whether clients are attending their programs. We then mistakenly assume that if people are performing assigned tasks, and clients are attending, then the program is accomplishing its function.

Attendance is not an outcome. Attendance rates going up or down are neither inherently good nor bad (e.g., attendance at a social rehabilitation program could be down because the program is so successful that the members are off at jobs or attendance could be down because members don't like the program and are staying away). Attendance is a measure of the process of service, nothing more. The same may be said of other "body count" measures. They show that processes of care are occurring and are useful for managing other processes of care (e.g., staffing patterns), but such measures do not provide information about the impact of the services on clients' lives.

Process measures will help a program manager order the processes of care, but only outcome measures can judge reliably a program's success and justify its funding. These outcome measures can be very crude: Do the target symptoms persist? Does the person have stable housing? Did the person get a job? Is the client satisfied with housing, activities, and relationships?

A program's essential goal (whether a community program with only three staff, a unit within a hospital, or a service system) is to *improve the quality of life* of the people for whom it exists. Managers may implement programmatic changes (changes in the processes of service) to make their programs function better, assuming that better functioning programs result in better clinical outcomes. The outcomes of these programmatic changes in processes need to be assessed to ensure that they produce the desired outcomes in program functioning. Therefore, *process* measures of clients' care (e.g., number of services given, number of clients seen in the community, waiting time prior to evaluation) can also be *outcome* measures for program functioning, which facilitate program management. The next important step, which is often omitted, is to measure whether the programmatic change has led to improved clinical outcomes.

The most well-intentioned process changes may backfire and not improve the efficacy of services. For example, if the utilization of restraints (a process of care) on one ward seems high and the desired programmatic outcome is to lower the utilization of restraints (a change in the process of care), the programmatic outcome might be accomplished but to the detriment of clients (e.g., via over-utilization of sedating medications). Similarly, a catchment area might have the

programmatic goal of reducing length of hospital stay (another measure of the process of care). Length of stay may be decreased desirably
by improving the community supports available, or undesirably by
discharging patients prematurely, or by a host of other factors. Only
by assessing client outcomes in relation to decreases of length of stay
can the value of the programmatic shift be judged.

Managers must constantly make decisions involving resource allocation and these decisions should be assisted by information on
client outcomes. Examples of such decisions would be: Who benefits most from a mobile crisis team? Who should be given access to
intensive case management? What are the costs and benefits of using therapists as case managers? What programs should provide
services at night? Where should respite care be located? Who should
have access to a group home?

Hard data on clinical outcome help to reduce disagreements about
resource allocation. Data can provide a consensual method for managers and clinicians to evaluate whether painful cutbacks are having
a negative impact on clients. Clinical impression may not correlate
with outcome. The New Hampshire Psychiatric Research Center recently described a study in which a popular day treatment program
was closed. Staff were redeployed to provide less costly individualized vocational placement and support. Despite dire predictions from
clinicians, careful outcome evaluation indicated that the vocational
intervention resulted in improved outcome and client satisfaction
(Drake, 1995).

HOW ARE OUTCOME DATA COLLECTED?

Outcome measures can be derived from a number of sources. Ideally,
an MCO and its provider network would all participate in a "clinical
information system" which tracks the episodes of care for each client.
In addition to collecting process measures relating to each encounter
(who did what, with whom, where, and when), a clinical information
system also records clinical data (e.g., symptomatology, level of functioning), which may serve as outcome measures.

Service systems without clinical information systems, rely on
three typical sources of outcome data: clinical records, formal client
self-report questionnaires, and clinician reports using standardized
measures. Some standardized measures (e.g., RAND 36-Item
Health Survey, RAND, 1992) are broad measures of health with
minimal emphasis on mental health.

Nevertheless, they can be a useful means of tracking changes in
health status over time. Others, such as the BASIS-32, are more specifically designed to measure mental health outcomes, but are
lengthy, and have not yet been shown to be useful in PSMC systems,
with clients with SPMI. Numerous products are currently being developed and marketed to meet the growing demand for sophisticated, sensitive, reliable, valid, standardized, and easy to administer
outcomes instruments. Providers must evaluate these tools carefully

with their own clients. They should seek consultation, if necessary, to determine which tools are best for their programs.

Families of patients may also serve as sources of data, both about their relatives under care and about their own perceptions of the outcomes of care. Family members may provide collateral information about patient outcome. They may also report on satisfaction with services, and family contributions and burdens. Most of the measures of the latter have been developed for individuals with severe mental disorders. Such measures are particulary important, given the findings of a recent study showing that "continuity of care," in the form of a case manager, reduced stress for family members who lived with a patient with SPMI (Tessler & Gamache, 1994).

Ideally, feedback from clients about changes in their lives should be a prime source of outcome data. Client-driven "report cards" have gained favor among payers, providers, and consumers both because of their face validity and because such measures are often relatively easy to collect. It is much easier to ask a client or family member to check off items in a simple survey than it is to have a clinician assess changes in symptoms and functioning over time. Such report cards must be brief or they will not be completed. As a result they may also seem overly simplistic and fail to measure important outcomes. Report cards or satisfaction surveys may be a particularly useful means of polling clients on domains of service accessibility (e.g., convenience, responsiveness, cultural appropriateness) but may not be good proxies for treatment outcomes.

People sometimes doubt whether clients with mental illnesses can complete such surveys. Our experience has been that all but the most severely mentally ill individuals are reliable informants. When conducting such surveys, one needs to be alert to the potential under-representation of people with the greatest cognitive impairments and the associated potential under reporting of information from people whose experiences with services might be different from that of most survey respondents.

WHAT SHOULD BE MEASURED?

Identify key outcomes. The global outcomes relevant to public sector managed care have to do with cost containment, access to care, changes in severity of illness, level of functioning, and client and family satisfaction.

Costs. When measuring costs, it is necessary to identify costs to whom. The State of California conducted a study of the costs of treating substance abuse and concluded that each dollar spent on treatment resulted in $7 of savings (Gerstein et al., 1994). The treatment costs were largely to the State of California Department of Alcohol and Drug Programs while the benefits were largely savings due to reductions in crime. This is a reminder that the organizations and individuals doing the spending might be very different than those realizing the savings. Therefore, it is important to monitor costs from the perspectives of all the relevant stakeholders.

Access. The definition of access also depends on who's asking and who is being asked: The NAMI primer for families and consumers defines access as: "The ability to obtain desired health care. Access is more than having insurance coverage or the ability to pay for services. It is also determined by the availability of services, acceptability of services, cultural appropriateness, location, hours of operation, transportation, and cost" (Malloy, 1995). NAMI's definition emphasizes the positive by specifying program characteristics associated with facilitating access. Other aspects of access include the absence of barriers to access such as the absence of policies that restrict admission (e.g., "not open to people who have started fires" or "must be compliant with medication") or rules designed to limit treatment (e.g., specifying a limit to the number of annual or life time admissions for treatment for substance abuse).

Clinical Improvement. When measuring the effectiveness of a managed care vendor, a provider, or a program operating within the public mental health sector, an evaluator must assess the impact of the services in question on *the lives of people with serious mental disorders.* Because mental illnesses affect many life domains, the scope of mental health services is very broad, particularly in the public sector. When evaluating a *system* of mental health care, outcomes in diverse domains are relevant: tenure in the community, symptomatology, medical status, housing, employment, education, social network, impact on others, victimization rates, substance abuse, quality of life. Hence, depending on the scope of responsibility of the entity being evaluated, outcome measures in each of these domains could be appropriate. Changes in the severity of a person's illness are inferred from changes in the person's functioning in these domains.

Managed mental health care vendors operating in the private sector typically manage the treatment of the more common acute psychiatric disorders (e.g., depression). Consequently, their outcome measures commonly focus on symptom relief and return to functioning within a short time frame. Because chronically disabled individuals are usually the responsibility of the public sector, these outcome measures have not had to span all of the domains relevant to public sector clients. As private sector MCOs begin to work in the public sector, it is important that their outcome targets (and the measures used to assess them) expand to include these additional domains.

Client/Family Satisfaction. An important correlate of the move toward consumer empowerment in the public sector is the increasing recognition that, even for the most severely ill, client preferences and choices must be seriously included in program and service design. Consequently, obtaining feedback from clients and families on the structure, process, and outcome of services has become as important in the public sector as in the private sector. Satisfaction is both a positive outcome and a guide for improving clinical outcomes through addressing structural and process causes of dissatisfaction. Satisfaction data is usually collected from brief, multiple choice or Likert scale self-report forms that are administered at discharge or at defined service intervals (e.g., after 4 initial outpatient visits or after every 6 months for clients in continuous treatment).

SETTLING ON MEASURES OF OUTCOME

Identifying presumed correlates of effectiveness. Measures of client satisfaction and client change are central to measures of effectiveness. As indicated above, all other measures are proxies for these outcomes. To assure that outcome measures are relevant it is important the clients and family members participate in selecting outcomes to be measured. This helps ensure that the program or system elements being measured do relate to consumers' satisfaction with services.

Narrowing the field. Picking what to measure involves specifying the responsibilities of the entity under consideration and deciding what measures will indicate that these responsibilities are being fulfilled. These "key indicators" may be part of the contract with the payer or part of the entity's internal quality management program. Structure, process, and outcome measures should be identified for each key area of responsibility, along with data sources and sampling plans. Identifying data sources and sampling plans up front helps to assure that collecting the selected measures is feasible. To save effort, these measures should piggy-back on normal business practices as much as possible. The next step is to establish thresholds for the measures which, when exceeded, trigger events such as increased monitoring, the creation of corrective action plans, and/ or the application of contractually specified penalties.

A program-level example. The following example is drawn from the program standards for case management services in the Connecticut Department of Mental Health and Addictions Services. The mission for the Department's case management programs is to maintain and improve the quality of clients' lives. Indicators of quality of life (outcome indicators) include: number of days homeless; number of days gainfully employed; number of legal involvements where client was alleged to have been at fault; number of incidents of victimization (e.g., client robbed, assaulted); number of months in which client had insufficient funds to meet basic needs; number of times client changed residences involuntarily; physical health status; average disposable income after costs of rent, utilities, and food. This list of outcome measures is long and detailed because case managers are expected to know about all of these aspects of the lives of any clients assigned to them. While these indicators would not be appropriate for a crisis program or a residential support program, it is part of the mission of a case management program to have this level of involvement with clients with serious mental disorders.

An example of a standard which emphasizes the structure of the case management programs is that assertive case management teams should have staff to client ratios of no less than 1:12. A related process measure requires that all clients have individual treatment plans which deal with all life areas important to the client (symptom stability, symptom education and management, housing, employment/daily structure, substance abuse, family/social relationships, finances, etc.). An audit would show whether client service plans are present and whether they contain key information, such as client preferences, strengths, and goals; services and activities needed by the client to achieve these goals; agency/program assigned to provide each service; and the planned intervention time frames.

A simple audit might be conducted by the case manager supervisor randomly picking treatment plans to review with case managers during supervision and noting whether these items were documented. By tallying the results of such audits, the supervisor could document the extent to which the standard was being met. At the other extreme, outside auditors (e.g., from the Department of Mental Health) could conduct the audit and note any areas of deficiency requiring corrective action.

One function of most case management programs is to provide continuity of care for clients. A measure aimed at determining whether the case managers provide continuity would be to measure whether case managers visit clients at least X days/hours after admission and at least Y times per week/month when the client is admitted to a hospital. Here, X and Y would vary according to the performance expectations for a particular program. A contract with a program might specify the following standard which, if not met, would result in a penalty: At least 90% of clients who are hospitalized will be seen by their case manager within 4 days of hospitalization, and at least 90% of clients discharged from a hospital will be seen by their case manager within 3 days of discharge. Having such process measures in place means that outliers with respect to meeting performance expectations can be identified. Programs can use such data to identify outlier case managers, and payers can use such information to identify outlier programs. In some systems, such outlier reports are easy to obtain because information systems contain data from case managers' service logs (what was done when and with whom) as well as hospital admission and discharge dates.

Measures for a managed care vendor. Introducing a managed care vendor into a system creates a new interface to monitor, even if the managed care vendor's functions previously had been performed within the State Mental Health Authority. Essock and Goldman (1995) note, for example, that when care requires prior authorization, the authorizer's decisions should be monitored via sampling to ensure that decisions are appropriately documented and adhere to the standards agreed upon for access. They note that, while the introduction of a managed mental health care vendor may decrease a State Mental Health Authority's information processing requirements in areas such as client tracking and billing, the new monitoring requirements do require the ability to track the vendor's performance in key domains and to audit the vendor's internal processes for managing and accomplishing these tasks. One of the great promises of private-sector managed care for public sector clients is the ability of organizations in the de-politicized private sector to take advantage of their access to capital for effective innovations which increase their levels of service integration and efficiency (Freeman & Trabin, 1994). Contracts with such vendors must have clearly defined performance expectations and external monitors so that, at the extreme, the fox is not left to guard the hen house.

Contracting with a managed care vendor to perform a broad range of coordinated mental health services for people with serious mental disorders means that the managed care vendor will be expected to perform appropriately in the following key domains: access, assessment, quality of the clinical care, risk management, utilization review (including a review of the quality, as well as the quantity, of care and intervening appropriately), appropriateness of the provider network, client and provider satisfaction, and grievance procedures. In each of these areas, measures can be defined, thresholds for performance set, and consequences for failing to meet the thresholds specified. Indeed, a State Mental Health Authority should have such performance expectations and means of monitoring their fulfillment whether a managed care vendor is employed or whether these tasks are part of internal quality-management procedures. What is new with a managed care vendor is the need to monitor the interface between the payer and the vendor as State agencies contract out for services. Because we tend to prepare for what we think we will be tested on, specifying performance expectations in important areas can help shape performance by creating incentives to provide good care. And, if more is specified than the payer (e.g., the State Mental Health Authority or the State Medicaid agency) can monitor, the payer can be selective about what among all of the items a contract specifies it actually will choose to monitor. A contract can specify that if quarterly audits by the payer find that the vendor is performing below any of the contractually agreed-upon standards, then the frequency of monitoring shall increase until the problem is corrected, with the increased cost of monitoring to be borne by the vendor. It is also useful to the payer to have the contract state that the managed care vendor's quality management system is subject to audit by the payer, and that the vendor must be able to demonstrate that its internal quality management system monitors the key domains spelled out in the contract and that corrective action is taken whenever problems are found. Auditing the vendor's quality management system is, at best, an efficient window into the functioning of key program components and, at worst, an alert that the vendor does not have at hand a means of monitoring the functioning of these program components. Both the good news and the bad news is important to the payer.

Specifying standards tied to the performance of individual clients keeps the standard focused on the system's central purpose: improving clients' lives. However, it is important to keep in mind that such client-focused standards may create incentives for dumping, for eliminating from the pool those who appear likely to be difficult to serve while still meeting the standards. Hence it is also important to build in "buffers", measures which create disincentives for dumping. For example, a clinical outcome measure addressing symptom stabilization after hospital admission is the rate of readmission within 30 days after discharge. A public sector payer can require its managed care vendor to decrease hospital utilization without a corresponding increase in early readmissions. However, many very difficult and non-compliant clients could be expected to have early readmissions. Treatment of those clients should not be discouraged. Consequently, the payer could set an outcome standard that allows a reasonable percentage (e.g., 10%) of clients to be readmitted during this early period, without penalty to the program. This margin for difficult clients could be coupled to the need to monitor service utilization to assure that access for these clients to hospitalization and hospital diversion services is not reduced relative to the access for other types of clients.

Often, however, measures of the structure or process of care do not create incentives for skimming and dumping (e.g., 80% of clients admitted to an emergency room will be evaluated by a network psychiatrist within X hours of admission is a process measure that is not influenced by the severity of clients' illnesses, hence does not create incentives for dumping). Hence, a mixture of measures to be used at the discretion of the payer helps dilute the incentive to game any particular measure. Wells, Astrachan, Tischler, and Unutzer (1995) have emphasized that we must tune our questions about the effects of managed care based on our understanding of the incentives created and how they are likely to affect patients.

CONCLUSION

The balance between the promise and the perils of public sector managed care is influenced by the ability to give accurate descriptions of the effectiveness, as well as the costs, of managed care providers in meeting the treatment needs of people with serious mental illnesses. Payers need these measures of effectiveness to hold the managed care vendors/providers accountable by incorporating such measures into contractually defined performance standards. Vendors and providers need these measures to insure the effectiveness of their approaches to service provision and to market their services. When monitoring performance, the greatest challenge is to make certain that the measures used create incentives for good care without narrowing providers' options for innovation and without creating incentives for underserving. One of the most attractive features of managed care to stakeholders is the "flexing" of benefits made possible when covered services are no longer confined to traditional inpatient and outpatient care. We must take care to insure that the monitoring of managed care vendors or other entities performing managed care functions promotes such flexibility and does not re-establish overly rigid, "one-size-fits-all" approaches to service delivery.

REFERENCES

Drake, R. (1995). *Integrating vocational rehabilitation into assertive case management teams*. Presentation at the American Psychiatric Association Institute on Psychiatric Services, Boston.

Essock, S.M., & Goldman, H.H. (1995). Health reform and changing state mental health systems: Why States are embracing managed care. *Health Affairs*, 34–44.

Freeman, M.A., & Trabin, T. (1994). *Managed behavioral healthcare: History, models, key issues, and future course*. Washington, DC: Center for Mental Health Services.

Gerstein, D.R., Johnson, R.A., Harwood, H.J., Fountain, D., Suter, N., & Malloy, K. (1994). *Evaluating recovery services: The California drug & alcohol treatment assessment (CALDATA) general report*. Sacramento: State of California, Health and Welfare Agency, Department of Alcohol and Drug Programs (under contract No. 92-001100).

Malloy, M. (1995). *Mental illness and managed care: A primer for families and consumers*. Arlington, VA: National Alliance for the Mentally Ill.

RAND (1992). *RAND 36-item Health Survey 1.0*. Santa Monica, CA: RAND Health Sciences Program.

Tesslor, R., & Gamache, G. (1994). Continuity of care, residence, and family burden in Ohio. *Milbank Quarterly 72*, 149–169.

Wells, K.B., Astrachan, B.M., Tisctrier, G.L., & Unutzer, J. (1995). Issues and approaches in evaluating managed mental health care. *Milbank Quarterly, 73*, 57–75.

24

Research: System, Program, and Clinician Level Measures

ALLAN BEIGEL, KENNETH MINKOFF, and MILES F. SHORE

INTRODUCTION

Public sector managed care (PSMC) initiatives have been implemented widely throughout the U.S. In spite of the urgent need to refine the technology of these initiatives in order to ensure quality outcomes and cost-effectiveness, there has been strikingly little research on managed mental health care in general, and public sector managed mental health care in particular, to provide a rational database to guide service system development.

This chapter will present a research agenda for managed mental health care in the public sector, organized around quality issues, public service system issues, and provider issues. This will be followed by a brief discussion of several methodological issues that affect the capacity to perform research in the public sector managed mental health care sector, and suggestions for addressing the methodological and financial barriers to conducting this research.

RESEARCH VERSUS OUTCOME EVALUATION

For the purpose of this discussion, it is important to distinguish research, per se, from outcome evaluation, which is discussed in the previous chapter by Essock and Goldman. Outcome evaluation involves assessing a particular intervention, program, or system of care to determine whether it achieves certain goals or results (outcomes). Research, in contrast, involves creating an experimental design which permits comparison of outcomes of two interventions (or comparison of an intervention with a control situation) in sufficiently controlled circumstances that one can determine whether one intervention is better than the other.

What determines a better intervention? To answer this question requires an understanding that in today's managed mental health care environment the central question is "value", not "quality". The difference between the two is based upon the insertion into the equation of the "cost" factor. Mathematically, the relationship may be expressed as "value equals quality divided by cost ($V = Q/C$)" (Santiago & Beigel, 1995).

Another way of approaching this concept is to recognize the differences between efficacy, effectiveness, and efficiency. For example, one may prove that a specific psychopharmacological agent is efficacious in carefully controlled clinical trials. However, this is not the same as proving that this same agent is effective when given to a large number of people within the community. Under these circumstances, the effectiveness of this same agent may depend on whether the patient takes the medication as prescribed, the physician is sufficiently knowledgeable about the medication to prescribe it properly, and/or the degree to which side effects may alter the way in which the medication is taken. Under any or all of these conditions, the medication may be ineffective while remaining efficacious.

In other circumstances, the relative value of an intervention may depend not on its efficaciousness or effectiveness, but on its efficiency. In this instance, two equally efficacious and effective medications may possess differing levels of efficiency, namely how many days it takes before a desired level of effectiveness is reached or the cost of each relative to the effectiveness achieved. Similarly, in a managed care system, a particular intervention (e.g., 24-hour telephonic precertification) may be efficacious in reducing the use of hospitalization in controlled circumstances, but its effectiveness at the systems level may relate to issues in the implementation of the precertification process (e.g., Do treatment delays due to the precertification process lead to increased symptoms prior to admission? Are there loopholes which permit subversion of the process?). Its efficiency may relate to the time and expense of implementing such a system relative to the potential savings.

Ultimately, the value of a given set of interventions may depend not on differences in efficacy, effectiveness, or efficiency, but on differences in cost. If they exist, then one of two equally efficacious, effective, and efficient approaches may have different degrees of value (cost/benefit ratio). Circumstances could also arise in which one intervention will have a higher value than another even though it is of less quality, simply because its cost, relatively speaking, is even lower than the comparison intervention and offsets any difference in quality (Garratini, 1993).

REVIEW OF PREVIOUS RESEARCH

With the notable exception of the Monroe-Livingston Capitation Study in the public sector (Babigian & Reed, 1987a; Babigian & Reed, 1987b; Babigian et al., 1991; Cole, Reed, Babigian, & Brown, 1994; Reed et al., 1994; Reed, Hennessy, & Babigian, 1995), and a few studies in the private sector (Mechanic & Aiken, 1989; Sturm et al., 1994), research on managed mental health care has been more a matter of research to be conducted than results to be reported. Despite the intense furor about managed care in academic psychiatric circles, there has been surprisingly little energy devoted to addressing scientific issues associated with managed care systems, as opposed to the political issues.

The Monroe-Livingston Study (in Rochester, New York) was funded by the New York State Office of Mental Health specifically to gather meaningful data on the impact of a case rate payment program on clinical outcomes for persons with SPMI. Utilizing different levels of case-based payments for clients with varying levels of service needs, and incorporating all funding (including income supports and rent subsidies), not just health-related funds, the study determined that capitaled patients had at least comparable outcomes, with reduced hospitalization and lower cost than the control group. Enhanced case management associated with the case rate seemed to correlate with the positive results.

Despite the limited applicability of this study to most contemporary managed care systems, which usually only manage health benefits, the study has provided methodological benchmarks for conducting cost-effectiveness research with public sector clients. It has also demonstrated the potential value of capitation or case rate payment systems for persons with SPMI and the utility of tiered (or differential) case rate systems associated with distinguishable levels of service needs.

THE RESEARCH AGENDA

1. Quality Outcomes Predictors

Quality oriented outcomes research in managed mental health care is the highest priority. It refers to the scientific study of which types of managed care interventions reliably produce desired outcomes with which types of clients and in which types of settings. The first question in designing such research is: What are the desired outcomes? For example, is the desired outcome the overall health of a population, e.g. changes in the incidence and prevalence of all or specific mental disorders, or the health of a specific individual? In the latter case, is the outcome to be assessed by determining changes in specific symptoms (e.g., depression, sleep disturbance, etc.) or is the outcome to be measured by determining changes in the level of functioning or disability (e.g., work related or family related), or both?

Similarly, an outcome related research question may be framed differently depending on whether social impact variables, such as the degree of utilization of welfare or public housing are considered important, or whether symptom relief is considered a sufficient outcome measure. As more complex outcome measures are used, the availability of the appropriate data sets becomes an increasingly significant methodological problem.

There are innumerable research questions related to quality and outcome of PSMC that need to be investigated. For the purposes of illustration, however, we have selected two representative research concerns to discuss in more detail.

Sample Issue 1: The Impact of utilization management on quality

Sample question: How does reduced access to inpatient care affect clinical outcome? Managed mental health care has achieved its financial success through sharp reductions in inpatient costs and utilization. As a result, legitimate questions have arisen regarding whether these reductions affect the short-term outcome for the patient, the overall cost of care for the entire treatment episode, or the long-term course of illness. If one assumes that a positive outcome is solely measured by the amount being spent on inpatient care, then the reductions in inpatient costs, measured annually, suggest a highly positive outcome. However, if one moves beyond this level of analysis to broader clinical outcome or cost − effectiveness (value) issues, then the research questions become more complex. To date, little research has been done in modern managed care settings on these more complex questions.

One method for conducting such research on a systems level is to use the system as its own control and to perform pre- and post-intervention comparisons of targeted outcomes. For example, is reduced inpatient utilization in the PSMC experimental condition associated with increased recidivism, suicide rates, corrections involvement, or homelessness in the target population compared with the control group? This type of design was used, in a non-rigorous fashion, as part of the outcome evaluation of MHMA's Medicaid program in Massachusetts (Callahan, Shepard, Beinecke, Larson, & Cavanaugh, 1994).

Sample Issue 2: Impact of preferred provider network composition on quality

Sample question: What are the outcome effects of using traditional public sector clinical settings instead of private office-based settings for PSMC clients? PSMC initiatives often lead to private sector providers suddenly competing with traditional public sector providers for contracts and referrals. While it is a commonly held belief that significantly disabled clients with SPMI have better outcomes in multidisciplinary public clinic settings, in which a broader array of services is available, there is little data to support this. Likewise, it is also assumed by some that "healthier" Medicaid clients prefer to receive services in private practice settings, with apparently more confidentiality and less stigma associated with the setting. This, too, is an unsubstantiated assertion. How can data which would resolve some of these questions be generated? Since it would be impossible and unethical to assign managed care clients into an experimental study, it may be possible to conduct research of this type using naturally occurring experimental conditions. For example, in a PSMC system which uses both private and public providers, one can retrospectively review all patients assigned to each type of provider, select matched populations for comparison, and compare outcomes. Outcome data can be obtained from utilization patterns, satisfaction surveys, clinical assessments, and standardized self-report instruments (e.g., SF-36 and BASIS-32). Of course, it is essential that the payer or MCO mandate that such data be collected in a standard or comparable way.

2. PSMC System Issues

A second priority for the research agenda is the investigation of the relationship of the design of the managed care arrangement (e.g., pricing, accountability, relationship to primary care system, benefit design, and provider type) to the overall outcome of the managed care project. Overall outcome refers not only to clinical and cost outcomes, but to the total system impact of implementation, and to the satisfaction of all stakeholders with the perceived results.

For example, an otherwise successful managed care program may still have a negative outcome, because of a perception of excess profit taken by the MCO. The central pricing mechanism utilized in the implementation of managed care has been the capitated approach, which is an actuarially based cost per covered life that generates a pool of funds from which the total costs of care are paid and profits or savings are realized. The risk faced when attempting to provide the contracted level of care within the funds allotted is personified by the individual whose service needs consistently require a level of care beyond available financial resources. At the population level, this risk is multiplied. For public systems attempting to introduce managed care into their environment, the high percentage of persons with SPMI within the population for which they have responsibility increases that risk. In addition, capitated public service systems, because of this responsibility, more often than private systems, face a choice between providing care to less seriously mentally ill persons with a higher potential for improvement and to more seriously mentally ill persons who require services of greater quantity and intensity.

Research questions suggested by these dilemmas include how to differentiate between levels of severity and the need for care among the mentally ill; how to determine the different case or capitation rates for the different levels of severity within this population; and how to assess what services should be recognized as contributing to these different rates (Reed et al., 1995). A related set of questions concerns the relationship of the degree of financial risk to the overall outcome. In a fully at-risk capitated system, there may be very strong incentives to undertreat. In a no-risk contract, there may be insufficient incentives to create appropriate system innovations. How can optimal risk corridors be determined by research? One research design might be to set up an initial managed care contract with variable risk components and to compare outcomes between the components to determine the best long-term structure.

A third set of systems questions involves the relative merits of systems integration. Traditionally, most public mental health systems have been organized and operated independently from other health care related delivery systems. In recent years, while there has been a more congenial administrative relationship, especially at the state level, between public mental health and public substance abuse systems, the integration of the two into a true behavioral health model has been accomplished in few states. An even smaller degree of integration has been achieved between behavioral health and general health care systems. As a result, PSMC systems face significant questions as to how to organize their managed care approaches within service and organizational environments that have not achieved a significant level of integration. With respect to integration of health and mental health, for example, different system approaches, as exemplified by "carve-out" and "carve-in" structures, represent a rich field for research that examines the impact of these different organizational and financing structures. The Oregon Health Plan (OHP), which has an integrated health and mental health benefit design, but regional variation in implementation, may be a natural experiment in which carve-in and carve-out models can be compared.

A fourth systems issue that warrants research regards the best methods by which public sector payers can define, operationalize, and monitor the accountability of contracted MCOs. Private sector MCOs, traditionally accountable for the bottom-line to their own stockholders and to the private companies for whom they do business, may have difficulty providing PSMC that is accountable for the broader range of performance issues and the greater diversity of stakeholders' concerns that are characteristic of the public sector. Similarly, public non-profit providers who take on managed care responsibilities must also be held accountable for performing what may be radically new functions. Public sector payers need to create contracting methodologies to assure this accountability. What are the best ways to do this: financial rewards, penalties, quality-based incentives, etc.? Public payers can create experimental designs by using a variety of accountability models within their contracting process and using independent evaluators to determine which models produce better results.

3. Provider Issues

In the earlier discussion of quality outcome research, we used an example about the composition of preferred provider networks and the relative value of matching certain types of clients to certain types of providers. This issue has broad implications, because developing networks and directing clients to specific providers is a common strategy for care management. However, there is very little research data to guide these types of decisions.

On the program level, significant research questions relate not only to type of provider (CMHC versus private practice group versus individual clinician), but also to comparisons between program models in providing a specific contracted service. For example, 24 hour triage and crisis intervention is a significant component of hospital diversion efforts in PSMC systems. MOCs often define very particular requirements for such service providers. How do these requirements affect service delivery? Are hospital-based crisis teams more successful than community-based teams in these efforts, and for which clients? Do credentialling standards which require crisis clinicians to be independently licensed affect quality? Should child and family or substance related crises require clinicians with training with those special populations?

At the provider level, PSMC raises a number of issues concerning the credentialling, the requirement for providers to have particular skills, and the mix of various types of clinical disciplines in system staffing patterns. Research is needed to address the question of licensure and certification requirements that correspond to the most effective and efficient use of personnel to achieve desired outcomes. For example, how do professionally trained, independently licensed case managers compare to experienced paraprofessionals or peer case managers in working with persons with SPMI? Should services by either of the latter two types of providers be allowed and "billable"? As this example indicates, substitutability of providers is an important issue. Managed mental health care may reduce costs by encouraging utilization of less costly providers in certain settings and under certain circumstances, or may mandate the use of more expensive providers at relatively low rates. Can these decisions be justified on the basis of value? For example, care delivered by psychiatrists is arguably the most expensive when calculated on a unit cost basis. Therefore, research questions arise as to whether the substitution of a provider whose unit cost is less results in overall cost reduction when measured on a per episode of illness or treatment basis, and for which clients.

In a similar vein, although there is emerging evidence that combining psychotherapy and pharmacotherapy in the treatment of certain mental disorders is more effective than utilizing either therapeutic intervention alone, little research data are available to indicate whether this "combined" therapy is delivered more efficiently by using two providers (a cheaper non-medical provider for the psychotherapy and a physician for the pharmacotherapy) or by utilizing a single provider (e.g., a psychiatrist) for the provision of the "combined" therapy.

Similarly, important questions arise about workforce supply. How many prescribing providers are necessary and sufficient for a particular population, as defined by diagnostic mix, acuity, disability, and demographics? What is the appropriate ratio of prescribing nurse practitioners to psychiatrists? What is the proper combination of nurses, psychologists, social workers, and other clinicians in providing services to public sector clients? There is little data to answer these questions, but the answers have profound implications for determining optimal capitation rates, as well as decisions about the direction of professional training and education (Beigel, 1995).

Finally, there are important questions concerning the role of primary care providers (PCPs). Within the managed care environment, increased reliance is being placed on PCPs to serve as gatekeepers to specialty services and as providers of services in instances where specialists had previously been used. Despite this shift in emphasis, there has been little research into how and when this strategy is most effectively used. Can the needs of persons with SPMI be addressed more effectively through capitated models that emphasize the use of PCPs who might not possess the skill level or the time necessary to deal with the complex problems of this specific population? Most recently, Sturm and Wells(1995) pointed out, using data from the Medical Outcomes Study, that there may be "less value per dollar" in using PCPs rather than mental health specialists in the treatment of depression. They found that established practice guidelines were more typically adhered to in specialty mental health practices rather than in general medical practices. Further, primary care and psychiatric training programs have devoted relatively little attention to how their curricula may need to be revised to better prepare mental health providers and PCPs to collaborate (See chapter by Pollack and Goetz). Some model training programs that have been established to examine these issues are now emerging. Studies of the effectiveness of these programs need to be expanded.

METHODOLOGICAL ISSUES

Difficulties of Research Design

Research in PSMC, as the earlier examples indicate, requires creativity in structuring designs in an in vivo system that does not permit random assignment or untreated controls. This may require proactive efforts by public payers to mandate MCOs to participate in research and to gather data for quality improvement.

DIFFICULTIES OF GATHERING AND ANALYZING DATA

1. Availability of Data Sets

Historically, managed care companies have been reluctant to share data with each other or to make data available for public review. The competitive managed care environment has reinforced the difficulty associated with achieving agreement as to what data sets are to be gathered and what standards are to be used to ensure that the available data from different sources are comparable, although some behavioral managed care organizations have recently indicated a willingness to collaborate in this area (AMBHA, 1995). Concerns about confidentiality also act as a barrier to large scale analyses of available data.

However, with the assumption of contracts in the public sector, the capacity of public agencies to insist on public accountability provides a countervailing force to the previous reluctance to share managed care data. Similarly, the demands from professional organizations and the consequences of litigation regarding managed care practices will also provide an impetus for managed care companies to share data. The ability to pursue a research agenda regarding the issues outlined in this chapter will depend on expanding the accessibility to data.

2. Specificity of Data Sets

Given the complexity of public care, especially that which is available for the severely and chronically mentally ill, it will be especially important to pursue the development of data sets that take into account the intricacies of the care giving system. Determining the effectiveness of public managed care will require the availability of data that go beyond that which will generally be under the control of the managed care company and will extend to data from related care systems such as housing and vocational rehabilitation organizations.

3. Determining Costs

An accurate determination of the costs of providing care is essential to the completion of studies that attempt to compare the effectiveness and efficiency of care across settings, among different practitioners, and between different types of service delivery structures.

One example of this methodological problem results from the administrative separation of the existing public mental health care system from other elements of the behavioral health system and from the general health care system. This separation creates significant methodological problems with regard to cost determination and cost-offset. These must be resolved to obtain, for example, appropriate data concerning optimal distribution of dollars for mental health care from the general health care resource pool.

Similar methodological problems associated with determining costs arise with regard to persons with dual diagnoses or SPMI who often require care in social welfare systems that are closely tied to the health care delivery system.

4. Determining Outcomes

Selecting reliable and valid measurable indicators that adequately reflect relevant outcomes is a significant challenge for any research or evaluation effort. See the chapter by Essock and Goldman for further discussion of how this can be accomplished.

5. Ensuring Impartiality

Impartiality in the collection and analysis of research data is a necessary component of producing valid and reproducible results. An active role for independent research entities, either within universities or the private sector, is essential. Only they will be able to provide the accountability and ensure the validity and objectivity of the research work being conducted.

The capacity of these independent entities to engage in this research requires a funding source. Public agencies that utilize managed care approaches to the provision of services will need to set aside funds for research and evaluation and develop mechanisms to ensure that these funds are placed in independent hands. Managed care companies may volunteer, or be required by contract, to contribute to the cost of these research endeavors (see below). Independent entities must be allowed to determine that the data provided is accurate and objective.

FUNDING AND IMPLEMENTING THE RESEARCH AGENDA

The agenda outlined in this chapter, and the methodological issues that need to be addressed, will require a collaborative effort between public sector agencies, MCOs, academic institutions, providers, families, and consumers. The principal vehicle for ensuring that a research agenda is incorporated into the evolution of managed mental health care in the public sector will be the contract between the public agency and the managed care company. The contract will also be a major tool for ensuring that the methodological issues, particularly as regards data collection, are addressed.

It is likely that these contracts will contain provisions that relate to the fee or profit margin for the managed care companies. To the extent that incentives are part of the fee arrangement, it is possible to include data collection and analytic requirements with which the managed care companies must comply before being eligible to either receive the basic fee or to collect incentive payments. Regardless of the method used to ensure that research and evaluation occur, the basic point is that it is less likely to occur unless the resources for its revision are part of the basic contractual relationship. In this regard, it will be useful to require managed care companies that are responding to requests for proposals to include within their submissions a clear plan for conducting research and evaluation on specific questions presented by the public contractor.

While it is important that each public managed mental health care contract contain appropriate funding for research and evaluation component, it is unlikely that it will be sufficient to address all of the relevant research issues. There will continue to be a significant role for the federal government and private foundations to play in supporting research into public sector managed mental health care. This role might be best carried out through a series of independent, academically based, research centers that are established to assess the key issues presented in this chapter. These entities would provide comparatively neutral settings to examine some of the most contentious and politically charged issues. They would also provide a path by which governing bodies, consumers, and other parties that are not directly involved in the contractual relationship between public service systems and managed care companies can obtain answers to questions of special relevance to them. In addition, these entities could support demonstration projects related to the quality, service system, and provider issues described in this chapter. In those instances, a research component could be built into the demonstration.

To date, the investment of both the federal government and foundations in managed mental health care research has been very limited. Hopefully, it will increase as greater understanding emerges regarding how important the issues discussed in this chapter will be to the future of public mental health care.

CONCLUSION

Managed care has burst upon the public mental health scene like a supersonic plane announced by a sonic boom, but unnoticed by most observers on the ground. As a result, relatively little investment has been made and few results achieved in accumulating data to answer many of the quality, system, and provider issues raised by its arrival. This chapter suggests a research agenda for PSMC. Critical methodological questions have been identified and some suggestions have been made as to how funding for this research agenda could be obtained.

Obtaining the answers will not easy in view of the urgency of the task and the relatively short amount of time available for completing it. A failure to develop a strategy to examine these issues will only intensify a dilemma that has been created by those who have moved forward because of instincts and reactions to crisis, rather than knowledge and rational planning.

REFERENCES

Babigian, H.M., & Reed, S.K. (1987a). Capitation systems for the chronic mentally ill. *Psychiatric Annals, 17,* 604–609.

Babigian, H.M., & Reed, S.K. (1987b). An experimental model: capitation payment system for the chronic mentally ill. *Psychiatric Annals, 17,* 599–602.

Babigian, H.M., Cole, R.E., Reed, S.K. et al. (1991). Methodology for evaluating the Monroe-Livingston capitation model. *Hospital and Community Psychiatry, 42,* 913–919.

Beigel, A. (1995). Psychiatric education in a changing medical education and health care environment. Rockville, MD: Substance Abuse and Mental Health Administration, Department of Health and Human Services.

Beigel, A., & Santiago, J.M. (1995). The evolution of private practice. In press.

Callahan Jr., J.J., Shepard, D.S., Beinecke, R.H., Larson, M.J., & Cavanaugh, D. (1994). *Evaluation of the Massachusetts Medicaid Mental Health/ Substance Abuse Program*. Unpublished Manuscript. Brandeis University, Heller School for Advanced Studies in Social Welfare, Waltham, Massachusetts.

Cole, R.E., Reed, S.K., Babigian, H.M., & Brown, S.W. (1994). A mental health capitation program: 1. patient outcomes. *Hospital and Community Psychiatry, 45*(11),1090–1096.

Garratini, S. (1993). A rational approach to pharmacotherapy. Milan: Instituto Recherche de Farmocologische Mario Negri.

Mechanic, D., & Aiken. L. (1989). Capitation in mental health: potentials and cautions. *New Directions for Mental Health Services, 43*, 5–18.

Reed, S.F., Hennessy, K.D., Mitchell, O.S., & Babigian, H.M. (1994). A mental health capitation program: 11. cost-benefit analysis. *Hospital and Community Psychiatry, 45*(11),1097–1103.

Reed, S.K., Hennessy, K.D., & Babigian, H.M. (1995). Setting capitation rates for comprehensive care of persons with disabling mental illness. *Psychiatric Services, 46*(2),127–129.

Sturm, R., McGlynn, E.A., Meridith, L.S. et al. (1994). Switches between prepaid and fee-for-service health systems among depressed outpatients. *Med Care, 32*,917–929.

Sturm, R., & Wells, K.B. (1995). How can care for depression become more cost effective? *Journal of the American Medical Association, 273*, 51–58.

25

Educational and Training Issues in Public Sector Managed Mental Health Care

ALLAN TASMAN AND KENNETH MINKOFF

INTRODUCTION

The enormous changes brought about by managed mental health care, in both public and private sector environments, have profound implications for the future of professional training in the mental health disciplines. The advent of public sector managed care (PSMC), in particular, makes the need to re-evaluate professional training even more urgent, as it becomes clear that trainees will be involved with managed care even when treating persons with SPMI, and even when working in "public" settings.

This chapter attempts to examine the major challenges facing professional training programs in the PSMC era, and to outline a strategy for change to help training become more relevant and to help training programs (and the disciplines they serve) survive. The recommendations made here are intended to augment, rather than replace, the curricula and educational experiences found in most training programs. Although this chapter is written by psychiatrists, and tends to focus more heavily on psychiatric residency training, the discussion is relevant to other mental health disciplines as well.

THE CHALLENGE OF PSMC

PSMC impacts training in two major ways. First, it impacts the *content* and relevance of traditional training: Are the clinical skills being taught truly applicable in the new health care system, or are new skills required? Do the settings (e.g., traditional inpatient and outpatient) in which training occurs reflect the true diversity of settings encountered in a PSMC system? If the answer to those questions is no, then radical change in the content of training is needed.

Second, PSMC impacts the *funding* of post-graduate training, particularly in hospital-based settings which support most residency programs and many psychology internship programs. When private-sector managed care began to decrease the reimbursement margins that supported many training programs, shifting training sites to capture public sector reimbursement became a useful survival strategy. In some cases, however, changes brought about by managed care occur so rapidly that programs cannot adapt. This was the situation when Timberlawn in Dallas, Texas, was forced to abruptly close its psychiatric residency. However, now that public sector reimbursement is also being affected (e.g., discounted inpatient rates, with inclusive physician charges), the funding base for many programs is significantly threatened. With regard to *all* mental health disciplines, perceived oversupply of professionals also has had a negative impact on the number of trainee applicants.

Consequently, the major challenge facing training programs can be stated as follows: How to enhance educational excellence by teaching the knowledge and skills necessary to function well in newer models of care delivery, while at the same time maintaining fiscal stability in a time of declining financial resources and support.

STRATEGIES FOR CHANGE

Successful programs will recognize that managed care represents the first phase of a profound revolution in the U.S. health care system, which will continue to evolve into more organized and integrated service delivery systems. Reorienting training so that the didactic and clinical experiences are designed to help trainees succeed in managed care practice environments is essential. There is near-universal agreement that some clinical experience should be gained in a managed care setting. Further, if a training institution operates its own managed care program, there is the potential to generate new revenue in the new system, which, in turn, can be used to subsidize training.

Unfortunately, at present, few psychiatry training programs have found that participation in managed care provides sufficient profit to defray the cost of educational programs. As systems continue to evolve, however, and educational institutions develop their own managed care oriented integrated delivery systems, there may be increased potential to retain such savings for training purposes.

In order for trainees to be well-prepared to succeed in managed care systems, comprehensive training should address each of the following: attitudes and assumptions; basic knowledge; clinical skills and experiences; and research and evaluation.

Survival Tips

Educational and Training Issues

Reorienting training so that the didactic and clinical experiences are designed to help trainees succeed in managed care practice environments is essential.

In order for trainees to be well-prepared to succeed in managed care systems, comprehensive training should address each of the following: attitudes and assumptions; basic knowledge; clinical skills and experiences; and research and evaluation.

The study of community mental health in general, and of population-based mental health systems in particular, is now more central to understanding the impact of health care delivery, outcomes, and payment methods.

PSMC clinical programs, with their emphasis on continuous treatment teams, are appropriate clinical settings for training programs to use for training experiences.

ATTITUDES AND ASSUMPTIONS

Managed mental health care in general, and PSMC in particular, challenge the conventional wisdom about how clinical care systems should be organized, and how training should be provided. From an academic perspective, managed care is a radical challenge to traditional orthodoxies about the organization, funding, and delivery of mental health care, which must be evaluated and understood in a spirit of academic inquiry. This attitude that managed care is a natural experiment may help us to learn more about how to provide better, more efficient, and more cost-effective treatment and needs to be conveyed to trainees through the design and content of the training program. The study of community mental health in general, and of population-based mental health systems in particular, once regarded as a somewhat peripheral or optional specialty area, is now more central to understanding the impact of health care delivery, outcomes, and payment methods.

Similar issues arise in the design of training experiences. For example, clinical training in psychiatry in the last several decades has started with 9–12 months (or more) of inpatient rotations, followed by outpatient and subspecialty training. Most training directors and department chairs now believe this model is not adequate. The increased emphasis within managed care programs on using non-hospital residential settings and intensive ambulatory treatment has significantly changed the educational balance, resulting in dramatic reductions in lengths of stay in hospitals. The shorter lengths of stay have reduced the opportunities for trainees in inpatient settings to follow patients through the course of an acute episode of illness.

Consequently, educational programs have struggled to design new models of clinical training, which will allow for optimal continuity of care experiences (Tasman, 1994). PSMC clinical programs, with their emphasis on continuous treatment teams, may provide just the kind of clinical settings that training programs are seeking to develop. With appropriate supervision, and appropriate definition of the clinical roles of the trainees, their participation as members of a managed care clinical team can provide important educational benefits. Positive experiences in such rotations will significantly help academicians to feel less suspicious about the general principles of managed care and more inclined to support the use of managed care programs as training sites. It is also important to recognize that many training programs have not provided sufficient experience for trainees to participate in the longitudinal care of patients with severe and persistent mental illnesses (SPMI). PSMC programs, often the predominant care providing organizations for persons with SPMI in some communities, provide tremendous potential for training and education in this area.

BASIC KNOWLEDGE

In order to reorient training to meet PSMC demands, programs must expand the core curriculum to incorporate a broader knowledge base regarding all aspects of mental health systems and reimbursement structures. This knowledge will become an infrastructure into which trainees can integrate their evolving clinical skills with the expectations of various reimbursement systems throughout their training.

Elements of a PSMC core curriculum are listed in Table 1.

As Table 1 indicates, there is already a substantial knowledge base that informs PSMC development. This body of knowledge should be used to prepare future mental health professionals to adequately understand the environment in which they will be practicing.

CLINICAL SKILLS AND EXPERIENCES

Because of the relatively short history of managed care programs, there is little literature available to define the necessary clinical skills and relevant training experiences for practice in a managed care en-

TABLE 1: PSMC Core Curriculum

Overview and history of health and mental health systems —
   public and private
Overview and history of health and mental financing and
   reimbursement
Community psychiatry and population-based mental health
   service delivery
History and evolution of managed care and PSMC
PSMC ideology and community mental health ideology
Managed care strategies and techniques
Examples of private and public system managed care models
Clinical and programmatic issues in capitated public delivery
   systems
Psychiatric roles in PSMC systems
Utilization management: case, program, systems level
Quality management: case, program, systems level
Development of a comprehensive care continuum:
      level of care determinations
      care management (case management)
      integration of services and programs
Program and outcome evaluation at the case, program, systems
   levels
Systems research strategies
Ethical issues in managed care and PSMC
Systems integration: psychiatric & addiction services; primary
   care & psychiatric care

---

vironment. Sabin (1994) has suggested that ethical managed care practice requires core skills: 1) a population-oriented practice management, 2) population-oriented program development, 3) application of an adult developmental model to treatment (e.g., building on strengths and fostering natural development, rather than regressive analytic reconstruction), 4) command of and access to a broad repertoire of treatment methodologies (e.g., brief treatment, behavioral treatment, psychopharmacology), 5) ethical and objective analysis of treatment effectiveness, and 6) patient advocacy within the care system.

Building upon Sabin's analysis, and incorporating elements from the earlier discussion of PSMC training issues, we have developed a more comprehensive list of core clinical skills to be developed in PSMC training, which are listed in Table 2. Most of the listed skills are already viewed as critical to the function of a psychiatrist (Langsley & Yager, 1988).

CORE COMPETENCIES

The concept of core competencies in professional training is not new. What is new in this discussion is that many skills, once thought

TABLE 2: Core Clinical Skills in PSMC Training

Primary Core Competencies
  Focused treatment planning and treatment prescription
  Utilization management and level of care determination
  Continuity of clinical case management in a variety of clinical
    settings
  Brief treatment, time-sensitive, and focused cognitive behavioral
    treatment methodologies
  Rehabilitative and recovery-oriented treatment approaches for
    persons with SPMI.
  Family and systems collaboration and involvement in
    treatment, including the primary care interface
  Responsible consumer and family advocacy

Ancillary Competencies
  Familiarity with a full range of hospital diversion and intensive
    outpatient programs
  Ability to collaborate with internal and external utilization
    reviewers
  Interdisciplinary teamwork in various clinical settings
  Population-oriented practice management
  Ability to practice in primary care settings and to provide
    consultation to outpatient primary care providers
  Ability to integrate psychiatric and substance disorder
    assessment, diagnosis, and treatment

to be of secondary importance, must now be incorporated into core educational experiences.

The ability to prescribe a specific course of treatment, to write a treatment plan with defined interventions and measurable outcomes, or to assess and articulate clinical criteria that determine a necessary level of care is no less important for PSMC competency than the ability to make an accurate diagnosis or to select the correct medication. Consequently, training programs need to incorporate the demonstration of those competencies into training, (by requiring, for example, that trainees write treatment plans or make level of care determinations on sample cases that are reviewed and critiqued), just as they require competency in the application of DSM-IV.

BRIEF OR TIME-SENSITIVE TREATMENT

With the advent of managed care, brief, focused, time-sensitive interventions, whether psychodynamic or cognitive-behavioral, have been emphasized as preferable first-line approaches to psychotherapy. In the short term, these approaches are often as effective and more efficient that costly longer-term, open-ended psychotherapies. Data on long-term efficacy of the briefer treatments awaits further study. A